Clinical Advances in Allergy and Asthma: Issues, Strategies, and Future Directions

Clinical Advances in Allergy and Asthma: Issues, Strategies, and Future Directions

Guest Editor

Laura Pini

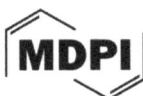

Basel • Beijing • Wuhan • Barcelona • Belgrade • Novi Sad • Cluj • Manchester

Guest Editor
Laura Pini
Department of Clinical and
Experimental Sciences
University of Brescia
Brescia
Italy

Editorial Office
MDPI AG
Grosspeteranlage 5
4052 Basel, Switzerland

This is a reprint of the Special Issue, published open access by the journal *Journal of Clinical Medicine* (ISSN 2077-0383), freely accessible at: https://www.mdpi.com/journal/jcm/special_issues/clinical_allergy_asthma.

For citation purposes, cite each article independently as indicated on the article page online and as indicated below:

Lastname, A.A.; Lastname, B.B. Article Title. *Journal Name* **Year**, *Volume Number*, Page Range.

ISBN 978-3-7258-4163-9 (Hbk)
ISBN 978-3-7258-4164-6 (PDF)
https://doi.org/10.3390/books978-3-7258-4164-6

© 2025 by the authors. Articles in this book are Open Access and distributed under the Creative Commons Attribution (CC BY) license. The book as a whole is distributed by MDPI under the terms and conditions of the Creative Commons Attribution-NonCommercial-NoDerivs (CC BY-NC-ND) license (https://creativecommons.org/licenses/by-nc-nd/4.0/).

Contents

Jordan Giordani, Alessandro Pini and Laura Pini
Evaluation of Long-Term Response to Biological Therapy in Severe Asthma and Considerations for Treatment Adjustment
Reprinted from: *J. Clin. Med.* **2025**, *14*, 2623, https://doi.org/10.3390/jcm14082623 1

Elisa Riccardi, Giuseppe Guida, Sonia Garino, Francesca Bertolini, Vitina Carriero, Mattia Brusamento, et al.
Biologics in T2 Severe Asthma: Unveiling Different Effectiveness by Real-World Indirect Comparison
Reprinted from: *J. Clin. Med.* **2024**, *13*, 4750, https://doi.org/10.3390/jcm13164750 5

Eusebi Chiner, María Murcia, Ignacio Boira, María Ángeles Bernabeu, Violeta Esteban and Eva Martínez-Moragón
Real-Life Clinical Outcomes of Benralizumab Treatment in Patients with Uncontrolled Severe Asthma and Coexisting Chronic Rhinosinusitis with Nasal Polyposis
Reprinted from: *J. Clin. Med.* **2024**, *13*, 4247, https://doi.org/10.3390/jcm13144247 25

Laura Pini, Diego Bagnasco, Bianca Beghè, Fulvio Braido, Paolo Cameli, Marco Caminati, et al.
Unlocking the Long-Term Effectiveness of Benralizumab in Severe Eosinophilic Asthma: A Three-Year Real-Life Study
Reprinted from: *J. Clin. Med.* **2024**, *13*, 3013, https://doi.org/10.3390/jcm13103013 37

Javier De Miguel-Díez, Ana Lopez-de-Andres, Francisco J. Caballero-Segura, Rodrigo Jimenez-Garcia, Valentin Hernández-Barrera, David Carabantes-Alarcon, et al.
Trends and Hospital Outcomes in HOSPITAL Admissions for Anaphylaxis in Children with and without Asthma in Spain (2016–2021)
Reprinted from: *J. Clin. Med.* **2023**, *12*, 6387, https://doi.org/10.3390/jcm12196387 55

Hisao Higo, Hirohisa Ichikawa, Yukako Arakawa, Yoshihiro Mori, Junko Itano, Akihiko Taniguchi, et al.
Switching to Dupilumab from Other Biologics without a Treatment Interval in Patients with Severe Asthma: A Multi-Center Retrospective Study
Reprinted from: *J. Clin. Med.* **2023**, *12*, 5174, https://doi.org/10.3390/jcm12165174 68

Ahmad R. Alsayed, Anas Abed, Mahmoud Abu-Samak, Farhan Alshammari and Bushra Alshammari
Etiologies of Acute Bronchiolitis in Children at Risk for Asthma, with Emphasis on the Human Rhinovirus Genotyping Protocol
Reprinted from: *J. Clin. Med.* **2023**, *12*, 3909, https://doi.org/10.3390/jcm12123909 80

Abdullah A. Alqarni, Abdulelah M. Aldhahir, Rayan A. Siraj, Jaber S. Alqahtani, Hams H. Alshehri, Amal M. Alshamrani, et al.
Prevalence of Overweight and Obesity and Their Impact on Spirometry Parameters in Patients with Asthma: A Multicentre, Retrospective Study
Reprinted from: *J. Clin. Med.* **2023**, *12*, 1843, https://doi.org/10.3390/jcm12051843 100

Agnieszka Barańska, Wiesław Kanadys, Artur Wdowiak, Maria Malm, Agata Błaszczuk, Urszula Religioni, et al.
Effects of Prenatal Paracetamol Exposure on the Development of Asthma and Wheezing in Childhood: A Systematic Review and Meta-Analysis
Reprinted from: *J. Clin. Med.* **2023**, *12*, 1832, https://doi.org/10.3390/jcm12051832 111

Jun Wen, Mohan Giri, Li Xu and Shuliang Guo
Association between Exposure to Selected Heavy Metals and Blood Eosinophil Counts in Asthmatic Adults: Results from NHANES 2011–2018
Reprinted from: *J. Clin. Med.* **2023**, *12*, 1543, https://doi.org/10.3390/jcm12041543 . . . . **122**

Shuwen Zhang, Xin Zhang, Ke Deng, Changyong Wang, Lisa G. Wood, Huajing Wan, et al.
Reduced Skeletal Muscle Mass Is Associated with an Increased Risk of Asthma Control and Exacerbation
Reprinted from: *J. Clin. Med.* **2022**, *11*, 7241, https://doi.org/10.3390/jcm11237241 . . . . **135**

Michiel A. G. E. Bannier, Sophie Kienhorst, Quirijn Jöbsis, Kim D. G. van de Kant, Frederik-Jan van Schooten, Agnieszka Smolinska and Edward Dompeling
Exhaled Breath Analysis for Investigating the Use of Inhaled Corticosteroids and Corticosteroid Responsiveness in Wheezing Preschool Children
Reprinted from: *J. Clin. Med.* **2022**, *11*, 5160, https://doi.org/10.3390/jcm11175160 . . . . **152**

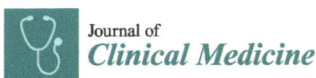 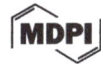

Editorial

Evaluation of Long-Term Response to Biological Therapy in Severe Asthma and Considerations for Treatment Adjustment

Jordan Giordani [1], Alessandro Pini [2] and Laura Pini [1,3,*]

[1] Department of Clinical and Experimental Sciences, University of Brescia, 25123 Brescia, Italy
[2] Department of Emergency, Anaesthesiological and Resuscitation Sciences, University Cattolica Sacro Cuore, 00168 Rome, Italy
[3] ASST Spedali Civili di Brescia, 25123 Brescia, Italy
* Correspondence: laura.pini@unibs.it; Tel.: +39-030-399-6263

Assessing long-term responses to biological therapies for severe asthma is critical for optimizing patient management and improving clinical outcomes. The literature provides a significant amount of data from long-term and real-life studies, which are essential for evaluating the durability, efficacy, and impact of these treatments over time. Long-term studies focus on the sustained effects of biological agents, while real-world studies offer insights into their effectiveness in everyday clinical settings, enhancing our understanding of treatment impacts on patient populations [1].

Recent advancements in the airway remodeling field have further refined the evaluation of biological therapies. Notably, Omalizumab, an anti-IgE monoclonal antibody, has been shown to inhibit IgE-mediated extracellular matrix (ECM) deposition and reduce reticular basement membrane thickness and fibronectin deposition [2]. Similarly, Mepolizumab, an anti-IL-5 agent, has improved airway remodeling by reducing eosinophil counts and tenascin expression [3]. Benralizumab, an anti-IL-5R agent, has been observed to diminish eosinophil counts associated with reductions in airway smooth muscle mass [4]. Dupilumab, an IL-4 receptor antagonist, has shown promise in preventing eosinophil infiltration into lung tissue, with ongoing studies evaluating its impact on lung function and structure [5]. At the same time, Tezepelumab, targeting thymic stromal lymphopoietin (TSLP), has demonstrated reductions in airway inflammation and remodeling in animal models, although human studies are still in progress [6].

An important recent therapeutic development is Depemokimab, a long-acting monoclonal antibody targeting IL-5. The phase III clinical trials SWIFT-1 and SWIFT-2 demonstrated that biannual Depemokimab administration led to a 54% reduction in exacerbations compared to placebo, along with the sustained suppression of type 2 inflammation, and improved the quality of life in patients with severe eosinophilic asthma [7].

In addition, more recent studies have investigated the use of Benralizumab during acute phases of severe asthma. A study published in *The Lancet Respiratory Medicine* showed that a single Benralizumab injection during an exacerbation reduced the need for additional treatments by 30% compared to oral steroids, with fewer side effects and the potential for at-home administration [8].

The long-term response to biological therapies can also be evaluated through their impact on the natural history of severe asthma. Patients who respond positively to treatment may experience two distinct outcomes upon discontinuation: a recurrence of symptoms or sustained remission. The XPORT study, a multicenter randomized controlled trial, reported that 33% of patients who discontinued Omalizumab experienced exacerbations compared to 52% in the placebo group, indicating a potential for sustained disease control [9]. Furthermore, a prospective study by Vennera et al. found that 60% of patients maintained long-term benefits up to four years after Omalizumab discontinuation [10]. Conversely, Haldar et al. reported an increase in exacerbations related to eosinophilia in patients who discontinued Mepolizumab after 12 months [11]. However, the COSMO study indicated that a 12-week Mepolizumab discontinuation did not significantly affect asthma control, as measured by the Asthma Control Questionnaire (ACQ5) [12]. These findings underline the variability in patient responses after biological therapy discontinuation.

Identifying candidates for biological therapy discontinuation necessitates a nuanced approach. When considering treatment adjustment or discontinuation, patients can be categorized into super-responders, partial responders, and non-responders. Super-responders may exhibit minimal residual symptoms, stable lung function without the need for oral corticosteroids (OCSs), and low fractional exhaled nitric oxide (FeNO) and eosinophil levels during treatment [13,14]. In contrast, partial and non-responders may require a reassessment of their treatment regimen. Real-world data from the ISAR registry and the CHRONICLE study indicated that approximately 79% of patients continued their current biologic therapy, while 10% discontinued and 11% switched to another biologic [15]. The decision to switch is often prompted by inadequate clinical response, adverse events, or patient preferences regarding treatment administration [16].

The assessment of response to biological therapy should be based on multiple outcomes: symptom improvement, rescue medication use, lung function, reduction in OCS, quality of life, and healthcare resource utilization [17]. A patient may be classified as a non-responder after 4–6 months of treatment if there is minimal clinical improvement, no steroid use reduction, and persistent eosinophilia or T2-low inflammation. Factors contributing to non-response may include disease mechanisms not targeted by the chosen biologic, comorbidities, poor adherence, or the presence of drug-neutralizing antibodies [18].

Currently, there are no specific guidelines on the timing and criteria for switching between biologics, but it is generally recommended that treatment is reassessed after 4–12 months. In many cases, switching directly from one biologic to another (e.g., from Omalizumab to Mepolizumab) has been shown to be safe, even without a wash-out period [19,20].

In conclusion, the long-term response to biological therapies has revolutionized the management of severe asthma, improving long-term outcomes and offering personalized treatment strategies. The Special Issue "Clinical Advances in Allergy and Asthma: Issues, Strategies, and Future Directions" primarily aims to provide innovative insights and increase readers' awareness of the new frontiers gradually opening up in treating severe asthma. In this context, biologic therapies are the most promising and clinically effective vanguard. The advances achieved so far and the possibility of tailored diagnostic and therapeutic approaches open up the possibility of leading patients toward the ambitious goal of clinical remission.

Author Contributions: Study design: J.G., A.P. and L.P.; data collection: J.G., A.P. and L.P.; initial draft: J.G., A.P. and L.P. All authors have read and agreed to the published version of the manuscript.

Funding: This research received no external funding.

Acknowledgments: Laura Pini, as Guest Editor of the Special Issue "Clinical Advances in Allergy and Asthma: Issues, Strategies, and Future Directions" would like to express her deep appreciation to all authors whose valuable work was published in this Issue and thus contributed to its success.

Conflicts of Interest: The authors declare no conflicts of interest.

References

1. Brusselle, G.G.; Koppelman, G.H. Biologic Therapies for Severe Asthma. *N. Engl. J. Med.* **2022**, *386*, 157–171. [CrossRef] [PubMed]
2. Domingo, C.; Mirapeix, R.M.; González-Barcala, F.J.; Forné, C.; García, F. Omalizumab in Severe Asthma: Effect on Oral Corticosteroid Exposure and Remodeling. A Randomized Open-Label Parallel Study. *Drugs* **2023**, *83*, 1111–1123. [CrossRef] [PubMed]
3. Varricchi, G.; Poto, R.; Lommatzsch, M.; Brusselle, G.; Braido, F.; Virchow, J.C.; Canonica, G.W. Biologics and airway remodeling in asthma: Early, late, and potential preventive effects. *Allergy* **2025**, *80*, 408–422. [CrossRef] [PubMed]
4. Visca, D.; Ardesi, F.; Zappa, M.; Grossi, S.; Pignatti, P.; Vanetti, M.; Pini, L.; Sotgiu, G.; Centis, R.; Migliori, G.B.; et al. The effect of benralizumab on inflammation in severe asthma: A real-life analysis. *Ther. Adv. Respir. Dis.* **2024**, *18*. [CrossRef] [PubMed]
5. Tajiri, T.; Suzuki, M.; Nishiyama, H.; Ozawa, Y.; Kurokawa, R.; Takeda, N.; Ito, K.; Fukumitsu, K.; Kanemitsu, Y.; Mori, Y.; et al. Efficacy of dupilumab for airway hypersecretion and airway wall thickening in patients with moderate-to-severe asthma: A prospective, observational study. *Allergol Int.* **2024**, *73*, 406–415. [CrossRef] [PubMed]
6. Diver, S.; Khalfaoui, L.; Emson, C.; Wenzel, S.E.; Menzies-Gow, A.; Wechsler, M.E.; Johnston, J.; Molfino, N.; Parnes, J.R.; Megally, A.; et al. Effect of tezepelumab on airway inflammatory cells, remodelling, and hyperresponsiveness in patients with moderate-to-severe uncontrolled asthma (CASCADE): A double-blind, randomised, placebo-controlled, phase 2 trial. *Lancet Respir. Med.* **2021**, *9*, 1299–1312, Erratum in *Lancet Respir. Med.* **2021**, *9*, e106. [CrossRef] [PubMed]
7. Jackson, D.J.; Wechsler, M.E.; Jackson, D.J.; Bernstein, D.; Korn, S.; Pfeffer, P.E.; Chen, R.; Saito, J.; de Luíz Martinez, G.; Dymek, L.; et al. SWIFT-1 and SWIFT-2 Investigators, SWIFT-1 Investigators, & SWIFT-2 Investigators. Twice-Yearly Depemokimab in Severe Asthma with an Eosinophilic Phenotype. *N. Engl. J. Med.* **2024**, *391*, 2337–2349. [PubMed]
8. Ramakrishnan, S.; Russell, R.E.K.; Mahmood, H.R.; Krassowska, K.; Melhorn, J.; Mwasuku, C.; Pavord, I.D.; Bermejo-Sanchez, L.; Howell, I.; Mahdi, M.; et al. Treating eosinophilic exacerbations of asthma and COPD with benralizumab (ABRA): A double-blind, double-dummy, active placebo-controlled randomised trial. *Lancet Respir. Med.* **2025**, *13*, 59–68. [CrossRef] [PubMed]
9. Ledford, D.; Busse, W.; Trzaskoma, B.; Omachi, T.A.; Rosén, K.; Chipps, B.E.; Luskin, A.T.; Solari, P.G. A randomized multicenter study evaluating Xolair persistence of response after long-term therapy. *J. Allergy Clin. Immunol.* **2017**, *140*, 162–169.e2. [CrossRef] [PubMed]
10. Vennera, M.D.C.; Sabadell, C.; Picado, C.; Spanish Omalizumab Registry. Duration of the efficacy of Omalizumab after treatment discontinuation in 'real life' severe asthma. *Thorax* **2018**, *73*, 782–784. [CrossRef] [PubMed]
11. Haldar, P.; Brightling, C.E.; Singapuri, A.; Hargadon, B.; Gupta, S.; Monteiro, W.; Bradding, P.; Green, R.H.; Wardlaw, A.J.; Ortega, H.; et al. Outcomes after cessation of mepolizumab therapy in severe eosinophilic asthma: A 12-month follow-up analysis. *J. Allergy Clin. Immunol.* **2014**, *133*, 921–923. [CrossRef] [PubMed]
12. Ortega, H.; Lemiere, C.; Llanos, J.P.; Forshag, M.; Price, R.; Albers, F.; Yancey, S.; Castro, M. Outcomes following mepolizumab treatment discontinuation: Real-world experience from an open-label trial. *Allergy Asthma Clin. Immunol.* **2019**, *15*, 37. [CrossRef] [PubMed]
13. Moore, W.C.; Kornmann, O.; Humbert, M.; Poirier, C.; Bel, E.H.; Kaneko, N.; Smith, S.G.; Martin, N.; Gilson, M.J.; Price, R.G.; et al. Stopping versus continuing long-term mepolizumab treatment in severe eosinophilic asthma (COMET study). *Eur. Respir. J.* **2022**, *59*, 2100396. [CrossRef] [PubMed]
14. Jeffery, M.M.; Inselman, J.W.; Maddux, J.T.; Lam, R.W.; Shah, N.D.; Rank, M.A. Asthma Patients Who Stop Asthma Biologics Have a Similar Risk of Asthma Exacerbations as Those Who Continue Asthma Biologics. *J. Allergy Clin. Immunol. Pract.* **2021**, *9*, 2742–2750.e1. [CrossRef] [PubMed]
15. Menzies-Gow, A.N.; McBrien, C.; Unni, B.; Porsbjerg, C.M.; Al-Ahmad, M.; Ambrose, C.S.; Dahl Assing, K.; von Bülow, A.; Busby, J.; Cosio, B.G.; et al. Real World Biologic Use and Switch Patterns in Severe Asthma: Data from the International Severe Asthma Registry and the US CHRONICLE Study. *J. Asthma Allergy* **2022**, *15*, 63–78. [CrossRef] [PubMed]
16. Nagase, H.; Suzukawa, M.; Oishi, K.; Matsunaga, K. Biologics for severe asthma: The real-world evidence, effectiveness of switching, and prediction factors for the efficacy. *Allergol. Int.* **2023**, *72*, 11–23. [CrossRef] [PubMed]
17. Roberts, G. Understanding the response to asthma biological therapy. *Clin. Exp. Allergy* **2020**, *50*, 992–993. [CrossRef] [PubMed]
18. Saco, T.; Ugalde, I.C.; Cardet, J.C.; Casale, T.B. Strategies for choosing a biologic for your patient with allergy or asthma. *Ann. Allergy Asthma Immunol.* **2021**, *127*, 627–637. [CrossRef] [PubMed]

19. Canonica, G.W.; Bagnasco, D.; Bondi, B.; Varricchi, G.; Paoletti, G.; Blasi, F.; Paggiaro, P.; Braido, F.; SANI Study Group. SANI clinical remission definition: A useful tool in severe asthma management. *J. Asthma* **2024**, *61*, 1593–1600. [CrossRef] [PubMed]
20. Chapman, K.R.; Albers, F.C.; Chipps, B.; Muñoz, X.; Devouassoux, G.; Bergna, M.; Galkin, D.; Azmi, J.; Mouneimne, D.; Price, R.G.; et al. The clinical benefit of Mepolizumab replacing Omalizumab in uncontrolled severe eosinophilic asthma. *Allergy* **2019**, *74*, 1716–1726. [CrossRef] [PubMed]

Disclaimer/Publisher's Note: The statements, opinions and data contained in all publications are solely those of the individual author(s) and contributor(s) and not of MDPI and/or the editor(s). MDPI and/or the editor(s) disclaim responsibility for any injury to people or property resulting from any ideas, methods, instructions or products referred to in the content.

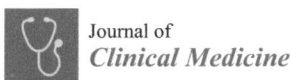

Article

Biologics in T2 Severe Asthma: Unveiling Different Effectiveness by Real-World Indirect Comparison

Elisa Riccardi [1,2,†], Giuseppe Guida [2,3,*,†], Sonia Garino [2], Francesca Bertolini [2], Vitina Carriero [2], Mattia Brusamento [4], Stefano Pizzimenti [3], Fabiana Giannoccaro [3], Erica Falzone [2], Elisa Arrigo [2], Stefano Levra [2] and Fabio Luigi Massimo Ricciardolo [2,3,5]

[1] Regional Hospital Parini, Pulmonology Unit, Aosta, 11100 Aosta, Italy; eli16riccardi@gmail.com
[2] Department of Clinical and Biological Sciences, University of Turin, Orbassano, 10043 Turin, Italy; sonia.garino@unito.it (S.G.); francesca.bertolini@unito.it (F.B.); vitina.carriero@unito.it (V.C.); erica.falzone@unito.it (E.F.); elisa.arrigo@unito.it (E.A.); stefano.levra@unito.it (S.L.); fabioluigimassimo.ricciardolo@unito.it (F.L.M.R.)
[3] Severe Asthma, Rare Lung Disease and Respiratory Pathophysiology, San Luigi Gonzaga University Hospital, Orbassano, 10043 Turin, Italy; pizzimentistefano@gmail.com (S.P.); fabiana.giannoccaro@gmail.com (F.G.)
[4] Re Learn S.R.L., 10122 Turin, Italy; bmattia92@gmail.com
[5] Institute of Translational Pharmacology, National Research Council (IFT-CNR), Section of Palermo, 90146 Palermo, Italy
* Correspondence: giuseppe.guida@unito.it; Tel.: +39-0119026776
† These authors contributed equally to this work.

Abstract: Background: Indirect comparison among biologics in severe asthma (SA) is a challenging but desirable goal for clinicians in real life. The aim of the study is to define characteristics of a biologic-treated T2-driven-SA population and to evaluate the effectiveness of biologic treatments in a real-world setting by variation in intra/inter-biologic parameters in an up to 4-year follow-up. **Methods**: Demographic, clinical, functional, and biological characteristics were evaluated retrospectively in 104 patients recruited until July 2022 at baseline (T0) and over a maximum of 4 years (T4) of biologic therapy (omalizumab/OmaG = 41, from T0 to T4, mepolizumab/MepoG = 26, from T0 to T4, benralizumab/BenraG = 18, from T0 to T2, and dupilumab/DupiG = 19, from T0 to T1). Variations of parameters using means of paired Delta were assessed. **Results**: At baseline, patients had high prevalence of T2-driven comorbidities, low asthma control test (ACT mean 17.65 ± 4.41), impaired pulmonary function (FEV$_1$ 65 ± 18 %pred), frequent exacerbations/year (AEs 3.5 ± 3), and OCS dependence (60%). DupiG had lower T2 biomarkers/comorbidities and AEs, and worse FEV$_1$ (57 ± 19 %pred) compared to other biologics ($p < 0.05$). All biologics improved ACT, FEV$_1$%, FVC%, AEs rate, and OCS use. FEV$_1$% improved in MepoG and BenraG over the minimal clinically important difference and was sustained over 4 years in OmaG and MepoG. A significant RV reduction in OmaG (T4) and DupiG (T1), and BenraG normalization (T2) of airflow limitation were found. We observed through inter-biologic parameters pair delta variation comparison a significant nocturnal awakenings reduction in BenraG vs. OmaG/MepoG, and neutrophils reduction in BenraG/DupiG vs. OmaG. **Conclusions**: Indirect comparison among biologics unveils clinical and functional improvements that may mark a different effectiveness. These results may highlight the preference of a single biologic compared to another with regard to specific treatable traits.

Keywords: severe asthma; indirect comparison; biologics; omalizumab; mepolizumab; dupilumab; benralizumab; precision medicine; treatable traits

1. Introduction

Severe asthma (SA) is a complex and heterogeneous disease presenting several clinical phenotypes driven by multiple molecular endotypes and affecting 5–10% of asthmatic patients [1]. At present, asthma phenotypes can be divided into two main groups based on the underlying inflammatory process: Type-2 (T2) High, representing approximately 70% of SA cases and associated with an eosinophilic inflammatory profile in induced sputum, and T2-Low [2]. The majority of all currently approved biologics for uncontrolled, moderate-to-severe asthma, target components of the T2 inflammatory pathway. Omalizumab suppresses the activity of IgE, mepolizumab binds IL-5, benralizumab blocks IL5Rα, whereas dupilumab inhibits the activity of IL-4 and IL-13. All biologics reached, in both a randomized controlled trial (RCT) and real-life studies (RLS), the expected outcomes in reducing airway eosinophilic inflammation, asthma exacerbation (AEs) rates, and improving lung function and symptoms scores [3]. Only recently, tezepelumab, a human monoclonal antibody that binds specifically to thymic stromal lymphopoietin (TSLP) and targets multiple disease pathways, including T2-low severe asthma, was adopted in clinical practice [4].

Although designed on different biologic targets, the indications for the clinical use of biologics to severe, T2, asthmatic patients frequently overlap, turning the choice for the best biologic treatment into a challenge [5]. At present no direct "head-to-head" trials of comparison between biologics in SA are available, while indirect methods, such as indirect treatment comparison (ITC), were explored. They compare the efficacy of each treatment based on selected endpoints in cohorts of patients with same defined selected clinical and inflammatory phenotypes, using different statistical methods. None of the studies using ITC succeeded in matching patient characteristics and many can be criticised because of arbitrary inclusion and exclusion criteria [6]. Moreover, ITC relied strictly on controlled data only from RCTs; accordingly, they are not generalizable and may underestimate the true treatment efficacies [7]. Recently, Taha Al-Shaikhly and colleagues demonstrated the relatively superior efficacy of Dupilumab in reducing AEs compared with anti-IL-5 and anti-IgE biologics in real life. However, head-to-head controlled RLS are still needed [8].

The great heterogeneity of T2 SA population supports the existence of distinct subtypes of T2 SA which could preferentially respond to a single biologic [9,10]. Pragmatic algorithms to guide the choice of biologic based on sub-endotypes of T2 asthma were suggested, remaining largely speculative from an evidence-based perspective [11]. With the upcoming of a great deal of data coming from RLS, the concept of clinical treatable traits within the T2, SA patients emerged, allowing a precision medicine approach [12]. A treatable trait is defined as a phenotypic or endotypic characteristic that can be successfully targeted with treatment. Each trait, such as comorbidities, lung function, or asthma symptoms could be a preferential target for one specific biologic. Thereafter, biomarkers in SA were explored with the aim of identifying the treatable trait and prediction of response to treatments [13]. Concomitantly, molecular phenotyping validated the recognition of biological endotypes that represent treatable mechanisms which need to be linked to biomarkers according to precision medicine approaches [14].

We aimed to compare retrospectively clinical, functional, and biological characteristics in a cohort of SA patients before and during treatment with four different biologic agents (omalizumab, mepolizumab, benralizumab, or dupilumab) in order to bring out those traits marking a different effectiveness. The evaluation of parameter variations over time for each biologic lets us define the "intra-biological" and the "inter-biological" changes in real life as a measure of indirect comparison.

2. Materials and Methods

2.1. Patients and Study Design

This monocentric, retrospective, observational, and real-life study was conducted at San Luigi Gonzaga University Hospital with the approval of the local ethical committee (Protocol number 4478/2017, approved on 20 March 2017) in accordance with the Declaration of Helsinki. The study involved 88 SA patients who gave written informed consent and who accessed our Severe Asthma and Rare Lung Disease Unit from January 2007 to July 2022. SA was defined according to ATS/ERS Guidelines [1]. All patients presented with T2 inflammation and were prescribed a biologic agent according to regional criteria for prescription (Table S1). T2 inflammation was defined if at least one of the following elements were present: peripheral blood eosinophils (PBE) $\geq$ 300/mcl, F_ENO $\geq$ 30 ppb, total IgE $\geq$ 100 UI/mL, or documented atopy through *prick test* or specific IgE measurement [15]. Patients were divided into four groups based on the biologic prescribed: omalizumab group (OmaG), mepolizumab group (MepoG), benralizumab group (BenraG), and dupilumab group (DupiG). Four patients included in the study were treated off-label with omalizumab, due to lack of available alternative biologics in the market at the time of prescription.

2.2. Baseline Descriptive Clinical, Functional, and Biological Characteristics

For each patient, we reported the following data: age, sex, age of asthma onset (<18 y/o: early-onset/>18 y/o: late-onset), BMI, history of smoke, comorbidities, atopy for seasonal or perennial allergens (animal dander or house dust mites), atopy for molds demonstrated by diagnostic tests (prick or specific IgE), HRCT characteristics (bronchiectasis, mucus plug, emphysema, and thickening of the bronchial walls), ER visits for asthma exacerbations, intubation due to asthma attacks, and number of exacerbations that required OCS burst in the previous year. We also reported maintenance treatment defining ICS dose, OCS dose, LABA, and LAMA. ICS was expressed as beclomethasone equivalent HFA (BDP HFA dose, mcg). OCS dependence patients were defined as patients who have at least one between the following characteristics: need of chronic treatment with OCS for more than 6 months in the previous year (chronic OCS) or number of asthma exacerbations that required at least 3 days of treatment with OCS $\geq$ 3/year in the previous year (OCS bursts $\geq$ 3/year). To assess asthma symptoms, an asthma control test (ACT) [16] was proposed to each patient at every follow-up visit. Activity limitations and nocturnal symptoms were evaluated through the first two questions of the ACT. Asthma was defined as "non controlled" if ACT score was $\leq$19 and as "controlled" if ACT was $\geq$20 [17]. Pulmonary function was assessed performing spirometry and/or plethysmography (Vmax Encore 62, Carefusion, Würzburg, Germany) with or without a post-bronchodilator test. The following spirometric data were collected: absolute FEV_1, FEV_1 %pred., absolute FVC, FVC %pred., absolute IT, IT %pred., absolute RV, RV %pred., absolute FVC post BD, absolute Delta FVC post BD, Delta FVC %post BD, absolute FEV_1 post BD, absolute Delta FEV_1 post BD, Delta FEV_1 %post BD, DLCO %pred., and DLCO/Va %pred. We also evaluated the percentage of patients that showed reversibility of FEV_1 (reversible) and the percentage of patients with fixed obstruction of the Tiffeneau index, after a bronchodilator test in accordance with ATS/ERS Guidelines [18]. Biological collected data included total IgE (UI/mL), total (cells/mcl), and percentage count of leukocytes, neutrophils, peripheral blood eosinophils PBE, fibrinogen levels (mg/dl) [19], and F_ENO values (ppb). F_ENO was measured with the single breath technique using F_ENO + (Medisoft, Sorinnes, Belgium). The presence of one or more biomarkers defining T2 inflammation, as defined in the methods section, was analyzed for each group of biologic-treated patients.

2.3. Collection of Variables for "Intra and Inter Biologics" Comparison over Time

We evaluated the variation in clinical, functional, and biological continuous variables in patients who were prescribed a biologic over 4 years (T1 = first year, T2 = second year, T3 = third year, and T4 = fourth year) in OmaG and MepoG, 2 years (T1 and T2) in BenraG, and 1 year (T1) in DupiG. OCS chronic treatment discontinuation or reduction over years was assessed.

Data from patients that switched from a biologic to another or more (N = 16) were collected before each start, so that a patient could be considered more than once in the analysis of comparison within and among biologics over years (N = 104). A wash-out period of 3 months was considered.

2.4. Statistical Analysis

Descriptive analysis and baseline comparisons were analysed using Graph Pad Prism software (version 9.0; GraphPad Software Inc., San Diego, CA, USA) and SPSS Statistic Version 28 (IBM Corp, Armonk, NY, USA). Descriptive analysis results are expressed as means ± SDs for continuous variables and as number/percentage for categorical variables. Python Version 3.8 was used for the A T paired sample test to evaluate the variation in Delta parameters for each year of treatment. The normality of the distributions was evaluated with D'Agostino and Pearson Test. The ROUT method detected outliers to be excluded. The Anova test (with Tukey post hoc test) or Kruskal–Wallis H-test (with Dunn post hoc test) were used to compare continuous variables, while the F Fisher test is used to compare categorical variables. Welch T test was performed to compare parameters at baseline between biologics, over years for each biologic and over years between biologics. p values of less than 0.05 were considered statistically significant.

3. Results

3.1. General Characteristics at Baseline of Severe Asthma Biologic-Treated Patients

The summary of general baseline characteristics is reported in Tables 1 and 2. At baseline the analysis of demographic characteristics did not show any significant difference between the groups.

Table 1. Baseline demographic and clinical characteristics of patients treated with different biologics. Results are expressed as mean ± standard deviation or as number with relative percentage.

	Demographic Characteristics				
	Overall	Omalizumab	Mepolizumab	Benralizumab	Dupilumab
N Patients (%)	88 (56.05%)	41 (46%)	23 (26.1%)	15 (17%)	9 (10%)
Sex: female n (%)/male n (%)	38(43.2%)/50 (56.8%)	16(39.0%)/25(61%)	10(43.5%)/13(56.5%)	9(60.0%)/6(40%)	3(33.3%)/6(66.7%)
Age (Years)	62.58 ± 11.92	64.24 ± 16.58	65.68 ± 14.82	60.87 ± 10.54	69.56 ± 16.0
BMI (Kg/m^2)	27.07 ± 5.44	28.4 ± 5.758	25.41 ± 4.39	27.76 ± 5.82	28.65 ± 4.46
Never smoker n (%)	48 (54.5%)	22 (53.7%)	13 (56.5%)	6 (40.0%)	7 (77.8%)
Current smoker n (%)	2 (2.3%)	1 (2.4%)	1 (4.3%)	0 (0.0%)	0 (0.0%)
Ex smoker n (%)	38 (43.2%)	18 (43.9%)	9 (39.1%)	9 (60.0%)	2 (22.2%)
P/Y (Current + ex)	17.8 ± 14.1	15.79 ± 11.84	12.70 ± 16.12	22.00 ± 12.19	37.00 ± 21.21
Early onset (year) n (%)	20 (22.7%)	13 (31.7%)	5 (21.7%)	1 (6.7%)	1 (11.1%)
Age of onset (years)	33.39 ±16.56	36.67 ± 15.89	31.96 ± 19.50	32.71 ± 19.09	39.33 ± 24.41
	Comorbidities				
ASA intolerance n (%)	16 (18.2%)	9 (22.0%)	5 (21.7%)	1 (6.7%)	1 (11.1%)
Rhinitis n (%)	68 (77.3%)	34 (82.9%) §§§	21 (91.3%) §§§	11 (73.3%) §	2 (22.2%)
Sinusitis (with or without polyps) n (%)	50 (56.8%)	25 (61.0%)	17 (73.9%)	8 (53.3%)	6 (66.7%)
Nasal polyposis n (%)	33 (37.5%)	11 (26.8%)	10 (43.5%)	7 (46.7%)	5 (55.6%)
Bronchiectasis n (%)	8 (9.1%)	2 (4.9%)	2 (8.7%)	4 (26.7%) *§	0 (0.0%)
GERD n (%)	20 (22.7%)	5 (12.2%)	5 (21.7%)	6 (40.0%)	4 (44.4%) *
OSAS n (%)	4 (4.5%)	1 (2.4%)	1 (4.3%)	1 (6.7%)	1 (11.1%)
Obesity n (%)	24 (27.3%)	8 (19.5%)	11 (47.8%) *	3 (20.0%)	2 (22.2%)
Diabetes n (%)	7 (8%)	3 (7.3%)	1 (4.3%)	1 (6.7%)	2 (22.2%)
Hypertension n (%)	24 (27.3%)	11 (26.8%)	8 (34.8%)	4 (26.7%)	1 (11.1%)
MI n (%)	3 (3.4%)	1 (2.4%)	0 (0.0%)	0 (0.0%)	2 (22.2%)
Heart failure n (%)	4 (4.5%)	1 (2.4%)	0 (0.0%)	1 (6.7%)	2 (22.2%)
Arrhythmias n (%)	6 (6.8%)	4 (9.8%)	0 (0.0%)	1 (6.7%)	1 (11.1%)

Table 1. Cont.

SAD n (%)	10 (11.4%)	6 (14.6%)	3 (13.0%)	0 (0.0%)	1 (11.1%)
VCD n (%)	2 (2.3%)	0 (0.0%)	0 (0.0%)	0 (0.0%)	2 (22.2%)
EGPA n (%)	0 (0%)	0 (0.0%)	0 (0.0%)	0 (0.0%)	0 (0.0%)
Osteoporosis n (%)	12 (13.6%)	8 (19.5%)	2 (8.7%)	1 (6.7%)	1 (11.1%)
Past pneumoniae n (%)	15 (17%)	6 (14.6%)	5 (21.7%)	3 (20.0%)	1 (11.1%)
ABPA n (%)	2 (2.3%)	2 (4.9%)	0 (0.0%)	0 (0.0%)	0 (0.0%)
Chronic pain n (%)	4 (4.5%)	2 (4.9%)	1 (4.3%)	0 (0.0%)	1 (11.1%)
Arthropathies n (%)	6 (6.8%)	1 (2.4%)	3 (13.0%)	2 (13.3%)	0 (0.0%)
Familiarity n (%)	16 (18.2%)	7 (17.1%)	2 (8.7%)	4 (26.7%)	3 (33.3%)
Atopy n (%)	64 (72.7%)	41 (100.0%)	12 (52.2%) ****	7 (46.7%) ****	4 (44.4%) ****
Monosesitize n (%)	12 (13.6%)	5 (12.2%)	3 (13.0%)	2 (13.3%)	2 (22.2%)
Polysensitized n (%)	52 (59.1%)	35 (85.4%)	9 (39.1%) ***	7 (46.7%) **	1 (11.1%) ****
Seasonal allergen n (%)	52 (59.1%)	33 (80.5%)	10 (43.5%) **	8 (53.3%) *	1 (11.1%) ****/#
Perennial allergen n (%)	49 (55.7%)	35 (85.4%)	6 (26.1%) ****	4 (26.7%) ****	4 (44.4%) **
Alternaria n (%)	7 (7.95%)	6 (14.6%)	1 (4.3%)	0 (0.0%)	0 (0.0%)
Aspergillus n (%)	16 (18.18%)	11 (26.8%)	4 (17.4%)	0 (0.0%) *	1 (11.1%)
Specific IgE n (%)	13 (14.8%)	8 (19.5%)	4 (17.4%)	0 (0.0%)	1 (11.1%)
Prick test n (%)	6 (6.8%)	6 (14.6%)	0 (0.0%)	0 (0.0%)	0 (0.0%)
Treatment/Clinical outcome					
BDP HFA dose, mcg	702.30 ± 216.00	673.17 ± 244.97	650.00 ± 174.93	783.33 ± 154.35 *°	757.89 ± 216.84
LABA n (%)	88 (100%)	41 (100%)	23 (100%)	15 (100%)	9 (100%)
LAMA n (%)	33 (37.5%)	12 (29.3%)	10 (43.5%)	6 (40.0%)	5 (55.6%)
Chronic OCS n (%)	24 (27.3%)	9 (22%)	8 (34.8%)	4 (26.7%)	3 (33.3%)
OCS bursts ≥ 3/year n (%)	44 (50%)	17 (41.5%)	15 (65.2%)	9 (60.0%)	3 (33.3%)
OCS bursts ≥ 3/year and Chronic OCS n (%)	15 (17.04%)	4 (9.7%)	6 (26.08%)	3 (20%)	2 (22.2%)
OCS dependence n (%)	53 (60.2%)	22 (53.7%)	17 (73.9%)	10 (66.7%)	4 (44.4%)
Biologic switches n (%)	16 (18%)	8 (19.5%)	5 (21.7%)	2 (13.3%)	1 (11.1%)
ACT score	17.65 ± 4.41	19.37 ± 2.97	16.69 ± 4.84 *	17.61 ± 4.98	15.42 ± 4.55 **
Controlled (ACT ≥ 20) n (%)	37 (42%)	26 (63.4%)	5 (21.7%) **	5 (33.3%)	1 (11.1%) **
Not controlled (ACT ≤ 19) n (%)	51 (58%)	15 (36.6%)	18 (78.3%) **	10 (66.7%)	8 (88.9%) **
Activity limitations	3.09 ± 1.24	3.19 ± 1.08	3.12 ± 1.24	3.44 ± 1.46	2.84 ± 1.21
Nocturnal symptoms	3.94 ± 1.40	4.52 ± 0.87	3.85 ± 1.46	3.82 ± 1.59	3.95 ± 1.58
Exacerbations/year	3.55 ± 2.94	3.15 ± 3.07	4.27 ± 2.91	4.00 ± 2.83	2.58 ± 1.95 °
ER visits n (%)	33 (37.5%)	13 (31.7%)	8 (34.8%)	7 (46.7%)	5 (55.6%)
Intubation n (%)	1 (1.1%)	1 (2.4%)	0 (0.0%)	0 (0.0%)	0 (0.0%)

BMI: Body mass index, P/Y: pack/years, ASA intolerance: Aspirin intolerance, GERD: gastroesophageal reflux disease, OSAS: obstructive sleep apnea syndrome, MI: myocardial infarction, SAD: social anxiety disorder; VCD: vocal cord dysfunction, EGPA: eosinophilic granulomatosis with polyangiitis, ABPA: allergic bronchopulmonary aspergillosis, BDP HFA dose: beclomethasone mcg equivalent dose hydrofluoroalkane, LABA: long acting beta agonist; LAMA: long-acting muscarinic antagonist, OCS: oral corticosteroids, ACT: asthma control test, and ER: emergency room. Significance vs. omalizumab: * < 0.05, ** < 0.001, *** < 0.0001, **** < 0.00001, significance vs. mepolizumab: ° < 0.05, significance vs. benralizumab: # < 0.05, and significance vs. dupilumab: § < 0.05, §§§ < 0.0001.

Table 2. Baseline functional and biological characteristics of patients treated with different biologics. Results are expressed as mean ±standard deviation.

	Functional Parameters/Biomarkers				
	Overall	Omalizumab	Mepolizumab	Benralizumab	Dupilumab
	T0	T0	T0	T0	T0
FVC abs. (L)	2.75 ± 1.01	2.76 ± 1.04	2.79 ± 1.05	2.95 ± 0.99	2.37 ± 0.60 #
FVC % pred.	86.88 ± 17.98	89.02 ± 18.91	83.50 ± 16.67	93.56 ± 22.56	83.05 ± 19.70
FEV_1 abs. (L)	1.701 ± 0.71	1.67 ± 0.63	1.72 ± 0.86	1.87 ± 0.75	1.32 ± 0.51 *#
FEV_1 % pred.	65.50 ± 17.73	65.08 ± 15.71	62.88 ± 19.41	72.67 ± 21.08	57.21 ± 18.89 #
IT abs.	59.43 ± 12.34	59.19 ± 13.47	58.59 ± 11.70	60.24 ± 14.47	53.58 ± 13.11
IT % pred.	72.74 ± 14.78	69.50 ± 13.71	74.46 ± 15.65	75.29 ± 18.95	67.78 ± 15.90
RV abs. (L)	3.09 ± 1.11	3.08 ± 1.04	3.18 ± 1.03	3.22 ± 1.45	3.13 ± 1.14
RV % pred.	147.70 ± 47.37	159.11 ± 46.37	148.73 ± 45.27	139.72 ± 49.73	150.94 ± 44.80
FVC post BD abs. (L)	3.02 ± 1.16	3.03 ± 1.2	2.95 ± 1.24	3.22 ± 1.11	2.57 ± 0.66 #
FVC Delta abs. post BD (L)	0.30 ± 0.24	0.33 ± 0.28	0.27 ± 0.21	0.25 ± 0.22	0.23 ± 0.17
FVC Delta % post BD	11.11 ± 8.3	11.92 ± 9.24	9.12 ± 7.18	7.36 ± 7.23	8.05 ± 9.17
FEV_1 post abs. (L)	1.93 ± 0.85	1.95 ± 0.76	1.82 ± 1.10	2.05 ± 0.85	1.53 ± 0.6 *#
FEV_1 Delta abs. post BD (L)	0.23 ± 0.19	0.24 ± 0.17	0.23 ± 0.19	0.18 ± 0.22	0.21 ± 0.18
FEV_1 Delta % post BD	15.01 ± 9.70	15.58 ± 8.35	15.66 ± 9.72	10.49 ± 12.76	16.16 ± 9.36
DLCO %	85.50 ± 20.16	87.71 ± 9.94	78.42 ± 23.13	85.38 ± 26.87	76.60 ± 13.94
DLCO/Va %	100.20 ± 22.13	102.86 ± 19.62	93.70 ± 20.64	101.30 ± 30.07	98.00 ± 22.40
F_ENO (ppb)	40.34 ± 29.42	35.47 ± 27.81	52.73 ± 33.00	39.96 ± 24.39	31.13 ± 22.94 °
Total IgE (UI/mL)	215.50 ± 180.40	323.45 ± 261.19	307.65 ± 421.13	466.07 ± 461.11	327.75 ± 649.39
Leucocytes absolute count (cells/mcl)	8124.00 ± 2121.00	8190.00 ± 1951.47	7771.65 ± 1822.44	8248.75 ± 1923.05	9152.63 ± 2546.82
Neutrophils (%)	55.00 ± 10.00	55.12 ± 9.19	52.95 ± 10.77	54.54 ± 8.11	58.55 ± 11.33
Neutrophils absolute count (cells/mcl)	4513.00 ± 1676.00	4588.46 ± 1583.27	4058.47 ± 1566.19	4570.62 ± 1274.58	5266.84 ± 1930.38
Eosinophils (%)	5.90 ± 4.45	5.44 ± 4.06	7.02 ± 4.13	7.00 ± 5.57	3.59 ± 2.59 °°#*
Eosinophils absolute count (cells/mcl)	436.30 ± 294.70	426.79 ± 310.28	560.38 ± 312.03	563.89 ± 468.83	296.84 ± 193.16 °#*
Fibrinogen (mg/dL)	355.00 ± 94.42	356.62 ± 95.72	363.40 ± 112.49	327.29 ± 86.61	366.86 ± 79.42

FEV_1: Forced expiratory volume in 1 s; FVC: forced vital capacity, abs: absolute, post BD: post bronchodilators, pred.: predicted, IT: Tiffeneau index, RV: residual volume, DLCO: diffusion capacity for carbon monoxide, and FeNO: exhaled nitric oxide. Significance vs. omalizumab: * < 0.05, Significance vs. Mepolizumab: ° < 0.05, °° < 0.001, significance vs. benralizumab: # < 0.05.

OmaG were all atopic with prevalent polysensitization to both seasonal and perennial allergens while it was about 50% for the other groups with a very low number (11.1%) of polysensitized in DupiG ($p < 0.00001$).

Concerning comorbidities, OmaG had less bronchiectasis on chest HRCT compared to BenraG ($p < 0.05$), less prevalence of obesity and GERD ($p < 0.05$) compared to MepoG, and presented a more controlled asthma of MepoG and DupiG ($p < 0.01$). DupiG had less rhinitis compared to other groups ($p < 0.001$) and a lesser mean number of AEs ($p < 0.05$ vs. MepoG). BenraG took higher doses of ICS compared to OmaG and MepoG ($p < 0.05$).

At baseline, DupiG had worse pulmonary function compared to OmaG and BenraG. In particular, FVC abs. and FEV_1 abs/ %pred. both pre and post BD were significantly inferior in DupiG ($p < 0.05$) compared to BenraG, while FEV_1 abs. pre and post BD were significantly inferior compared to OmaG ($p < 0.05$).

Lower basal F_ENO values compared to MepoG ($p < 0.05$) and lower count of PBE as compared to others ($p < 0.05$) were reported in DupiG.

3.2. T2 Phenotyping Patients

The majority of patients (86.3%) had at least two positive T2 biomarkers at baseline. DupiG patients reported a significantly lower rate of 3–4 T2 positive biomarkers compared to BenraG and MepoG (Table 3).

Table 3. Distribution of expression of T2 biomarkers in patients treated with different biologics.

(n)	T2 Biomarkers				
	Overall (88)	Omalizumab (41)	Mepolizumab (23)	Benralizumab (15)	Dupilumab (9)
1–2 biomarker n (%)	39 (44.3%)	20 (48.8%)	7 (30.4%)	5 (33.3%)	7 (77.7%) °#
3–4 biomarkers n (%)	49 (55.6%)	21 (51.2%)	16 (69.5%)	10 (66.6%)	2 (22.2%) °#

Significance vs. mepolizumab: ° < 0.05, significance vs. benralizumab: # < 0.05.

3.3. Analysis of "Intra-Biologic" Parameters over Years

The number of SA patients for each bio group decreased over time, as shown in Table S2, for lost in follow-up, outbreak of pandemic SARS-CoV-2, or different starting point of biologics. The number and sequence of switches from a biologic to another is represented in Figure S1.

As shown in Table 4, OmaG showed a significant reduction in ICS mean dose ($p < 0.05$) at T4, an improvement in ACT, a significant reduction in AEs (from 3.15 to 1.0; $p < 0.001$ at T1), and an increase in FEV_1 and FVC % pred. already evident from T1 (from 65.08 to 72.87 and from 89.02 to 97.02, respectively $p < 0.05$). A reduction in RV %pred. emerged at T4 (from 159.11 to 113.0, $p < 0.05$). Anti-IgE did not affect F_ENO values nor PBE count, while total IgE levels increased.

MepoG showed from T1 a significant progressive improvement in ACT ($p < 0.000.1$ at T3), activity limitations ($p < 0.0001$ at T3), and nocturnal symptoms ($p < 0.05$). MepoG dramatically reduced the number of AEs at T1 (from 4.27 to 1.08, $p < 0.0001$) with greater effects to T4 (0.44) and improved pulmonary function starting from T2 with the highest value at T3 (ΔFEV_1 %pred. 24%; $p < 0.01$, absolute delta +610 mL, and FVC %pred. $p < 0.00001$). At T4 post-FVC BD reversibility decreased ($p < 0.001$). MepoG significantly reduced PBE count at T1 ($p < 0.00001$) with further reduction over years, while it did not affect F_ENO values nor total IgE.

BenraG increased ACT at T1 ($p < 0.05$) and reduced AEs (4.0 vs. 0.89, $p < 0.001$). An improvement of FEV_1 (+850 mL/+25.4%) and IT (from 60.2 to 72.0) was clearly evident at T2 with normalization of IT abs. ($p < 0.05$). Anti IL5-Rα did not influence F_ENO or total IgE values, while it reduced PBE count starting from T1 with a total suppression at T2 ($p < 0.00001$). We also observed a significant mean reduction in the neutrophils absolute count at T2 (from 4570 to 3115, delta −955/mcl; $p < 0.001$) and a trend toward a concomitant reduction in fibrinogen values (from 327.3 to 294.0).

Table 4. "Intra-biologic" analysis of functional and biological characteristics of patients treated with a biologic therapy over years.

	Omalizumab					Mepolizumab					Benralizumab				Dupilumab	
	T0	T1	T3	T4	T0	T1	T2	T3	T4	T0	T1	T2	T0	T1
BDP HFA dose, mcg	673.17 ± 244.97	662.50 ± 258.88	558.06 ± 293.00	500.00 ± 258.20 *	650.00 ± 174.93	580.00 ± 261.41	600.00 ± 215.21	600.00 ± 181.50	688.89 ± 247.21	783.33 ± 154.35	766.67 ± 123.67	650.00 ± 232.99	757.89 ± 216.84	800.00 ± 240.37
ACT score	19.37 ± 2.97	20.70 ± 2.56 *	20.83 ± 3.44	21.57 ± 2.92 *	16.69 ± 4.84	20.67 ± 3.41 °°	20.40 ± 4.67 °	21.83 ± 3.00 °°°	22.22 ± 3.42 °°	17.61 ± 4.28 #	21.94 ± 4.28 #	21.00 ± 3.96	15.42 ± 4.55	20.00 ± 3.86 §§
Activity limitation	3.19 ± 1.08	4.05 ± 0.90 *	4.17 ± 1.20 *	4.50 ± 1.16 *	3.12 ± 1.24	3.92 ± 0.97 °	3.95 ± 1.19 °	4.39 ± 0.78 °°°	4.56 ± 0.73 °°	3.44 ± 1.46	4.17 ± 1.25	4.38 ± 0.74 #	2.84 ± 1.21	3.95 ± 1.13 §
Nocturnal symptoms	4.52 ± 0.87	4.82 ± 0.50	4.76 ± 0.97	4.93 ± 0.27	3.85 ± 1.46	4.83 ± 0.64 °	4.30 ± 1.38	4.67 ± 0.77 °	4.67 ± 1.00	3.82 ± 1.59	4.61 ± 1.04	4.88 ± 0.35 #	3.95 ± 1.58	4.26 ± 1.15
Exacerbations/year	3.15 ± 3.07	1.00 ± 1.47 ***	1.22 ± 1.70 **	1.13 ± 1.58 **	4.27 ± 2.91	1.08 ± 1.35 °°°	0.75 ± 0.91 °°°	0.61 ± 0.70 °°°	0.44 ± 0.73 °°°	4.00 ± 2.83	0.89 ± 0.90 ##	1.12 ± 1.25 ##	2.58 ± 1.95	0.42 ± 0.96 §§§
FVC abs. (L)	2.76 ± 1.04	3.04 ± 1.12	2.94 ± 1.07	2.78 ± 1.03	2.79 ± 1.05	3.02 ± 1.19	2.88 ± 0.86	3.39 ± 1.34	2.81 ± 0.72	2.95 ± 0.99	3.11 ± 1.11	3.44 ± 1.22	2.37 ± 0.60	2.54 ± 0.69
FVC % pred.	89.02 ± 18.91	97.72 ± 16.27	95.55 ± 16.57	99.08 ± 18.92	83.50 ± 16.67	91.61 ± 25.16	99.12 ± 27.29	108.40 ± 16.15 °°°	98.71 ± 18.51	93.56 ± 22.56	96.61 ± 23.09	105.00 ± 23.00	83.05 ± 19.70	85.71 ± 21.93
FEV₁ abs. (L)	1.67 ± 0.63	1.87 ± 0.72	1.87 ± 0.63	1.90 ± 0.71	1.81 ± 0.73	2.01 ± 1.04	1.82 ± 0.73	2.33 ± 1.15	1.89 ± 0.57	1.87 ± 0.75	2.11 ± 1.00	2.72 ± 0.95 #	1.32 ± 0.51	1.58 ± 0.65
FEV₁ % pred.	65.08 ± 15.71	72.97 ± 17.64 *	75.30 ± 16.93 *	76.70 ± 21.90 *	62.88 ± 19.41	73.62 ± 28.37	76.06 ± 28.78	86.73 ± 20.79 °°	81.43 ± 18.61	72.67 ± 21.08	79.06 ± 28.85	98.12 ± 20.57 #	57.21 ± 18.89	64.47 ± 19.23
IT abs.	59.19 ± 13.47	61.69 ± 9.19	63.43 ± 9.53	63.97 ± 11.01	58.59 ± 11.70	61.18 ± 12.54	60.10 ± 12.97	64.33 ± 13.04	65.99 ± 8.27	62.21 ± 14.24	79.06 ± 28.85	72.00 ± 5.63 #	53.58 ± 13.11	59.56 ± 13.12
IT % pred.	69.50 ± 13.71	77.82 ± 11.10 *	78.85 ± 12.5 *	75.96 ± 13.12	74.46 ± 15.65	76.77 ± 15.77	73.88 ± 16.09	80.67 ± 17.22	79.43 ± 8.89	75.29 ± 18.95	79.94 ± 19.59	94.14 ± 8.13 ##	67.78 ± 15.90	73.33 ± 15.43
RV abs. (L)	3.08 ± 1.04	2.63 ± 0.78	2.79 ± 0.82	2.18 ± 0.85 *	3.18 ± 1.03	2.85 ± 0.97	3.08 ± 0.83	2.55 ± 0.56	2.44 ± 0.73	3.22 ± 1.4	2.78 ± 1.17	3.25 ± 2.08	3.13 ± 1.14	2.47 ± 0.07 §
RV % pred.	159.11 ± 46.37	127.15 ± 38.82 *	132.64 ± 44.90	113.00 ± 28.21 **	148.73 ± 45.27	143.13 ± 51.42	154.36 ± 36.97	127.58 ± 31.77	121.20 ± 41.03	139.72 ± 49.73	142.71 ± 50.81	105.43 ± 46.24	150.94 ± 44.80	125.33 ± 41.85
FVC post BD abs.(L)	3.03 ± 1.21	3.48 ± 1.26	3.03 ± 0.63	2.82 ± 1.23	2.95 ± 1.24	3.13 ± 1.08	3.02 ± 0.96	3.62 ± 1.29	3.21 ± 0.46	3.22 ± 1.11	3.30 ± 1.08	3.35 ± 1.52	2.57 ± 0.66	2.69 ± 0.73
FVC Delta abs. post BD (L)	0.33 ± 0.28	0.15 ± 0.21 *	0.22 ± 0.29	0.16 ± 0.21	0.27 ± 0.21	0.15 ± 0.12	0.20 ± 0.22	0.17 ± 0.19	0.08 ± 0.03 °	0.25 ± 0.22	0.24 ± 0.33	0.16 ± 0.14	0.23 ± 0.17	0.19 ± 0.16
FVC Delta % post BD	11.92 ± 9.24	6.48 ± 9.08	8.95 ± 13.60	4.00 ± 6.22 *	9.12 ± 7.18	4.93 ± 4.25	6.62 ± 5.84	5.75 ± 6.95	2.42 ± 1.25 °°	7.36 ± 7.23	5.87 ± 6.96	5.62 ± 3.74	8.05 ± 9.17	9.91 ± 8.58
FEV₁ post abs. (L)	1.95 ± 0.76	2.06 ± 0.84	1.84 ± 0.49	2.01 ± 0.79	1.82 ± 1.10	2.26 ± 0.95	2.01 ± 0.88	2.58 ± 1.10	2.38 ± 0.21	2.05 ± 0.85	2.20 ± 0.82	2.56 ± 1.24	1.53 ± 0.63	1.60 ± 0.62
FEV₁ Post BD abs. (L)	0.24 ± 0.17	0.17 ± 0.12	0.15 ± 0.15	0.21 ± 0.17	0.23 ± 0.19	0.16 ± 0.10	0.10 ± 0.46	0.17 ± 0.16	0.13 ± 0.14	0.18 ± 0.22	0.17 ± 0.20	0.13 ± 0.15	0.21 ± 0.18	0.17 ± 0.06
FEV₁ Delta % post BD	15.58 ± 8.35	10.60 ± 8.24	8.38 ± 7.67 *	11.55 ± 6.71	15.66 ± 9.72	7.52 ± 2.91	1.72 ± 33.20	8.37 ± 10.17	6.55 ± 7.31	10.49 ± 12.76	10.49 ± 9.79	6.13 ± 5.31	16.16 ± 9.36	13.75 ± 9.05
DLCO %	87.71 ± 9.94	98.75 ± 21.87	105.50 ± 17.68	97.00 ± 22.00	78.42 ± 23.13	64.00 ± 46.67	41.99 ± 30.12	88.20 ± 15.06		85.38 ± 26.87	92.67 ± 24.01	94.50 ± 17.68	76.60 ± 13.94	89.00 ± 19.37
F_ENO (ppb)	35.47 ± 27.81	31.54 ± 21.89	42.64 ± 34.23	48.11 ± 51.61	52.73 ± 33.00	56.87 ± 50.08	41.99 ± 30.12	59.75 ± 50.89	641.95 ± 833.04	39.96 ± 24.39	50.84 ± 60.13	53.60 ± 40.48	31.13 ± 22.94	29.48 ± 17.17
Total IgE (UI/mL)	323.45 ± 261.19	792.33 ± 649.35 *	606.55 ± 419.06 *	576.06 ± 519.86	307.65 ± 421.13	236.91 ± 152.03	197.13 ± 213.36	149.00 ± 49.50		466.07 ± 461.11	613.67 ± 793.41		327.75 ± 649.39	221.05 ± 280.84
Leukocytes absolute count (cells/mcl)	8190.00 ± 1951.47	7357.42 ± 1952.10	7977.14 ± 3673.14	7321.50 ± 2063.33	7771.65 ± 1822.44	7977.39 ± 1870.07	7325.56 ± 2491.86	7248.82 ± 2038.64	7220.00 ± 1464.66	8248.75 ± 1923.05	7551.76 ± 2973.69	6182.86 ± 1190.44 ##	9152.63 ± 2546.82	8011.25 ± 1772.18
Neutrophils %	55.12 ± 9.19	59.48 ± 11.54	58.88 ± 8.09	56.07 ± 7.01	52.95 ± 10.77	57.99 ± 8.98	55.28 ± 10.03	60.73 ± 11.93	56.89 ± 7.43	54.54 ± 8.11	58.46 ± 10.16	49.07 ± 9.79	58.55 ± 11.33	53.83 ± 5.49

Table 4. Cont.

	Omalizumab					Mepolizumab					Benralizumab			Dupilumab		
	T0	T1	T2	T3	T4	T0	T1	T2	T3	T4	T0	T1	T2	T0	T1
Neutrophils absolute count (cells/mcl)	4588.46 ± 1583.27	4246.47 ± 1556.59	5072.31 ± 2982.80	4062.31 ± 1195.96	4072.22 ± 1414.37	4058.47 ± 1566.19	4574.55 ± 1522.37	4115.00 ± 1994.25	4817.65 ± 2309.18	4085.71 ± 821.52	4570.62 ± 1274.58	4490.00 ± 2040.00	3115.00 ± 299.25 ##	5266.84 ± 1930.38	4304.50 ± 1610.92
Eosinophils %	5.44 ± 4.06	4.59 ± 3.71	5.17 ± 4.76	5.35 ± 3.44	5.03 ± 2.97	7.02 ± 4.13	1.43 ± 1.16 °°°°	1.50 ± 1.25 °°°°	1.29 ± 1.37 °°°°	1.04 ± 0.59 °°°°	7.00 ± 5.57	0.53 ± 2.00 ###	0.00 ± 0.00 ####	3.59 ± 2.59	5.94 ± 6.57
Eosinophils absolute count (cells/mcl)	426.79 ± 310.28	341.68 ± 271.28	363.29 ± 271.66	396.40 ± 231.73	403.12 ± 218.90	560.38 ± 312.03	108.26 ± 79.98 °°°°	105.00 ± 81.47 °°°°	85.88 ± 81.17 °°°°	74.29 ± 38.23 °°°°	563.89 ± 468.83	47.06 ± 188.94 ###	0.00 ± 0.00 ####	296.84 ± 193.16	527.06 ± 613.29
Fibrinogen (mg/dl)	356.62 ± 95.72	344.33 ± 100.47	330.67 ± 73.95	429.40 ± 88.71		363.40 ± 112.49		369.25 ± 95.12	404.22 ± 101.63	419.75 ± 129.64	327.29 ± 86.61	327.67 ± 92.39	294.00 ± 75.36	366.86 ± 79.42	382.50 ± 98.99

BDP HFA dose: beclomethasone mcg equivalent dose hydrofluoroalkane, FEV₁: forced expiratory volume in 1 s; FVC: forced vital capacity, abs: absolute, post BD: post bronchodilators, pred.: predicted, IT: Tiffenau index, RV: residual volume, DLCO: diffusion capacity for carbon monoxide, and FeNO: exhaled nitric oxide. Results are expressed as mean ±standard deviation significance vs. T0 in omalizumab: * < 0.05, ** < 0.001, *** < 0.0001, significance vs. T0 in mepolizumab: ° < 0.05, °° < 0.001, °°° < 0.0001, °°°° < 0.00001, significance vs. T0 in benralizumab: # < 0.05, ## < 0.001, ### < 0.0001, #### < 0.00001, and significance vs. T0 in dupilumab: § < 0.05, §§ < 0.001, §§§ < 0.0001,. Empty cells: not enough values for calculation.

DupiG improved ACT score, activity limitations and nocturnal symptoms ($p < 0.001$) at T1. It was able to decrease the number of AEs (2.58 vs. 0.42, $p < 0.0001$) and RV abs (delta −660 mL; $p < 0.05$). An improvement in delta changes in FEV_1 was observed, although not statistical significance (+260 mL, +7.26%). It did not affect F_ENO or IgE values while showing an increase in PBE count which was not statistically significant.

3.4. Analysis of "Inter-Biologic" Parameters over Years

Table 5 shows the "inter-biologic" comparison of means of paired Delta change for each variable over years.

BenraG and DupiG improved ACT at T1 more than OmaG ($p < 0.05$, $p < 0.001$, respectively), while MepoG improved ACT at T3 more than OmaG (Figure 1A). BenraG reduced nocturnal asthma symptoms more than both OmaG and MepoG at T2 ($p < 0.05$, Figure 1B). The AEs reduction was similar among biologics but more pronounced at T3 in favor of MepoG vs. OmaG ($p < 0.05$, Figure 1F) of MepoG than DupiG at T1. OmaG improved more IT% pred. from T2 to T4 ($p < 0.01$ at T3) compared to MepoG with a trend of amelioration with regard to FVC %pred. in favor of MepoG to OmaG at T3 (Figure 1C, E). Only DupiG showed an improved FVC Delta% post BD at T1 compared to OmaG (Figure 1D). We observed a significant downward trend in the neutrophil count both for BenraG and DupiG compared to OmaG at T1 (Figure 1G, $p < 0.05$). Finally, PBE was significantly reduced starting from T1 for MepoG and BenraG while augmented in DupiG (Figure 1H).

Table 5. "Inter-biologic" analysis of functional and biological characteristics of patients treated with a biologic therapy over years.

	Omalizumab				Mepolizumab				Benralizumab		Dupilumab
	Delta T1	Delta T2	Delta T3	Delta T4	Delta T1	Delta T2	Delta T3	Delta T4	Delta T1	Delta T2	Delta T1
BDP HFA dose, mcg	−17.50 ±169.29	−69.70 ±251.85	−87.10 ±301.93	−100.00 ±263.00	−72.00 ±279.17	−40.00 ±270.28	−16.67 ±214.89	55.56 ±278.89	−16.67 ±161.79	−37.50 ±346.15	42.11 ±254.55
ACT score	1.40 ± 3.42	1.48 ± 3.78	1.17 ± 3.75	1.96 ± 3.97	3.88 ± 3.78	3.45 ± 4.66	4.22 ± 4.98 *	6.33 ± 7.07	4.33 ± 5.76 *	5.12 ± 3.09 *	4.58 ± 4.03 **
Activity limitation	0.81 ± 1.36	1.14 ± 1.56	0.77 ± 1.24	1.38 ± 1.19	0.75 ± 1.07	0.75 ± 1.33	1.06 ± 1.30	1.67 ± 1.41	0.72 ± 1.71	1.12 ± 1.25	1.11 ± 1.05
Nocturnal symptoms	0.29 ± 1.06	0.07 ± 1.07	0.08 ± 0.76	0.50 ± 0.76	0.92 ± 1.35	0.30 ± 1.38	0.67 ± 1.46	0.78 ± 1.86	0.76 ± 1.64	1.71 ± 1.38 *°	0.32 ± 1.38
Exacerbations/year	−2.28 ±2.80	−2.06 ± 3.74	−1.90 ±3.32	−2.57 ± 3.54	−3.38 ±2.63	−3.55 ±2.31	−4.00 ±3.22 *	−4.78 ±3.46	−3.11 ±2.78	−4.00 ±2.78	−2.16 ±1.61 *
FVC abs. (L)	0.24 ±0.39	0.22 ±0.38	0.26 ±0.46	0.16 ±0.64	0.15 ±0.54	0.14 ±0.47	0.29 ±0.44	−0.02 ± 0.31	0.16 ±0.47	0.26 ±0.49	0.15 ±0.39
FVC % pred.	6.94 ±15.91	5.55 ±14.80	8.76 ±16.62	8.04 ±23.81	6.57 ±21.27	14.94 ±23.08	18.53 ±16.82	17.29 ±22.34	3.06 ±14.95	8.14 ±14.58	3.47 ±15.99
FEV1 abs. (L)	0.19 ±0.42	0.23 ±0.35	0.28 ±0.39	0.19 ±0.47	0.21 ±0.45	0.14 ±0.40	0.31 ±0.45	0.04 ±0.29	0.24 ±0.46	0.41 ±0.47	0.23 ±0.46
FEV1 % pred.	7.17 ±18.52	9.93 ±13.72	13.60 ±16.68	12.23 ±20.58	9.50 ±17.37	12.94 ±19.21	16.00 ±16.27	13.86 ±18.40	6.39 ±14.97	13.12 ±15.53	7.35 ±19.54
IT abs. (L)	2.28 ±10.81	4.67 ±9.42	5.75 ±10.92	4.18 ±10.99	2.38 ±4.56	1.44 ±6.38	2.26 ±4.69	2.53 ±5.71	2.28 ±5.47	3.00 ±7.14	5.27 ±10.61
IT % pred.	6.67 ±13.42	9.46 ±11.87	12.75 ±11.80	7.88 ±12.41	2.82 ±6.62	−0.06 ±8.76 *	1.73 ± 7.82 **	−2.14 ±7.67 *	3.50 ±7.31	4.43 ±8.92	5.00 ±8.43
RV abs. (L)	−0.37 ±1.33	−0.29 ±0.68	−0.86 ±0.88	−0.94 ±0.47	−0.77 ±1.55	0.34 ±0.76	−0.37 ±0.47		−0.12 ±0.62	−0.29 ±0.24	−0.52 ±1.00
RV % pred.	−35.08 ±59.49	−9.50 ±36.03	−42.29 ±38.81	−54.00 ±17.11	−12.00 ±55.61	8.60 ±32.42	−17.80 ±19.69		10.57 ±46.88 *	−17.29 ±16.10	−21.40 ±35.64
FVC post BD abs. (L)	0.16 ±0.25	0.22 ±0.41	0.24 ±0.60	0.32 ±0.86	0.28 ±0.55	0.14 ±0.47	−0.03 ±0.53		0.11 ±0.33	0.19 ±0.37	−0.04 ±0.47

Table 5. Cont.

	Omalizumab				Mepolizumab				Benralizumab		Dupilumab
	Delta T1	Delta T2	Delta T3	Delta T4	Delta T1	Delta T2	Delta T3	Delta T4	Delta T1	Delta T2	Delta T1
FVC Delta abs. post BD (L)	−0.08 ±0.19	−0.12 ±0.23	−0.25 ±0.30	−0.36 ±0.52	−0.04 ±0.24	0.01 ±0.17	−0.09 ±0.07		−0.01 ±0.49	−0.29 ±0.26	−0.02 ±0.27
FVC Delta % post BD	−3.25 ±6.19	−0.07 ±18.79	−9.68 ±7.88	−6.86 ±9.04	−3.19 ±8.45	1.18 ±8.32	−2.62 ±2.29		−2.42 ±11.01	−9.49 ±9.19	5.33 ±8.18 *
FEV$_1$ post abs. (L)	0.07 ±0.35	0.12 ±0.16	0.41 ±0.53	0.52 ±0.66	0.27 ±0.51	0.11 ±0.48	0.01 ±0.41		0.14 ±0.30	0.28 ±0.27	0.13 ±0.48
FEV$_1$ Delta post BD abs. (L)	−0.02 ±0.17	−0.03 ±0.09	−0.04 ±0.14	−0.02 ±0.08	−0.07 ±0.15	−0.15 ±0.42	−0.10 ±0.12		−0.02 ±0.29	−0.18 ±0.18	−0.00 ±0.16
FEV$_1$ Delta % post BD	−1.33 ±10.02		17.00 ±5.66		2.00 ±18.38		−0.67 ±3.06		−12.50 ±17.68		−8.00 ±11.31
DLCO %	−1.42 ±8.01	−4.22 ±8.82	−7.19 ±10.01	−5.29 ±5.61	−6.75 ±9.06	−17.80 ±36.10	−4.87 ±6.36		0.63 ±15.24	−8.10 ±8.80	−0.23 ±10.56
F$_E$NO (ppb)	−1.34 ±23.16	4.77 ±36.86	−9.32 ±27.86	4.11 ±46.58	4.36 ±45.94	−7.94 ±21.08	4.61 ±31.11		13.68 ±58.70	−12.65 ±44.47	−0.61 ±29.36
Total IgE (UI/mL)	433.87 ± 469.39	244.41 ± 296.61	280.61 ± 267.28	336.62 ± 362.71	−150.81 ±335.34 *	−510.51 ±727.59	37.50 ±26.16 *	−245.20 ±361.76	138.75 ± 425.38		
Leukocytes absolute count (cells/mcl)	−613.20 ±1861.53	637.65 ±3656.95	−202.00 ±1700.98	−103.33 ±2191.77	235.52 ±2347.21	−25.72 ±3029.60	−591.18 ±2212.59	−637.14 ±1793.19	−359.33 ±2304.89	−531.43 ±933.82	−1332.50 ±2656.25
Neutrophils %	2.65 ± 6.80	5.56 ± 4.21	1.35 ± 4.89	−2.47 ±1.56	2.09 ±12.31	−2.95 ±11.22 *	4.55 ±9.29	−6.78 ±8.06	5.71 ±10.29	−3.03 ±11.69	−4.32 ±9.67 *#
Neutrophils absolute count (cells/mcl)	14.62 ± 1092.97	512.86 ± 557.37	8.00 ± 505.64		376.92 ± 2331.59	−546.70 ±2450.23	507.78 ± 2400.87	−1500.00 ± 608.11	218.00 ± 1553.83	−631.67 ±1050.17 *	−1056.75 ±2574.46

Table 5. *Cont.*

	Omalizumab					Mepolizumab				Benralizumab		Dupilumab
	Delta T1	Delta T2	Delta T3	Delta T4	Delta T1	Delta T2	Delta T3	Delta T4		Delta T1	Delta T2	Delta T1
Eosinophils %	−1.33 ±3.15	−1.87 ±3.53	−2.66 ±4.00	−2.03 ±3.08	−5.70 ±4.39 **	−5.83 ±4.07 *	−6.93 ±3.98 **	−6.27 ±5.19		−6.49 ±6.79 *	−5.94 ±2.89 *	2.49 ±6.97 °°##
Eosinophils absolute count (cells/mcl)	−94.72 ±236.97	−128.50 ±349.03	−128.50 ±261.76	−125.38 ±298.07	−463.91 ±329.31 ****	−471.50 ±308.17 **	−537.65 ±312.28 **	−465.71 ±338.62 *		−520.59 ±560.21 **	−367.14 ±148.74 *	231.18 ±674.46 °°°##
Fibrinogen (mg/dL)	0.00 ±0.00	16.75 ±25.58	54.00 ±119.25			22.88 ±46.77	−20.00 ±23.61	−38.00 ±11.31		1.64 ± 30.03	15.00 ± 41.01	−38.33 ±44.66

BDP HFA dose: beclomethasone mcg equivalent dose hydrofluoroalkane, FEV$_1$: forced expiratory volume in 1 s; FVC: forced vital capacity, abs: absolute, post BD: post bronchodilators, pred.: predicted, IT: Tiffenau index, RV: residual volume, DLCO: diffusion capacity for carbon monoxide, and FeNO: exhaled nitric oxide. Values represent the variation in parameters from each time point (e. T1, T2, T3, and T4) to T0 (paired Delta). Delta are expressed as mean ± standard deviation significance vs. omalizumab: * < 0.05, ** < 0.001, **** < 0.00001, significance vs. mepolizumab: ° < 0.05, °° < 0.001, °°° < 0.0001, significance vs. benralizumab: # < 0.05, ## < 0.001. Empty cells: not enough values for calculation.

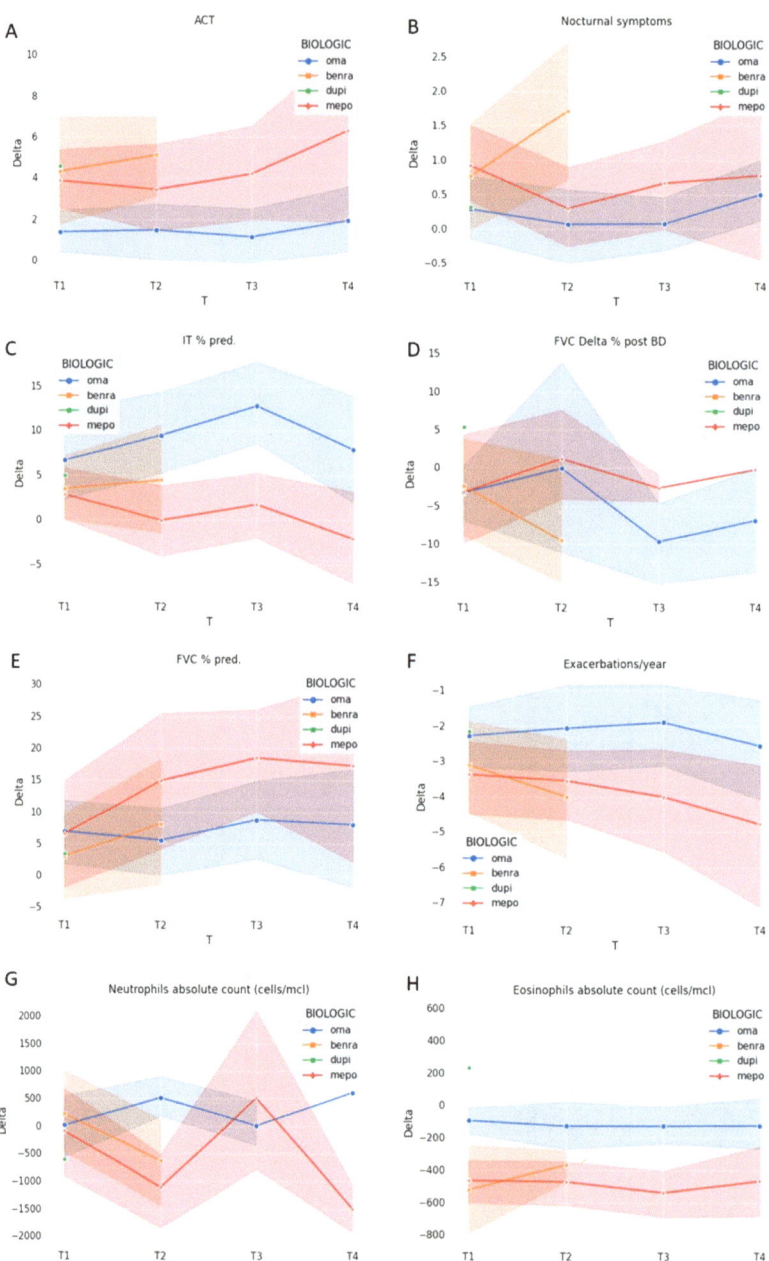

Figure 1. Solid lines represent the trend of mean paired Delta values calculated from each time point towards T0. Shaded areas cover 95% IC. (**A**) ACT: asthma control test, (**B**) nocturnal symptoms, (**C**) TI % pred.: Tiffeneau index, (**D**) FVC Delta % post BD, (**E**) FVC% pred., (**F**) exacerbations/year, (**G**) neutrophils, and (**H**) eosinophils absolute count.

3.5. OCS Chronic Treatment

At baseline, there were no differences in the prevalence of patients with chronic OCS treatment (Table 1). Overall, at T1, discontinuation of OCS was reached of 16/31 (51.6%), with the best yield for OmaG (66%) and MepoG (63.6%). At T4, 60% (N = 5) of patients in the OmaG withdrew OCS, while all patients interrupted OCS maintenance treatment at T3 in MepoG and at T2 in BenraG. The proportion of patients interrupting chronic OCS in DupiG was 28.5% at T1, while 28.5% reduced chronic OCS therapy by 50% (Figure 2A–D and Table S3).

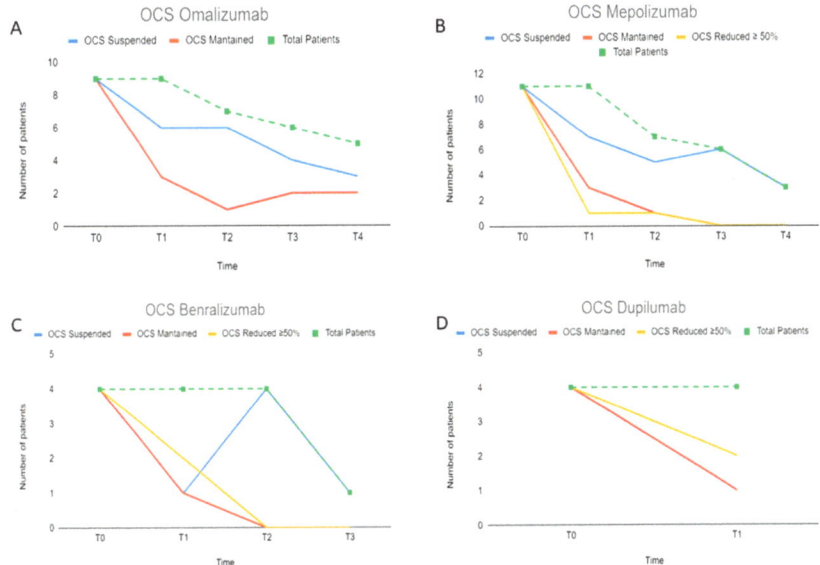

Figure 2. (**A**–**D**) Graphics showing for each biologic agent the number of patients who suspended/maintained OCS chronic treatment over years (T0–T4). (**A**) Omalizumab, (**B**) mepolizumab, (**C**) benralizumab, and (**D**) dupilumab.

4. Discussion

This retrospective study compared clinical, functional, and biological characteristics in a cohort of SA patients before and during treatment with omalizumab, mepolizumab, benralizumab, and dupilumab. Baseline characteristics of SA biologic-treated patients revealed that DupiG likely included more patients with mixed phenotype (77% of patients with only 1 or 2 T2-positive biomarkers) compared to other groups, maybe due to less stringent prescription criteria with respect to T2 biomarkers. Actually, DupiG had less rhinitis and high GERD at baseline. The "intra-biologic" analysis confirmed, as in other RLS, the effect of all biologics on the expected outcomes; in all the four groups, AEs decreased significantly, ACT, FEV$_1$%, and FVC% improved, while OCS were progressively withdrawn from T1 to T4.

In our study, omalizumab ameliorated ACT, although not reaching MID (improvement of ≥ 3) [20] activity limitations and decreased AEs already at T1. We observed a lung function improvement from T1 and RV reduction at T4, in line with observations from the INNOVATE study and RLS [21,22]. Other clinical observations regarding RV reduction are inconclusive [23]. Omalizumab seems to have a "deflating" action that occurs after a prolonged period of therapy (T4). In fact, IgE stimulates bronchial epithelial cells to synthesise growth factors involved in airway remodeling, such as TGF-β, smooth muscle cells proliferation, the release and production of pro-inflammatory agents, extracellular matrix proteins, and the synthesis of type I and III collagen [24,25]. We also observed progressive FVC improvement, but FVC Delta abs./% post bronchodilator reduced, which is explained by the limited further "reversibility" effect after normalization of lung function. Omalizumab did not affect F_ENO values nor PBE count. Anti-IgE real-life experiences are now more than 5 years and, in some studies, associated with an observed F_ENO reduction. However systematic review showed conflicting data on F_ENO modulation by omalizumab, remaining unclear [26]. The increase in total IgE, occurred due to the formation of IgG-IgE immune complexes, which are erroneously considered in the count by the automatic counter.

Mepolizumab showed a significant effect on ACT already at T1, which was long lasting until T4. The effect on AEs reduction was dramatically positive from T1 with further improvement up to T4, in line with both RCT and RLS results [27–30]. We showed an increase already at T2 in FVC absolute value. The effect of mepolizumab on lung function is controversial and generally slight. According to MENSA and MUSCA trials, mepolizumab improved FEV_1 when compared to placebo at 24 and 32 weeks, respectively [27,31], while in RLS, it showed an increase in FEV_1 abs. of 230 mL at 12 months [32]. Although not statistically significant, the progressive decrease in RV suggests a slow improvement in dynamic hyperinflation. This anti-remodeling action is likely due to the reduction in TGF-β1 eosinophil BAL-derived synthesis mediated by mepolizumab [33]. ICS, F_ENO, and total IgE values did not variate over years. In RLS, the effect of mepolizumab on F_ENO was slow and mild with a mean reduction of 14.33 ppb [32] but, similarly to the current study, it was not evident in other studies [34].

In what regards benralizumab, ACT and AEs ratio improved already at T1. At T2, a significant increase in FEV_1 and IT was evident. Despite RCT reporting an increase in FEV_1 ranging from 80 mL at 3 months to 125 mL at 14th months [35,36], RLS extended this finding to +300 mL and +400 mL improvement at 48 and 96 weeks, respectively [37]. We confirmed this evidence reporting even a more pronounced effect at T2, this corresponding to a reversion from fixed obstruction to normal function (IT from 60 to 72). To our knowledge, our observation is one of the few regarding normalization of lung function with biologics [38]. These results prove the role of IL-5 in guiding the SA demodeling effect [39]. Total F_ENO and IgE values did not change significantly during treatment, while PBE reduced to zero at T2, as expected. A significant mean reduction in neutrophil count and fibrinogen value was observed at T2, suggesting an anti-inflammatory long-term effect of Benralizumab. Recent studies demonstrated that IL-5R shares the β-chain with the GM-CSF receptor and was found on neutrophils infiltrating lungs and other anatomical sites of mice as well as on neutrophils in the BAL of children with refractory asthma [40,41]. We hypothesised that neutrophils reduction might be explained by benralizumab-induced direct killing of these cells through FcγRIIIa receptor-mediated binding to NK cells, and by GM-CSF receptor inhibition at a progenitor cell level.

The observation of dupilumab was limited at 1 year. ACT improvement was significant, as well as the AEs reduction, in line with previous RLS and RCT [29,42,43]. An improvement in lung function is present with a concomitant significant reduction in absolute RV. Based on our observation, dupilumab may have a predominant effect in demodeling, blocking IL-13 pathways. IL-13 causes contraction and proliferation of smooth muscle cells and is the main inducer of subepithelial fibrosis due to fibroblast proliferation and collagen production [44]. Surprisingly, at T1, no significant improvement in F_ENO was observed. However, approximately 50% of DupiG are "switchers" with possibly reduced baseline F_ENO values compared to naïve patients.

Here, we add during our Intra-biologic observation relevant and new effects on lung function. Some biologics give an improvement in FEV_1% over the minimal clinically important difference [45] or are sustained for a very long time. Others have desufflating effects, as suggested from RV improvement. In our study, all patients received a high ICS dose at baseline (Table 1) that remained unchanged during the follow-up, therefore not significantly influencing the effects of biologics on lung function.

The "inter-biologic" analysis by comparing means of paired Delta change for each variable represents an indirect method of comparison. It is, to our knowledge, a never-explored method of comparison among biologics in SA. Benralizumab and dupilumab improved ACT at T1 and mepolizumab at T3, more than omalizumab, probably because OmaG showed higher ACT values at baseline. In addition, benralizumab reduced nocturnal asthma symptoms more than both omalizumab and mepolizumab at T2, this could be considered a specific "biologic-treated treatable trait". The effect on AEs reduction is significant for all biologics with the only differences at T3 in favor of mepolizumab vs. omalizumab and at T1 of mepolizumab vs. dupilumab. This latter finding can be explained by the presence of numerous "switchers" in DupiG, presenting at baseline a lesser number of AEs. Dupilumab improved FVC Delta% post BD at T1 more than OmaG, sustaining the anti-remodelling action on small airways with partial recovery of FVC reversibility post BD [44]. On the contrary, benralizumab-induced increase in RV at T1 compared with OmaG, could be explained by a lesser effect on small airway disease in severe asthma in a real-life setting [46].

Discontinuation of OCS chronic treatment is an expected goal of biologic treatment in SA. Overall, it was reached in about 50% of patients. OmaG discontinued OCS up to T4 in 60% of patients. As far as RLS are concerned, approximately 50% of patients discontinued OCS chronic therapy at 1 or 4 years [22,47]. In what regards mepolizumab, at T1, 63.63% of patients discontinued OCS, up to 100% at T3. The OCS-sparing effect of mepolizumab is attested also in RLS with a 62% chronic OCS-treated patients reduction at 2 years [33]. In our study, the discontinuation rate at T3 is higher than data reported in literature. All BenraG OCS-treated patients discontinued therapy at T2, confirming the 82% complete OCS cessation at 36 months of therapy previously observed [30]. Here, only 28.5% DupiG suspended OCS at T1, definitively less than expected [43]; it is likely that OCS maintenance in this cluster is a clue of a more difficult-to-treat asthma in a potentially overlapped phenotype, often switching from an unsuccessful different biologic [8].

Our study presents some limitations. First, the present study is retrospective. Results from RLS of biologic-treated SA patients are strongly dependent on the population selected and on the physician attitudes in the choice of treatment. Patients' and physicians' preferences may regard less frequent dosing, SC administration, and faster onset, as well as cost/insurance coverage and convenience issues. In the present study, the group of physicians was the same over years and patients were always involved in the treatment choice [48]. The choice of a biologic was not generally guided according to predefined specific biomarker level (although the presence of high blood peripheral eosinophils may often lead to the use of IL-5 or IL-5R inhibitors, as well as high F_ENO to anti IL4/IL-13 R). The reduction in the number of patients over years due to different starting time, loss in follow-up (pandemic SARS-CoV-2), or interruption, has limited statistical yield.

5. Conclusions

Our study underlined the differential beneficial effects of biologic treatments towards peculiar clinical, functional, and biological outcomes over years. The particularity of this work resides in the comparison between biologics using means of paired Delta, an indirect method of comparison able to unveil the superiority of a peculiar pathway targeting treatment in regard to a specific "trait". This method could be useful to identify a specific "biologic-treated treatable trait" that can guide the choice among different biologics at baseline. The identification of different patient groups or traits with greater expected efficacy for a biologic remains as one of the greatest unmet needs in SA treatment.

Supplementary Materials: The following supporting information can be downloaded at https://www.mdpi.com/article/10.3390/jcm13164750/s1, Table S1: Regional criteria for prescription of biologic treatment; Table S2: Number of evaluated patients at T1, T2, T3, T4 for each biologics and the total number of patients at each Time point; Table S3: Number of evaluated patients at T1, T2, T3, T4 for each biologics and the total number of patients at each Time point. Figure S1: Number and sequence of treatments for all biologic switchers (N = 16).

Author Contributions: Conceptualization, E.R., G.G., F.L.M.R., F.B., V.C. and S.P.; methodology, E.R., G.G., F.B. and V.C.; software, E.R., G.G. and M.B.; formal analysis: G.G., F.B. and M.B.; data curation, E.R., G.G., S.G., F.B., V.C., M.B. and S.L.; investigation, E.R., G.G., S.G., S.P., F.G., E.F., E.A. and S.L.; writing original draft preparation, E.R., G.G., F.L.M.R., F.B., V.C. and S.L.; writing review and editing, E.R., G.G., S.G., F.B., V.C., M.B., S.P., F.G., E.F., E.A., S.L. and F.L.M.R.; supervision, E.R., G.G. and F.L.M.R. Project administration, F.L.M.R.; resources, F.L.M.R. All authors have read and agreed to the published version of the manuscript.

Funding: This research did not receive any specific grant from funding agencies in the public, commercial, or not-for-profit sectors.

Institutional Review Board Statement: The patients signed informed consent to participate in this study. The San Luigi Gonzaga University Hospital Ethical Review Board approved the study (protocol number:4478/2017, approved on 20 March 2017), in accordance with the Declaration of Helsinki.

Informed Consent Statement: Informed consent was obtained from all subjects involved in the study.

Data Availability Statement: Data are available on request from the authors.

Acknowledgments: We thank Laura Gibson for the English language revision.

Conflicts of Interest: G.G. reports fee as speaker for AstraZeneca; F.L.M.R. reports grants, personal fees, and other compensation from AstraZeneca, Boehringer Ingelheim, Chiesi, GSK, and Novartis, and personal fees and grants to support scientific research from Sanofi, all outside of the submitted work. M.B. is an employer of Re Learn S.R.L. that has no conflict of interest related to the contents of this manuscripts. All the other authors declare no conflict of interest.

References

1. Chung, K.F.; Wenzel, S.E.; Brozek, J.L.; Bush, A.; Castro, M.; Sterk, P.J.; Adcock, I.M.; Bateman, E.D.; Bel, E.H.; Bleecker, E.R.; et al. International ERS/ATS guidelines on definition, evaluation and treatment of severe asthma. *Eur. Respir. J.* **2014**, *43*, 343–373. [CrossRef]
2. Wenzel, S.E. Asthma phenotypes: The evolution from clinical to molecular approaches. *Nat. Med.* **2012**, *18*, 716–725. [CrossRef]
3. Shah, P.A.; Brightling, C. Biologics for severe asthma—Which, when and why? *Respirology* **2023**, *28*, 709–721. [CrossRef]
4. Panettieri, R., Jr.; Lugogo, N.; Corren, J.; Ambrose, C.S. Tezepelumab for Severe Asthma: One Drug Targeting Multiple Disease Pathways and Patient Types. *J. Asthma Allergy* **2024**, *17*, 219–236. [CrossRef]
5. Ito, A.; Miyoshi, S.; Toyota, H.; Suzuki, Y.; Uehara, Y.; Hattori, S.; Takeshita, Y.; Sakasegawa, H.; Kuramochi, M.; Kobayashi, K.; et al. The overlapping eligibility for biologics in patients with severe asthma and phenotypes. *Arerugi* **2022**, *71*, 210–220. (In Japanese) [CrossRef]
6. Pavord, I.D.; Hanania, N.A.; Corren, J. Controversies in Allergy: Choosing a Biologic for Patients with Severe Asthma. *J. Allergy Clin. Immunol. Pract.* **2022**, *10*, 410–419. [CrossRef]
7. Menzies-Gow, A.; Steenkamp, J.; Singh, S.; Erhardt, W.; Rowell, J.; Rane, P.; Martin, N.; Llanos, J.P.; Quinton, A. Tezepelumab compared with other biologics for the treatment of severe asthma: A systematic review and indirect treatment comparison. *J. Med. Econ.* **2022**, *25*, 679–690. [CrossRef]
8. Al-Shaikhly, T.; Norris, M.R.; Dennis, E.H.; Liu, G.; Craig, T.J. Comparative Impact of Asthma Biologics: A Nationwide US Claim-Based Analysis. *J. Allergy Clin. Immunol. Pract.* **2024**, *12*, 1558–1567. [CrossRef]
9. Ricciardolo, F.L.; Guida, G.; Bertolini, F.; Di Stefano, A.; Carriero, V. Phenotype overlap in the natural history of asthma. *Eur. Respir. Rev.* **2023**, *32*, 220201. [CrossRef]
10. Frøssing, L.; Silberbrandt, A.; Von Bülow, A.; Backer, V.; Porsbjerg, C. The Prevalence of Subtypes of Type 2 Inflammation in an Unselected Population of Patients with Severe Asthma. *J. Allergy Clin. Immunol. Pract.* **2021**, *9*, 1267–1275. [CrossRef]
11. Papadopoulos, N.G.; Barnes, P.; Canonica, G.W.; Gaga, M.; Heaney, L.; Menzies-Gow, A.; Kritikos, V.; Fitzgerald, M. The evolving algorithm of biological selection in severe asthma. *Allergy* **2020**, *75*, 1555–1563. [CrossRef] [PubMed]
12. McDonald, V.M.; Clark, V.L.; Cordova-Rivera, L.; Wark, P.A.B.; Baines, K.J.; Gibson, P.G. Targeting treatable traits in severe asthma: A randomised controlled trial. *Eur. Respir. J.* **2020**, *55*, 1901509. [CrossRef] [PubMed]
13. Guida, G.; Bagnasco, D.; Carriero, V.; Bertolini, F.; Ricciardolo, F.L.M.; Nicola, S.; Brussino, L.; Nappi, E.; Paoletti, G.; Canonica, G.W.; et al. Critical evaluation of asthma biomarkers in clinical practice. *Front. Med.* **2022**, *9*, 969243. [CrossRef] [PubMed]
14. Chen, C.-Y.; Wu, K.-H.; Guo, B.-C.; Lin, W.-Y.; Chang, Y.-J.; Wei, C.-W.; Lin, M.-J.; Wu, H.-P. Personalized Medicine in Severe Asthma: From Biomarkers to Biologics. *Int. J. Mol. Sci.* **2023**, *25*, 182. [CrossRef] [PubMed]
15. Ricciardolo, F.L.M.; Sprio, A.E.; Baroso, A.; Gallo, F.; Riccardi, E.; Bertolini, F.; Carriero, V.; Arrigo, E.; Ciprandi, G. Characterization of T2-Low and T2-High Asthma Phenotypes in Real-Life. *Biomedicines* **2021**, *9*, 1684. [CrossRef] [PubMed]

16. van Dijk, B.C.P.; Svedsater, H.; Heddini, A.; Nelsen, L.; Balradj, J.S.; Alleman, C. Relationship between the Asthma Control Test (ACT) and other outcomes: A targeted literature review. *BMC Pulm. Med.* **2020**, *20*, 79. [CrossRef]
17. Nathan, R.A.; Sorkness, C.A.; Kosinski, M.; Schatz, M.; Li, J.T.; Marcus, P.; Murray, J.J.; Pendergraft, T.B. Development of the asthma control test: A survey for assessing asthma control. *J. Allergy Clin. Immunol.* **2004**, *113*, 59–65. [CrossRef] [PubMed]
18. Graham, B.L.; Steenbruggen, I.; Miller, M.R.; Barjaktarevic, I.Z.; Cooper, B.G.; Hall, G.L.; Hallstrand, T.S.; Kaminsky, D.A.; McCarthy, K.; McCormack, M.C.; et al. Standardization of Spirometry 2019 Update. An Official American Thoracic Society and European Respiratory Society Technical Statement. *Am. J. Respir. Crit. Care Med.* **2019**, *200*, e70–e88. [CrossRef] [PubMed]
19. Carriero, V.; Bertolini, F.; Sprio, A.E.; Bullone, M.; Ciprandi, G.; Ricciardolo, F.L.M. High levels of plasma fibrinogen could predict frequent asthma exacerbations. *J. Allergy Clin. Immunol. Pract.* **2020**, *8*, 2392–2395.e7. [CrossRef]
20. Schatz, M.; Kosinski, M.; Yarlas, A.S.; Hanlon, J.; Watson, M.E.; Jhingran, P. The minimally important difference of the Asthma Control Test. *J. Allergy Clin. Immunol.* **2009**, *124*, 719–723.e1. [CrossRef]
21. Humbert, M.; Beasley, R.; Ayres, J.; Slavin, R.; Hébert, J.; Bousquet, J.; Beeh, K.; Ramos, S.; Canonica, G.W.; Hedgecock, S.; et al. Benefits of omalizumab as add-on therapy in patients with severe persistent asthma who are inadequately controlled despite best available therapy (GINA 2002 step 4 treatment): INNOVATE. *Allergy* **2005**, *60*, 309–316. [CrossRef] [PubMed]
22. Bousquet, J.; Humbert, M.; Gibson, P.G.; Kostikas, K.; Jaumont, X.; Pfister, P.; Nissen, F. Real-World Effectiveness of Omalizumab in Severe Allergic Asthma: A Meta-Analysis of Observational Studies. *J. Allergy Clin. Immunol. Pract.* **2021**, *9*, 2702–2714. [CrossRef] [PubMed]
23. Paganin, F.; Mangiapan, G.; Proust, A.; Prudhomme, A.; Attia, J.; Marchand-Adam, S.; Pellet, F.; Milhe, F.; Melloni, B.; Bernady, A.; et al. Lung function parameters in omalizumab responder patients: An interesting tool? *Allergy* **2017**, *72*, 1953–1961. [CrossRef] [PubMed]
24. Roth, M.; Zhong, J.; Zumkeller, C.; S'ng, C.T.; Goulet, S.; Tamm, M. The role of IgE-receptors in IgE-dependent airway smooth muscle cell remodelling. *PLoS ONE* **2013**, *8*, e56015. [CrossRef] [PubMed]
25. Riccio, A.M.; Negro, R.W.; Micheletto, C.; De Ferrari, L.; Folli, C.; Chiappori, A.; Canonica, G.W. Omalizumab modulates bronchial reticular basement membrane thickness and eosinophil infiltration in severe persistent allergic asthma patients. *Int. J. Immunopathol. Pharmacol.* **2012**, *25*, 475–484. [CrossRef] [PubMed]
26. Pianigiani, T.; Alderighi, L.; Meocci, M.; Messina, M.; Perea, B.; Luzzi, S.; Bergantini, L.; D'alessandro, M.; Refini, R.M.; Bargagli, E.; et al. Exploring the Interaction between Fractional Exhaled Nitric Oxide and Biologic Treatment in Severe Asthma: A Systematic Review. *Antioxidants* **2023**, *12*, 400. [CrossRef]
27. Ortega, H.G.; Liu, M.C.; Pavord, I.D.; Brusselle, G.G.; Fitzgerald, J.M.; Chetta, A.; Humbert, M.; Katz, L.E.; Keene, O.N.; Yancey, S.W.; et al. Mepolizumab treatment in patients with severe eosinophilic asthma. *N. Engl. J. Med.* **2014**, *371*, 1198–1207. [CrossRef] [PubMed]
28. Khurana, S.; Brusselle, G.G.; Bel, E.H.; FitzGerald, J.M.; Masoli, M.; Korn, S.; Kato, M.; Albers, F.C.; Bradford, E.S.; Gilson, M.J.; et al. Long-term Safety and Clinical Benefit of Mepolizumab in Patients with the Most Severe Eosinophilic Asthma: The COSMEX Study. *Clin. Ther.* **2019**, *41*, 2041–2056.e5. [CrossRef] [PubMed]
29. Charles, D.; Shanley, J.; Temple, S.; Rattu, A.; Khaleva, E.; Roberts, G. Real-world efficacy of treatment with benralizumab, dupilumab, mepolizumab and reslizumab for severe asthma: A systematic review and meta-analysis. *Clin. Exp. Allergy* **2022**, *52*, 616–627. [CrossRef]
30. Fyles, F.; Nuttall, A.; Joplin, H.; Burhan, H. Long-Term Real-World Outcomes of Mepolizumab and Benralizumab Among Biologic-Naive Patients with Severe Eosinophilic Asthma: Experience of 3 Years' Therapy. *J. Allergy Clin. Immunol. Pract.* **2023**, *11*, 2715–2723. [CrossRef]
31. Chupp, G.L.; Bradford, E.S.; Albers, F.C.; Bratton, D.J.; Wang-Jairaj, J.; Nelsen, L.M.; Trevor, J.L.; Magnan, A.; Brinke, A.T. Efficacy of mepolizumab add-on therapy on health-related quality of life and markers of asthma control in severe eosinophilic asthma (MUSCA): A randomised, double-blind, placebo-controlled, parallel-group, multicentre, phase 3b trial. *Lancet Respir. Med.* **2017**, *5*, 390–400. [CrossRef]
32. Li, H.; Zhang, Q.; Wang, J.; Gao, S.; Li, C.; Wang, J.; Zhang, S.; Lin, J. Real-world Effectiveness of Mepolizumab in Severe Eosinophilic Asthma: A Systematic Review and Meta-analysis. *Clin. Ther.* **2021**, *43*, e192–e208. [CrossRef]
33. Flood-Page, P.; Menzies-Gow, A.; Phipps, S.; Ying, S.; Wangoo, A.; Ludwig, M.S.; Barnes, N.; Robinson, D.; Kay, A.B. Anti-IL-5 treatment reduces deposition of ECM proteins in the bronchial subepithelial basement membrane of mild atopic asthmatics. *J. Clin. Investig.* **2003**, *112*, 1029–1036. [CrossRef] [PubMed]
34. Ricciardolo, F.L.M.; Silkoff, P.E. Perspectives on exhaled nitric oxide. *J. Breath Res.* **2017**, *11*, 047104. [CrossRef]
35. Ferguson, G.T.; FitzGerald, J.M.; Bleecker, E.R.; Laviolette, M.; Bernstein, D.; LaForce, C.; Mansfield, L.; Barker, P.; Wu, Y.; Jison, M.; et al. Benralizumab for patients with mild to moderate, persistent asthma (BISE): A randomised, double-blind, placebo-controlled, phase 3 trial. *Lancet Respir. Med.* **2017**, *5*, 568–576. [CrossRef]
36. FitzGerald, J.M.; Bleecker, E.R.; Nair, P.; Korn, S.; Ohta, K.; Lommatzsch, M.; Ferguson, G.T.; Busse, W.W.; Barker, P.; Sproule, S.; et al. Benralizumab, an anti-interleukin-5 receptor α monoclonal antibody, as add-on treatment for patients with severe, uncontrolled, eosinophilic asthma (CALIMA): A randomised, double-blind, placebo-controlled phase 3 trial. *Lancet* **2016**, *388*, 2128–2141. [CrossRef] [PubMed]

37. Menzella, F.; Bargagli, E.; Aliani, M.; Bracciale, P.; Brussino, L.; Caiaffa, M.F.; Caruso, C.; Centanni, S.; D'amato, M.; Del Giacco, S.; et al. ChAracterization of ItaliaN severe uncontrolled Asthmatic patieNts Key features when receiving Benralizumab in a real-life setting: The observational rEtrospective ANANKE study. *Respir. Res.* **2022**, *23*, 36. [CrossRef]
38. Vitale, C.; Maglio, A.; Pelaia, C.; D'amato, M.; Ciampo, L.; Pelaia, G.; Molino, A.; Vatrella, A. Effectiveness of Benralizumab in OCS-Dependent Severe Asthma: The Impact of 2 Years of Therapy in a Real-Life Setting. *J. Clin. Med.* **2023**, *12*, 985. [CrossRef]
39. Guida, G.; Riccio, A.M. Immune induction of airway remodeling. *Semin. Immunol.* **2019**, *46*, 101346. [CrossRef]
40. Gorski, S.A.; Lawrence, M.G.; Hinkelman, A.; Spano, M.M.; Steinke, J.W.; Borish, L.; Teague, W.G.; Braciale, T.J. Expression of IL-5 receptor alpha by murine and human lung neutrophils. *PLoS ONE* **2019**, *14*, e0221113. [CrossRef]
41. Tavernier, J.; Devos, R.; Cornelis, S.; Tuypens, T.; Van der Heyden, J.; Fiers, W.; Plaetinck, G. A human high affinity interleukin-5 receptor (IL5R) is composed of an IL5-specific α chain and a β chain shared with the receptor for GM-CSF. *Cell* **1991**, *66*, 1175–1184. [CrossRef] [PubMed]
42. Castro, M.; Corren, J.; Pavord, I.D.; Maspero, J.; Wenzel, S.; Rabe, K.F.; Busse, W.W.; Ford, L.; Sher, L.; Fitzgerald, J.M.; et al. Dupilumab Efficacy and Safety in Moderate-to-Severe Uncontrolled Asthma. *N. Engl. J. Med.* **2018**, *378*, 2486–2496. [CrossRef]
43. Rabe, K.F.; Nair, P.; Brusselle, G.; Maspero, J.F.; Castro, M.; Sher, L.; Zhu, H.; Hamilton, J.D.; Swanson, B.N.; Khan, A.; et al. Efficacy and Safety of Dupilumab in Glucocorticoid-Dependent Severe Asthma. *N. Engl. J. Med.* **2018**, *378*, 2475–2485. [CrossRef]
44. Pelaia, C.; Heffler, E.; Crimi, C.; Maglio, A.; Vatrella, A.; Pelaia, G.; Canonica, G.W. Interleukins 4 and 13 in Asthma: Key Pathophysiologic Cytokines and Druggable Molecular Targets. *Front. Pharmacol.* **2022**, *13*, 851940. [CrossRef]
45. Louis, R.; Satia, I.; Ojanguren, I.; Schleich, F.; Bonini, M.; Tonia, T.; Rigau, D.; Brinke, A.T.; Buhl, R.; Loukides, S.; et al. European Respiratory Society Guidelines for the Diagnosis of Asthma in Adults. *Eur. Respir. J.* **2022**, *60*, 2101585. [CrossRef]
46. Chan, R.; Lipworth, B.J. Real-life effects of benralizumab on airway oscillometry in severe eosinophilic asthma. *BMJ Open Respir. Res.* **2023**, *10*, e001472. [CrossRef]
47. Papaioannou, A.I.; Mplizou, M.; Porpodis, K.; Fouka, E.; Zervas, E.; Samitas, K.; Markatos, M.; Bakakos, P.; Papiris, S.; Gaga, M.; et al. Long-term efficacy and safety of omalizumab in patients with allergic asthma: A real-life study. *Allergy Asthma Proc.* **2021**, *42*, 235–242. [CrossRef]
48. Gelhorn, H.L.; Balantac, Z.; Ambrose, C.S.; Chung, Y.N.; Stone, B. Patient and physician preferences for attributes of biologic medications for severe asthma. *Patient Prefer. Adherence* **2019**, *13*, 1253–1268. [CrossRef]

Disclaimer/Publisher's Note: The statements, opinions and data contained in all publications are solely those of the individual author(s) and contributor(s) and not of MDPI and/or the editor(s). MDPI and/or the editor(s) disclaim responsibility for any injury to people or property resulting from any ideas, methods, instructions or products referred to in the content.

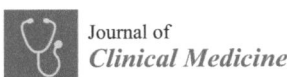

Article

Real-Life Clinical Outcomes of Benralizumab Treatment in Patients with Uncontrolled Severe Asthma and Coexisting Chronic Rhinosinusitis with Nasal Polyposis

Eusebi Chiner [1], María Murcia [1], Ignacio Boira [1,*], María Ángeles Bernabeu [2], Violeta Esteban [1] and Eva Martínez-Moragón [3]

1. Pulmonology Department, University Hospital of Saint John of Alicante, 03550 Alicante, Spain; echinervives@gmail.com (E.C.); maria.murcia11@goumh.umh.es (M.M.); violeta_er@hotmail.com (V.E.)
2. Pharmacy Department, University Hospital of Saint John of Alicante, 03550 Alicante, Spain; bernabeu_marmar@gva.es
3. Pulmonology Department, Doctor Peset University Hospital, 46017 Valencia, Spain; evamartinezmoragon@gmail.com
* Correspondence: nachoboiraenrique@hotmail.es; Tel.: +34-965-16-94-00

Abstract: Background: The objective of this study was to evaluate, the clinical benefit of benralizumab in patients with uncontrolled severe asthma associated with chronic rhinosinusitis with nasal polyposis (CRSwNP). **Methods:** The study included patients with uncontrolled severe asthma associated with CRSwNP who started therapy with benralizumab. Pulmonary function, eosinophilia, IgE, comorbidity, changes in the Asthma Control Test (ACT), Asthma Control Questionnaire (ACQ), Visual Analogue Scale (VAS), Quality of Life (AQLQ), VAS (obstruction, drip, anosmia, facial pressure), SNOT-22, decrease or withdrawal of steroids and other medication, hospital admissions and emergency visits were analysed. The FEOS scale and EXACTO were employed in the assessment of response. **Results:** We analyzed 58 patients who completed minimal treatment at 12 months. After treatment with benralizumab, exacerbations were reduced by 82% ($p < 0.001$), steroid cycles by 84% ($p < 0.001$), emergencies visit by 83% $p < 0.001$) and admissions by 76% ($p < 0.001$), improving all the scales for asthma control, ($p < 0.001$). In terms of lung function, differences were observed in FVC% ($p < 0.001$), FEV1% ($p < 0.001$), and FEV1/FVC% (69.5 ± 10 vs. 74 ± 10, $p < 0.001$). In relation to CRSwNP, differences were observed in SNOT-22 (54.66 ± 17 vs. 20.24 ± 9, $p < 0.001$), VAS obstruction (7.91 ± 1 vs. 1.36 ± 1, $p < 0.001$), VAS drip (7.76 ± 1 vs. 1.38 ± 1, $p < 0.001$), VAS anosmia (7.66 ± 1 vs. 1.38 ± 1, $p < 0.001$) and VAS facial pressure (7.91 ± 1 vs. 1.22 ± 1, $p < 0.001$). The mean FEOS score after treatment was 73 ± 14. A complete response/super response was achieved in 33 patients (57%), good response in 16 (28%) and partial response in 9 (15%). **Conclusions:** The administration of benralizumab to patients with uncontrolled severe asthma associated with CRSwNP has been demonstrated to improve nasal symptoms, asthma control and lung function. This resulted in a reduction in the need for oral steroids, maintenance and rescue medication, emergency room visits, and hospital admissions, with 57% of patients achieving the clinical remission criteria.

Keywords: asthma; benralizumab; polyposis; rhinosinusitis

1. Introduction

Despite improvements in the diagnosis and treatment of asthma, approximately 5–10% of patients develop a severe form of the disease, of whom 50% are considered uncontrolled [1,2].

Chronic rhinosinusitis (CRS) affects the nasosinusal mucosa, which may or may not present with nasal polyposis (NP). This is characterised by chronic inflammation with hyperplasia of the sinus mucosa into the nasal cavity. Up to 40% of patients with uncontrolled severe asthma associate chronic rhinosinusitis with nasal polyposis (CRSwNP), with higher severity, more exacerbations and poorer quality of life compared to those without polyposis [3,4].

These two disorders frequently coexist on a common anatomical, immunological, histopathological and pathophysiological basis. Typically, type 2 (T2) inflammation, defined by augmented tissue and peripheral blood eosinophil levels, is the underlying mechanism in asthma with CRSwNP. This process is mediated by T lymphocytes (predominantly T helper type 2), innate lymphoid cells (ILC2) and mast cells, which activate the production of interleukin-5 (IL-5) and the proliferation and differentiation of its receptor (IL-5R). The IL-5R receptor is a heterodimer comprising an IL-5Rα ligand-specific α-subunit and a β-subunit that is common to other cytokine receptors [5].

The differentiation of asthma phenotypes has gained increasing importance due to the progress in individualized treatment approaches and the emergence of biological agents. T2 asthma is triggered by allergens, pollutants, and microorganisms that are captured by dendritic cells leading to the release of interleukin (IL)-25, IL-33, and thymic stromal lymphopoietin (TSLP) from bronchial epithelial cells. These cytokines activate type 2 innate lymphoid cells (ILC2), which play a crucial role in initiating type 2 immune responses. Elevated levels of T helper 2 cell (Th2)-related cytokines such as IL-4, IL-5, IL-13 along with immunoglobulin E (IgE) characterize T2 asthma. Non-T2 asthma lacks clear biomarkers [1].

The discovery of the molecular mechanisms involved in the pathogenesis of asthma has enabled the development of anti-eosinophilic biologic therapies targeting IL-5 (mepolizumab and reslizumab) or its receptor (benralizumab). Dupilumab is a kind of humanized monoclonal antibody that specifically targets the α subunit of the IL-4 and IL-13 receptors, effectively inhibiting the immune effects mediated by IL-4 and IL-13. Tezepelumab's role in management of type-2 low asthma and potentially non-type 2 asthma is an exciting prospect, however, further studies need to be conducted to explore the mechanisms of these improvements and determine the efficacy of treatment. These therapies have been shown to be efficacy in patients with uncontrolled severe asthma, improving quality of life by reducing exacerbations, improving lung function and reducing systemic corticosteroids (SCS) consumption. Furthermore, they have a good safety profile [6,7].

Benralizumab is a humanised monoclonal antibody that binds to the α-subunit of the IL-5 receptor through its Fab domain, thereby competing against IL-5 binding to its receptor. Furthermore, the afucosylated Fc domain enables binding to the Fc region of the RIIIa receptor on NK cells, macrophages and neutrophils. This results in the activation of cellular cytotoxicity directed at eosinophils, which induces their apoptosis and causes a near-complete depletion [8]. This depleting effect has also been confirmed in induced sputum in a real-life study in which 85% of patients presented a sputum eosinophil count of <3% after 6 months of treatment. [9].

Given that suboptimal control of CRSwNP is associated with reduced asthma control and quality of life, there is a need for the development of new therapeutic approaches. A systematic review evidenced that dupilumab, mepolizumab and benralizumab produced sustained long-term improvement in smell in patients with CRSwNP [10].

Benralizumab has been demonstrated to be effective in the control of uncontrolled severe asthma associated with CRSwNP. A randomised, double-blind, placebo-controlled trial, despite a small sample size, suggested a positive effect in the treatment of CRSwNP with benralizumab. This was evidenced by a statistically significant reduction in nasal polyp size, sinus occupancy, symptoms and improved sense of smell in the majority of patients (83%) [11]. In another study, quality of life and lung function were significantly improved in asthmatic patients with CRSwNP compared to patients with asthma without polyposis [12]. Furthermore, in the CALIMA study, it was concluded that the association of T2 asthma with NP was a predictor of response to anti-IL-5 antibodies in asthma [13]. The phase III OSTRO evaluated the efficacy of benralizumab in symptomatic CRSwNP despite intranasal corticosteroid therapy and a history of CRS or NP surgery evidenced a reduction in nasal obstruction and improvement in olfaction compared to placebo in patients with CRSwNP [14]. Similarly, the subgroup of patients in the ANDHI study with nasal polyps and asthma treated with benralizumab developed an improvement in both asthma and 22-item Sino-Nasal Outcome Test (SNOT-22), with greater improvements observed in patients with higher scores (greater NP involvement) [15].

The objective of this study was to evaluate, in real life, the clinical benefit of benralizumab in patients with uncontrolled severe asthma associated with CRSwNP. Specifically, we assessed the impact of benralizumab on nasal obstruction parameters, as well as on the reduction of hospitalisations, emergency room visits, asthma control and lung function. In addition, we aimed to estimate the clinical remission of severe asthma in patients with CRSwNP-associated asthma after treatment.

2. Materials and Methods

2.1. Type of Study

A single-centre, observational, prospective and real-life study was conducted on patients with uncontrolled severe asthma who initiated treatment with benralizumab through a joint dispensing protocol with a hospital pharmacy service.

2.2. Study Period

January 2019 to September 2023.

2.3. Population

The study included all patients ≥ 18 years old with eosinophilic uncontrolled severe asthma and CRSwNP. who were prescribed benralizumab. Uncontrolled severe asthma was defined as a condition that necessitates high-dose inhaled corticosteroids (ICS)/long-acting ß2-adrenergic agonists (LABA) or adjunctive medications such as leukotriene modulators and oral corticosteroids (OCS) for adequate control [1,3].

The following sociodemographic characteristics were assessed: age, sex, body mass index (BMI), smoking status, age of asthma onset, and atopy. Additionally, the levels of immunoglobulin E (IgE) and other biologics previously administered for un-controlled severe asthma were evaluated.

2.4. Inclusion Criteria

All patients met the criteria for uncontrolled severe asthma with CRSwNP and received 30 mg benralizumab subcutaneously every 4 weeks for the first 3 doses and then every 8 weeks, starting at T0, for at least 12 months (T12). All patients were clinically assessed in their usual visit regimen at periods between 3 and 6 months between the baseline visit (T0) and the final evaluation visit (T12). All patients had eosinophil counts of ≥ 150 cells per microlitre (μL) with maintenance treatment with oral glucocorticoids or a history of at least 300 eosinophils/μL in the previous 12 months. Benralizumab was administered when patients had at least two exacerbations in the year prior to onset and uncontrolled severe asthma symptoms.

Exacerbations were defined as a loss of control requiring the administration of oral glucocorticoids for at least three days and/or emergency department visits and/or hospitalisations and/or primary care consultations due to respiratory symptoms. In patients on maintenance oral glucocorticoids, exacerbation was defined as a doubling of the maintenance steroid dose for three days. All patients received a combination of high-dose inhaled corticosteroids (IGCs) and a long-acting beta agonist (LABAs) or a triple regimen of IGCs, LABAs and long-acting antimuscarinics (LAMAs), which could include a leukotriene inhibitor. All patients used an additional controller (short-acting β2-agonists [SABA]) on demand.

CRSwNP was diagnosed by an ear, nose and throat (ENT) specialist in accordance with the Spanish Consensus on the Management of Chronic Rhinosinusitis with Nasal Polyps (POLINA Guide 2023) as the presence of two or more symptoms, one of which must be nasal congestion and/or anterior/posterior rhinorrhoea, plus facial pain/pressure or reduced/loss of smell, for more than 12 weeks [16]. Furthermore, endoscopic signs of nasal polyps and/or mucopurulent discharge and/or oedema in the middle meatus and/or computed tomography (CT) changes of the middle meatus or sinuses were observed.

All patients underwent nasal examination, endoscopy and sinus computed tomography (CT) when appropriate and had a history of sinus surgery. All patients were using IGC and nasal antihistamines.

2.5. Efficacy Monitoring

The assessment of asthma symptom control, oral glucocorticoid dose, exacerbations and forced expiratory volume in 1 s (FEV1) was conducted at baseline and at scheduled visits at 6 and 12 months after baseline. Spirometry was performed in accordance with the Spanish Society of Pulmonology and Thoracic Surgery (SEPAR) criteria [17], with reversibility testing conducted in all patients prior to benralizumab initiation.

The self-administered Asthma Control Test (ACT) [18] and Asthma Control Questionnaire (ACQ) [18] were employed to monitor symptoms at baseline and throughout the course of treatment, while the mini–Asthma Quality of Life Questionnaire (miniAQLQ) was utilized to assess quality of life.

The SNOT-22 questionnaire [19] was used to assess the response in CRSwNP. SNOT-22 was developed for use in chronic rhinosinusitis and assesses the symptoms and functional and emotional consequences of chronic rhinosinusitis through responses to 22 items using a 6-category scale, from 0 (no problem) to 5 (problem as bad as it can be). Greater scores indicate a poorer outcome (range 0–110).

A visual analogue scale (VAS) was also employed to assess nasal obstruction, rhinorrhea, anosmia, and facial pressure. The scale ranged from 0 to 10, with 0–3 being classified as mild, >3–7 moderate, and >7–10 severe. The higher the score, the greater the subjective burden of CRSwNP symptoms, and the lower the score, the lesser the burden [16].

The response to biological treatment between T0 and T12 was evaluated using the FEOS scale [20] and the degree of asthma control using the multidimensional EXACTO scale, which classifies patients into four categories: non-response, partial response, good response, and complete response/super-responder, based on exacerbations, ACT, oral glucocorticoids, and FEV1 according to changes from T0 [21].

2.6. Statistical Study

A statistical study was conducted to analyse the data. The baseline or outcome numerical variables were presented as mean and standard deviation or as median and interquartile range. All differences were assessed by comparing values at T0 with T12 using either the Student's *t*-test (for paired data) or the Wilcoxon test, depending on the normality of the data. A *p*-value of less than 0.05 was considered statistically significant for all parameters recorded. All statistical analyses were conducted using SPSS version 18.

2.7. Ethical Considerations

The study was conducted in accordance with the ethical principles. Written informed consent was obtained from all patients included in the study. The study was approved by the ethics committee.

3. Results

Fifty-eight patients were analysed in the study, all of whom completed treatment with benralizumab at 12 months. Of the patients studied, 6 (10%) had previously been treated with omalizumab. The baseline characteristics of the patients are shown in Table 1.

An overall 93% of patients had at least one comorbidity, with rhinitis being the most frequent (Figure 1).

Twenty-two patients (37.9%) were identified as current smokers. The treatment administered to patients consisted of one or more drugs. All patients were prescribed high-dose IGCs, 98% LABAs, 88% SABAs, 45% montelukast, 45% LAMAs, 21% antihistamines, 57%

anti-leukotrienes, 1.7% xanthines and 5% maintenance oral glucocorticoids. In total, 76% of patients received nasal corticosteroids in combination with local and/or systemic antihistamines. In terms of lung function, a comparison of baseline and after treatment values revealed statistically significant improvements in FVC%, FEV1% and FEV1/FVC% (Figure 2).

Table 1. General characteristics of the patients included in the study (n = 58). BMI: Body Mass Index. IgE: Inmunoglobulin E. FEV1: forced expiratory volume in 1 s. FVC: Forced Vital Capacity. ACT: Asthma Control Test. ACQ: Asthma Control Questionnaire. VAS: Visual Analogue Scale. SNOT-22: 22-item Sino-Nasal Outcome Test. AQLQ: Asthma Quality of Life Questionnaire. ENT: Ear, Nose and Throat.

Baseline Characteristics	Value/Mean ± Standard Deviation
Mean age (years)	55 ± 14
BMI (Kg/m^2)	27 ± 8
Sex	64% women, 36% men
Eosinophils, cel/µL	786 ± 504
IgE (UI/mL)	361 ± 807
Atopy/allergy	17 patients
FEV1 (Liters and %) FEV1/FVC (%) FVC (liters and %)	2.45 ± 0.8 (84 ± 18%) 69.5 ± 10 (%) 3.47 ± 1.01 (97 ± 16%)
ACT // ACQ// VAS	15 ± 2 // 3 ± 1 // 7.5 ± 1
SNOT-22	55 ± 17
VAS: Obstruction Runny nose Anosmia Facial pressure	 8 ± 1 7.8 ± 1 7.6 ± 1 7.8 ± 1
Mini-AQLQ	2.4 ± 0.4
Number emergency visits / year	2.62 ± 2.7
Number of hospital admissions/year	0.84 ± 2
Days of hospital admission	3 ± 8
Global exacerbations	5.6 ± 5
Oral glucocorticoid cycles	3.16 ± 3
Time of treatment (months)	14.4 ± 8
Previous ENT surgery (one or more)	Total: 55% (32) One: 47% (15) Two: 31% (10) Three or more: 22% (7)

Moreover, significant changes were also observed in punctuation of ACQ (3.19 ± 1 vs. 1.1 ± 0.81, $p < 0.001$), ACT (15.33 ± 1.59 vs. 22.48 ± 2, $p < 0.001$), mini-AQLQ (2.4 ± 0.38 vs. 5.3 ± 0.84, $p < 0.001$) and VAS (7.57 ± 1 vs. 2.1 ± 1, $p < 0.001$) and VAS (7.57 ± 1 vs. 2.1 ± 1, $p < 0.001$) (Figure 3).

With regard to CRSwNP, significant differences were observed in the punctuation of SNOT-22 after the treatment (55 ± 17 vs. 20 ± 9, $p < 0.001$). Furthermore, there was a significant improvement in VAS obstruction, VAS drip, VAS anosmia and VAS facial pressure (8 ± 1 vs. 1 ± 1, $p < 0.001$).

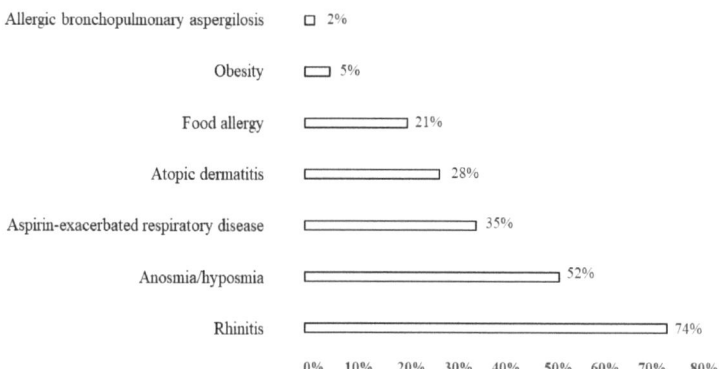

Figure 1. Comorbidities of the patients under study.

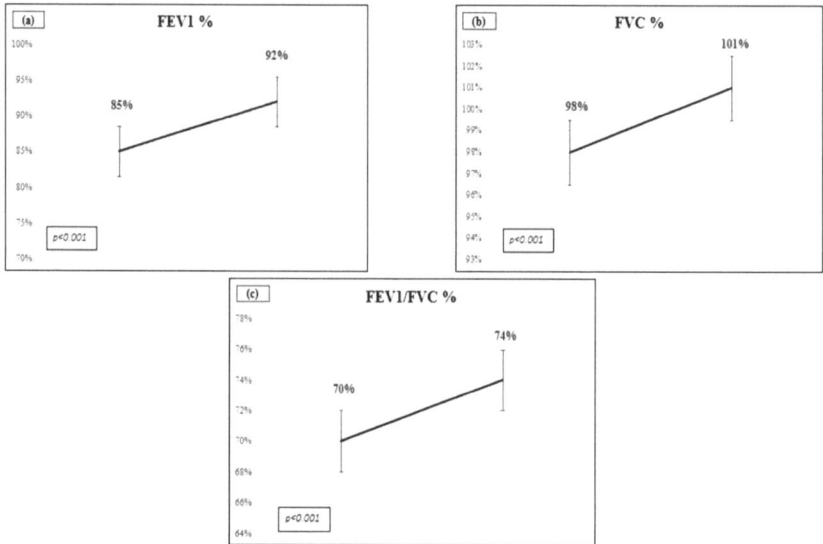

Figure 2. A comparison of respiratory function before and after treatment. (a) FVC% (Forced Vital Capacity expressed in %); (b) FEV1% (Forced Expiratory Volume in the 1st second expressed in %) and (c) FEV1/FVC ratio in %.

We compared post-treatment SNOT-22 response by groups with response < 40 points or a difference of less than 12 points from baseline, according to the presence of atopy or not, and by eosinophil level < 500 cells/μL or greater than 500 cells/μL.

In this regard, 35 patients (60%) had negative and 23 (40%) positive pricks or RAST and 16 patients (29%) had less than 500 eosinophils and 42 (71%) more than 500 eosinophils). When comparing the two groups, 8 patients (15%) had a score over 40 post treatment, of which 7 (30%) were atopic and 1 (3%) non-atopic (chi square 4.705, $p = 0.032$), indicating a better response in non-atopic patients.

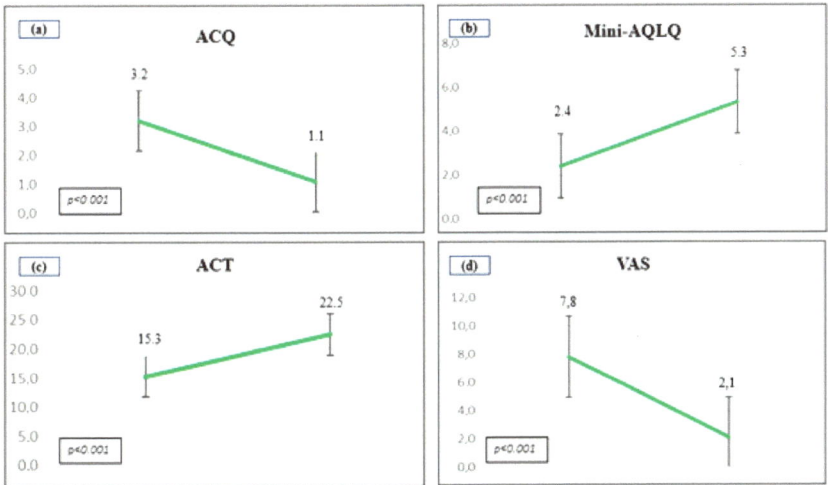

Figure 3. Changes in punctuation of the scales after the treatment. (**a**) ACQ (Asthma Control Questionnaire); (**b**) Mini-AQLQ (Asthma Quality of Life Questionnaire); (**c**) ACT (Asthma Control Test) and (**d**) VAS (Visual Analogue Scale).

Regarding eosinophils, with less than 500 cells/μL, 9 (56%) presented change in SNOT-22 < 12 versus 6 (14%) in the group with more than 500 cells/μL (chi square 4.214, $p = 0.04$), indicating better response with greater eosinophilia.

In the year prior to the initiation of benralizumab, 33% of patients had been hospitalised, 70% had visited the emergency department, and 72% had received courses of oral glucocorticoids. The mean number of exacerbations per patient per year was 5.6 ± 5. After treatment with benralizumab, exacerbations were reduced by 82% (5.6 ± 5 vs. 1 ± 2.5, $p < 0.001$), the number of steroid cycles by 84% (3, 16 ± 3 versus 0.5 ± 1, $p < 0.001$), emergency department visits by 83% (2.62 ± 2.7 versus 0.45 ± 1, $p < 0.001$) and hospital admissions by 76% (0.84 ± 1 versus 0.2 ± 0.8, $p < 0.001$) (Figure 4).

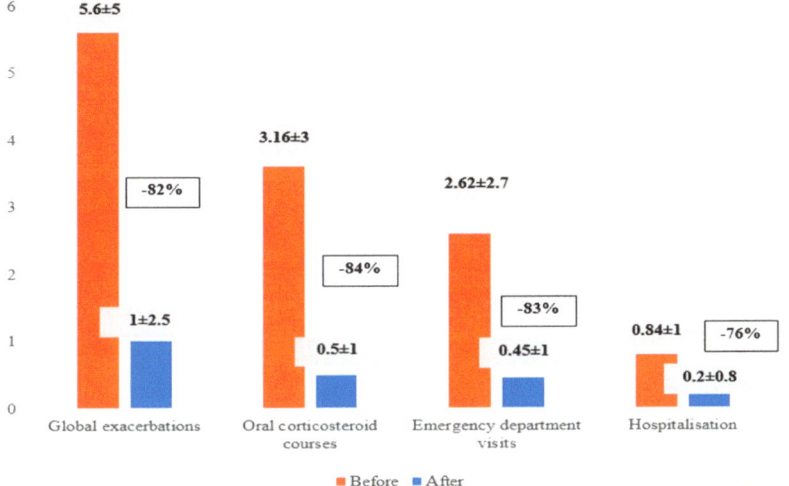

Figure 4. A comparison of the incidence of global exacerbations, the number of oral corticosteroid courses administered, the number of emergency department visits and the number of hospitalisations before and after benralizumab treatment.

The mean FEOS score after treatment was 73 ± 14. According to the multidimensional EXACTO scale, 33 patients (57%) achieved a complete or super-response, 16 (28%) a good response, and 9 (15%) a partial response (Figure 5).

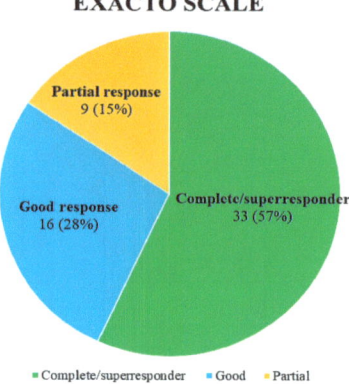

Figure 5. Consensus response EXACTO (Exacerbations, ACT, systemic corticosteroids and FEV1-Obstruction) to benralizumab treatment: partial response, good response or complete/superresponder.

The adverse effects observed were minor: transient fever in 5 patients, odynophagia in 4, headache in 2, with no major adverse effects requiring discontinuation of treatment.

4. Discussion

The coexistence of uncontrolled severe asthma and CRSwNP has been demonstrated to exert a deleterious influence on asthma control and quality of life. This highlights the necessity for the development of novel additional treatment options to provide adequate control of uncontrolled severe asthma associated with CRSwNP [1].

In the case of CRSwNP, the POLINA guidelines recommend the use of individual or global assessment scores of nasal symptoms to measure the response to treatment. These may be measured using a VAS or a semi-qualitative score, as well as a register of exacerbations and measurement of SNOT-22. In contrast, with regard to uncontrolled severe asthma, the Spanish Guideline on the Management *of* Asthma (GEMA) indicate that the response to treatment should be evaluated based on the number of exacerbations, the reduction or withdrawal of pharmacological treatment necessary for control (especially oral glucocorticoids), subjective asthma control rating scales (ACT, ACQ, VAS and AQLQ), and the impact on lung function as measured by FEV1 [1]. These criteria have been evaluated in this study and found to be comparable to those of published trials such as CANONICA [2] and OSTRO [14], as well as other real-life studies [22,23].

The characteristics of the patients in our study were similar to those of recently published studies. Specifically, our population had a mean age of 56 years and a higher percentage of women, as in OSTRO [14] and CANONICA [2], as well as elevated levels of eosinophils and IgE. This is consistent with the findings of the aforementioned studies, which suggest that eosinophils may play an important role in the pathogenesis of uncontrolled severe asthma with CRSwNP, representing a potential therapeutic target. With regard to lung function, the mean FEV1 was found to be compatible with obstructive pathology, and ACQ was elevated, indicating poor asthma control. It was noteworthy that a high proportion of patients were receiving oral corticosteroids and that there was a significantly increased annual exacerbation rate and SNOT-22.

In relation to uncontrolled severe asthma, our study demonstrated a statistically significant improvement in lung function, subjective asthma control and quality of life, as well as a reduction in the annual global exacerbation rate of 82%. These findings are comparable to those of the CANONICA study, which observed a 0.5 L improvement in FEV1, a reduction in ACQ of 1.69 points, and a significant reduction in annual asthma exacerbations [2]. With regard to the response of asthma to biologic therapy, a notably high score was achieved on the FEOS scale, as well as on the multidimensional EXACTO scale. Furthermore, in terms of clinical remission, 57% of patients exhibited a complete response or super-response. These results are comparable to those obtained in a recently published article on the response and remission of uncontrolled severe asthma with biologic therapy [24]. With respect to CRSwNP, a reduction of 25 points was observed on the SNOT-22 scale, with a mean value of 20 points after treatment. This is higher than that shown in studies such as OSTRO (−6.23 points) [14] and similar to that of CANONICA (−20 points) [2]. Although the POLINA guidelines do not establish a specific SNOT-22 value to be considered a response to treatment with a biologic, most authors use a reduction of 8.9 points with respect to baseline and SNOT-22 below 30 points as an important variation in terms of response to treatment, which is consistent with the findings of our study [2,16,25]. In our study, patients with a higher degree of eosinophilia and a lower component of atopy presented better nasal response, although without differences in asthma control.

Patients with uncontrolled severe asthma typically require treatment with oral glucocorticoids, which, in the case of association with CRSwNP, may be increased and persistent. Given that long-term administration of oral glucocorticoids may lead to adverse effects, it is important to reduce their consumption. Regarding to the impact of benralizumab on oral corticosteroid consumption, the ZONDA trial demonstrated that benralizumab administration resulted in a 75% reduction in oral glucocorticoids use [26]. The results demonstrated a more favourable outcome, with a reduction of 84% in the maintenance oral glucocorticoid use compared to those observed in the ANANKE real-life study, where a 64% reduction in oral glucocorticoid use was observed [22].

An essential aspect of our study is that it is a real-life study, which allows us to complement the information collected in the literature to date. This is because our work includes a heterogeneous group of patients who have been followed and treated in a way that is adjusted to daily clinical practice. In our case, the study included a large number of patients (n = 58) collected in a single centre and with a uniform work system throughout the follow-up of patients during the study, which can be interpreted as a strength.

This can be compared with other multicentre real-life studies. On the one hand, two Italian studies with a small patient sample: one comprising 59 patients with uncontrolled severe asthma of which 34 had CRSwNP [27] and another with 10 patients with uncontrolled severe asthma and CRSwNP [28]. Additionally, there are larger-scale real-life studies with greater patient numbers, such as the ANANKE study with 110 patients [22], Nolasco et al. with 79 patients [29] and Pini et al. with 108 patients [30]. Despite the differences in the samples, all of the studies presented similar results and conclusions regarding the efficacy of benralizumab in patients with uncontrolled severe asthma and CRSwNP.

Given that the results of our study show a very significant efficacy in the control of uncontrolled severe asthma NCSA and associated CRSwNP, other published clinical trials such as SIROCCO [31] and CALIMA [13], as well as real-life studies comparing the efficacy of benralizumab in asthma patients with and also agree that nasal polypo-sis is a consistent predictor of response to benralizumab in terms of asthma control outcomes, with better outcomes in patients with associated CRSwNP. Additionally, benralizumab has shown to be demonstrated more cost-effective (52.21 quali-ty-adjusted life years [QALYs]) than mepolizumab (51.39 QALYs) and dupilumab (51.30 QALYs) [32].

Limitations of our study include the fact that the only information we have on CRSwNP in patients is their diagnosis by an ENT specialist, although we do not have precise information on imaging techniques before and after the study, but the number of previous nasal surgical treatments.

ENT specialist also work in real life and the study was not designed as a prospective study including all objective data such as imaging techniques or smell tests but as a clinical study carried out in routine clinical practice and this should be taken into con-sideration.

In conclusion, benralizumab demonstrated efficacy in improving nasal symptoms as measured by SNOT-22, as well as in reducing obstruction, drip, anosmia and facial pressure parameters. Furthermore, it was associated with a significant reduction in the number of hospital admissions and emergency department visits, as well as a reduction in oral corticosteroid consumption. Additionally, benralizumab was associated with improved lung function in patients with uncontrolled severe asthma with CRSwNP, with two-thirds of patients achieving complete asthma remission.

Author Contributions: Conceptualization, E.C., M.M., I.B., M.Á.B., V.E. and E.M.-M.; Methodology, E.C., M.M., I.B., M.Á.B., V.E. and E.M.-M.; Software, E.C., M.M., I.B., M.Á.B., V.E. and E.M.-M.; Validation, E.C., M.M., I.B., M.Á.B., V.E. and E.M.-M.; Formal Analysis, E.C., M.M., I.B., M.Á.B., V.E. and E.M.-M.; Investigation, E.C., M.M., I.B., M.Á.B., V.E. and E.M.-M.; Resources, E.C., M.M., I.B., M.Á.B., V.E. and E.M.-M.; Data Curation, E.C., M.M., I.B., M.Á.B., V.E. and E.M.-M.; Writing—Original Draft Preparation, E.C., M.M., I.B., M.Á.B., V.E. and E.M.-M.; Writing—Review & Editing, E.C., M.M., I.B., M.Á.B., V.E. and E.M.-M.; Visualization, E.C., M.M., I.B., M.Á.B., V.E. and E.M.-M.; Supervision, E.C., M.M., I.B., M.Á.B., V.E. and E.M.-M.; Project Administration, E.C., M.M., I.B., M.Á.B., V.E. and E.M.-M. All authors have read and agreed to the published version of the manuscript.

Funding: This research received no external funding.

Institutional Review Board Statement: The study was conducted in accordance with the Declaration of Helsinki, and approved by the or Ethics Committee of Research Involving Medicines of the General University Hospital of Elda (protocol code 2023/04 and date of approval on 26 June 2023).

Informed Consent Statement: Informed consent was obtained from all subjects involved in the study.

Data Availability Statement: Data are contained within the article.

Conflicts of Interest: The authors declare no conflict of interest.

References

1. Plaza, V.; Alobid, I.; Álvarez, C.; Blanco, M.; Ferreira, J.; García, G.; Gómez-Outes, A.; Garín Escrivá, N.; Gómez, F.; Hidalgo, A.; et al. GEMA 5.3. Spanish Guideline on the Management of Asthma. *Open Respir. Arch.* **2023**, *5*, 100277. [CrossRef] [PubMed]
2. Canonica, G.W.; Harrison, T.W.; Chanez, P.; Menzella, F.; Louis, R.; Cosio, B.G.; Lugogo, N.L.; Mohan, A.; Burden, A.; Garcia, E. Benralizumab improves symptoms of patients with severe, eosinophilic asthma with a diagnosis of nasal polyposis. *Allergy* **2022**, *77*, 150–161. [CrossRef] [PubMed]
3. Bagnasco, D.; Paggiaro, P.; Latorre, M.; Folli, C.; Testino, E.; Bassi, A.; Milanese, M.; Heffler, E.; Manfredi, A.; Riccio, A.M.; et al. Severe asthma: One disease and multiple definitions. *World Allergy Organ. J.* **2021**, *14*, 100606. [CrossRef] [PubMed]
4. Alobid, I.; Benítez, P.; Bernal-Sprekelsen, M.; Roca, J.; Alonso, J.; Picado, C.; Mullol, J. Nasal polyposis and its impact on quality of life: Comparison between the effects of medical and surgical treatments. *Allergy* **2005**, *60*, 452–458. [CrossRef] [PubMed]
5. Kusano, S.; Kukimoto-Niino, M.; Hino, N.; Ohsawa, N.; Ikutani, M.; Takaki, S.; Sakamoto, K.; Hara-Yokoyama, M.; Shirouzu, M.; Takatsu, K.; et al. Structural basis of interleukin-5 dimer recognition by its α receptor. *Protein Sci.* **2012**, *21*, 850–864. [CrossRef] [PubMed]
6. McGregor, M.C.; Krings, J.G.; Nair, P.; Castro, M. Role of Biologics in Asthma. *Am. J. Respir. Crit. Care Med.* **2019**, *199*, 433–445. [CrossRef]
7. Agache, I.; Beltran, J.; Akdis, C.; Akdis, M.; Canelo-Aybar, C.; Canonica, G.W.; Casale, T.; Chivato, T.; Corren, J.; Del Giacco, S.; et al. Efficacy and safety of treatment with biologicals (benralizumab, dupilumab, mepolizumab, omalizumab and reslizumab) for severe eosinophilic asthma. A systematic review for the EAACI Guidelines—Recommendations on the use of biologicals in severe asthma. *Allergy* **2020**, *75*, 1023–1042. [CrossRef] [PubMed]
8. Dávila, G.I.; Moreno, B.F.; Quirce, S. Benralizumab: A New Approach for the Treatment of Severe Eosinophilic Asthma. *J. Investig. Allergol. Clin. Immunol.* **2019**, *29*, 84–93. [CrossRef] [PubMed]
9. Schleich, F.; Moermans, C.; Seidel, L.; Kempeneers, C.; Louis, G.; Rogister, F.; Tombu, S.; Pottier, L.; Poirrier, A.L.; Ziant, S.; et al. Benralizumab in severe eosinophilic asthma in real life: Confirmed effectiveness and contrasted effect on sputum eosinophilia versus exhaled nitric oxide fraction—PROMISE. *ERJ Open Res.* **2023**, *9*, 00383–02023. [CrossRef]

10. Barroso, B.; Valverde-Monge, M.; Betancor, D.; Gómez-López, A.; Villalobos-Vilda, C.; González-Cano, B.; Sastre, J. Improvement in Smell Using Monoclonal Antibodies Among Patients With Chronic Rhinosinusitis With Nasal Polyps: A Systematic Review. *J. Investig. Allergol. Clin. Immunol.* **2023**, *33*, 419–430. [CrossRef]
11. Tversky, J.; Lane, A.P.; Azar, A. Benralizumab effect on severe chronic rhinosinusitis with nasal polyps (CRSwNP): A randomized double-blind placebo-controlled trial. *Clin. Exp. Allergy* **2021**, *51*, 836–844. [CrossRef] [PubMed]
12. Matsuno, O.; Minamoto, S. Rapid effect of benralizumab for severe asthma with chronic rhinosinusitis with nasal polyps. *Pulm. Pharmacol. Ther.* **2020**, *64*, 101965. [CrossRef] [PubMed]
13. FitzGerald, J.M.; Bleecker, E.R.; Nair, P.; Korn, S.; Ohta, K.; Lommatzsch, M.; Ferguson, G.T.; Busse, W.W.; Barker, P.; Sproule, S.; et al. Benralizumab, an anti-interleukin-5 receptor α monoclonal antibody, as add-on treatment for patients with severe, uncontrolled, eosinophilic asthma (CALIMA): A randomised, double-blind, placebo-controlled phase 3 trial. *Lancet* **2016**, *388*, 2128–2141. [CrossRef] [PubMed]
14. Bachert, C.; Han, J.K.; Desrosiers, M.Y.; Gevaert, P.; Heffler, E.; Hopkins, C.; Tversky, J.R.; Barker, P.; Cohen, D.; Emson, C.; et al. Efficacy and safety of benralizumab in chronic rhinosinusitis with nasal polyps: A randomized, placebo-controlled trial. *J. Allergy Clin. Immunol.* **2022**, *149*, 1309–1317. [CrossRef]
15. Harrison, T.W.; Chanez, P.; Menzella, F.; Canonica, G.W.; Louis, R.; Cosio, B.G.; Lugogo, N.L.; Mohan, A.; Burden, A.; McDermott, L.; et al. Onset of effect and impact on health-related quality of life, exacerbation rate, lung function, and nasal polyposis symptoms for patients with severe eosinophilic asthma treated with benralizumab (ANDHI): A randomised, controlled, phase 3b trial. *Lancet Respir. Med.* **2021**, *9*, 260–274. [CrossRef] [PubMed]
16. Alobid, I.; Colás, C.; Castillo, J.A.; Arismendi, E.; Del Cuvillo, A.; Gómez-Outes, A.; Sastre, J.; Mullol, J. Spanish Consensus on the Management of Chronic Rhinosinusitis With Nasal Polyps (POLIposis NAsal/POLINA 2.0). *J. Investig. Allergol. Clin. Immunol.* **2023**, *33*, 317–331. [CrossRef] [PubMed]
17. García-Río, F.; Calle, M.; Burgos, F.; Casan, P.; Del Campo, F.; Galdiz, J.B.; Giner, J.; González-Mangado, N.; Ortega, F.; Puente, L. Spirometry. *Arch. Bronconeumol.* **2013**, *9*, 388–401. [CrossRef]
18. Jia, C.E.; Zhang, H.P.; Lv, Y.; Liang, R.; Jiang, Y.Q.; Powell, H.; Fu, J.J.; Wang, L.; Gibson, P.G.; Wang, G. The Asthma Control Test and Asthma Control Questionnaire for assessing asthma control: Systematic review and meta-analysis. *J. Allergy Clin. Immunol.* **2013**, *131*, 695–703. [CrossRef]
19. Liu, M.; Liu, J.; Weitzel, E.K.; Chen, P.G. The predictive utility of the 22-item sino-nasal outcome test (SNOT-22): A scoping review. *Int. Forum Allergy Rhinol.* **2022**, *12*, 83–102. [CrossRef]
20. Pérez de Llano, L.; Dávila, I.; Martínez-Moragón, E.; Domínguez-Ortega, J.; Almonacid, C.; Colás, C.; García-Rivero, J.L.; Carmona, L.; García de Yébenes, M.J.; Cosío, B.G. Development of a Tool to Measure the Clinical Response to Biologic Therapy in Uncontrolled Severe Asthma: The FEV1, Exacerbations, Oral Corticosteroids, Symptoms Score. *J. Allergy Clin. Immunol. Pract.* **2021**, *9*, 2725–2731. [CrossRef]
21. Alvarez-Gutiérrez, F.J.; Blanco-Aparicio, M.; Casas-Maldonado, F.; Plaza, V.; González-Barcala, F.J.; Carretero-Gracia, J.Á.; Castilla-Martínez, M.; Cisneros, C.; Diaz-Pérez, D.; Domingo-Ribas, C.; et al. Documento de consenso de asma grave en adultos. Actualización 2022 [Consensus document for severe asthma in adults. 2022 update]. *Open Respir Arch.* **2022**, *4*, 100192. [CrossRef] [PubMed]
22. D'Amato, M.; Menzella, F.; Altieri, E.; Bargagli, E.; Bracciale, P.; Brussino, L.; Caiaffa, M.F.; Canonica, G.W.; Caruso, C.; Centanni, S.; et al. Benralizumab in Patients With Severe Eosinophilic Asthma With and Without Chronic Rhinosinusitis With Nasal Polyps: An ANANKE Study post-hoc Analysis. *Front. Allergy.* **2022**, *3*, 881218. [CrossRef] [PubMed]
23. Martinez-Moragon, E.; Chiner, E.; Suliana Mogrovejo, A.; Palop Cervera, M.; Lluch Tortajada, I.; Boira, J.; Sánchez Vera, A.F. Real-world clinical remission of severe asthma with benralizumab in Spanish adults with severe asthma. *J. Asthma.* **2024**, *4*, 1–15. [CrossRef] [PubMed]
24. Valverde-Monge, M.; Sánchez-Carrasco, P.; Betancor, D.; Barroso, B.; Rodrigo-Muñoz, J.M.; Mahillo-Fernández, I.; Arismendi, E.; Bobolea, I.; Cárdaba, B.; Cruz, M.J.; et al. Comparison of Long-term Response and Remission to Omalizumab and Anti-IL-5/IL-5R Using Different Criteria in a Real-life Cohort of Severe Asthma Patients. *Arch. Bronconeumol.* **2024**, *60*, 23–32. [CrossRef]
25. Padilla-Galo, A.; Moya Carmona, I.; Ausín, P.; Carazo Fernández, L.; García-Moguel, I.; Velasco-Garrido, J.L.; Andújar-Espinosa, R.; Casas-Maldonado, F.; Martínez- Moragón, E.; Martínez Rivera, C.; et al. Achieving clinical outcomes with benralizumab in severe eosinophilic asthma patients in a real-world setting: Orbe II study. *Respir. Res.* **2023**, *24*, 235. [CrossRef] [PubMed]
26. Nair, P.; Wenzel, S.; Rabe, K.F.; Bourdin, A.; Lugogo, N.L.; Kuna, P.; Barker, P.; Sproule, S.; Ponnarambil, S.; Goldman, M. Oral Glucocorticoid- Sparing Effect of Benralizumab in Severe Asthma. *N. Engl. J. Med.* **2017**, *376*, 2448–2458. [CrossRef]
27. Bagnasco, D.; Brussino, L.; Bonavia, M.; Calzolari, E.; Caminati, M.; Caruso, C.; D'Amato, M.; De Ferrari, L.; Di Marco, F.; Imeri, G.; et al. Efficacy of Benralizumab in severe asthma in real life and focus on nasal polyposis. *Respir. Med.* **2020**, *171*, 106080. [CrossRef]
28. Lombardo, N.; Pelaia, C.; Ciriolo, M.; Della Corte, M.; Piazzetta, G.; Lobello, N.; Viola, P.; Pelaia, G. Real-life effects of benralizumab on allergic chronic rhinosinusitis and nasal polyposis associated with severe asthma. *Int. J. Immunopathol. Pharmacol.* **2020**, *34*, 2058738420950851. [CrossRef] [PubMed]
29. Nolasco, S.; Crimi, C.; Pelaia, C.; Benfante, A.; Caiaffa, M.F.; Calabrese, C.; Carpagnano, G.E.; Ciotta, D.; D'Amato, M.; Macchia, L.; et al. Benralizumab Effectiveness in Severe Eosinophilic Asthma with and without Chronic Rhinosinusitis with Nasal Polyps: A Real-World Multicenter Study. *J. Allergy Clin. Immunol. Pract.* **2021**, *9*, 4371–4380.e4. [CrossRef]

30. Pini, L.; Bagnasco, D.; Beghè, B.; Braido, F.; Cameli, P.; Caminati, M.; Caruso, C.; Crimi, C.; Guarnieri, G.; Latorre, M.; et al. Unlocking the Long-Term Effectiveness of Benralizumab in Severe Eosinophilic Asthma: A Three-Year Real-Life Study. *J. Clin. Med.* **2024**, *13*, 3013. [CrossRef]
31. Bleecker, E.R.; FitzGerald, J.M.; Chanez, P.; Papi, A.; Weinstein, S.F.; Barker, P.; Sproule, S.; Gilmartin, G.; Aurivillius, M.; Werkström, V.; et al. Efficacy and safety of benralizumab for patients with severe asthma uncontrolled with high-dosage inhaled corticosteroids and long-acting β2-agonists (SIROCCO): A randomised, multicentre, placebo-controlled phase 3 trial. *Lancet* **2016**, *388*, 2115–2127. [CrossRef] [PubMed]
32. Mareque, M.; Climente, M.; Martinez-Moragon, E.; Padilla, A.; Oyagüez, I.; Touron, C.; Torres, C.; Martinez, A. Cost-effectiveness of benralizumab versus mepolizumab and dupilumab in patients with severe uncontrolled eosinophilic asthma in Spain. *J. Asthma.* **2023**, *60*, 1210–1220. [CrossRef] [PubMed]

Disclaimer/Publisher's Note: The statements, opinions and data contained in all publications are solely those of the individual author(s) and contributor(s) and not of MDPI and/or the editor(s). MDPI and/or the editor(s) disclaim responsibility for any injury to people or property resulting from any ideas, methods, instructions or products referred to in the content.

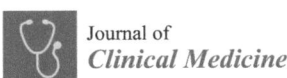

Article

Unlocking the Long-Term Effectiveness of Benralizumab in Severe Eosinophilic Asthma: A Three-Year Real-Life Study

Laura Pini [1,2,*], Diego Bagnasco [3], Bianca Beghè [4], Fulvio Braido [3], Paolo Cameli [5], Marco Caminati [6,7], Cristiano Caruso [8], Claudia Crimi [9], Gabriella Guarnieri [10], Manuela Latorre [11], Francesco Menzella [12], Claudio Micheletto [13], Andrea Vianello [10], Dina Visca [14,15], Benedetta Bondi [3], Yehia El Masri [2], Jordan Giordani [2], Andrea Mastrototaro [6], Matteo Maule [7], Alessandro Pini [16], Stefano Piras [2], Martina Zappa [14], Gianenrico Senna [6,7], Antonio Spanevello [14,15], Pierluigi Paggiaro [17], Francesco Blasi [18,19], Giorgio Walter Canonica [20,21] and on behalf of the SANI Study Group [†]

1. ASST Spedali Civili of Brescia, 25123 Brescia, Italy
2. Department of Clinical and Experimental Sciences, University of Brescia, 25122 Brescia, Italy
3. Allergy and Respiratory Diseases Clinic, IRCCS Policlinico San Martino, 16132 Genova, Italy
4. Department of Medical and Surgical Sciences, Maternal, Infant and Adult, University of Modena and Reggio Emilia, 41124 Modena, Italy
5. Respiratory Diseases Unit, Department of Medical Sciences, Azienda Ospedaliera-Universitaria Senese, 53100 Siena, Italy
6. Department of Medicine, University of Verona, 37134 Verona, Italy
7. Asthma Center and Allergy Unit, Verona University Hospital, 37126 Verona, Italy
8. Allergologic Unit, Policlinico Agostino Gemelli, 00168 Rome, Italy
9. Respiratory Medicine Unit, Policlinico "G. Rodolico-San Marco" University Hospital, 95123 Catania, Italy
10. Department of Cardiac, Thoracic and Vascular Sciences, University of Padova, 35122 Padova, Italy
11. Pneumologic Unit, Department of Medical Specialties, Nuovo Ospedale delle Apuane, 54100 Massa, Italy
12. Pneumologic Unit, Ospedale di Montebelluna, 31044 Montebelluna, Italy
13. Pneumologic Unit, Ospedale Borgo Trento, 37126 Verona, Italy
14. Department of Medicine and Surgery, Respiratory Diseases, University of Insubria, 21100 Varese, Italy
15. Department of Cardio-Respiratory Medicine and Rehabilitation, Division of Pulmonary Rehabilitation, Istituti Clinici Scientifici Maugeri, IRCCS, 21049 Tradate, Italy
16. Department of Emergency, Anaesthesiological and Resuscitation Sciences, University Cattolica Sacro Cuore, 29122 Rome, Italy
17. Department of Surgery, Medicine, Molecular Biology and Critical Care, University of Pisa, 56124 Pisa, Italy
18. Department of Pathophysiology and Transplantation, University of Milano, 20122 Milan, Italy
19. Respiratory Unit and Cystic Fibrosis Center, Fondazione IRCCS Cà Granda Ospedale Maggiore Policlinico di Milano, 20122 Milan, Italy
20. Personalized Medicine Center, Asthma and Allergology, Humanitas Research Hospital, 20089 Rozzano, Italy
21. Department of Biomedical Sciences, Humanitas University, 20090 Pieve Emanuele, Italy
* Correspondence: laura.pini@unibs.it
† Severe Asthma Network in Italy (SANI). Additional members of SANI are listed in Supplementary Materials.

Abstract: Background: Benralizumab has been shown to restore good control of severe eosinophilic asthma (SEA). Robust data on benralizumab effectiveness over periods longer than 2 years are scarce. **Methods:** This retrospective multicentric study was conducted on 108 Italian SEA patients treated with benralizumab for up to 36 months. Partial and complete clinical remission (CR) were assessed. Data were analyzed with descriptive statistics or using linear, logistic, and negative binomial mixed-effect regression models. **Results:** At 36 months, benralizumab reduced the exacerbation rate by 89% and increased the forced expiratory volume in 1 second (FEV_1) (+440 mL at 36 months, $p < 0.0001$). Benralizumab improved asthma control as well as sinonasal symptoms in patients with chronic rhinosinusitis with nasal polyposis (CRSwNP). Up to 93.33% of patients either reduced or discontinued OCS; benralizumab also decreased ICS use and other asthma medications. Overall, 84.31% of patients achieved partial or complete CR. **Conclusions:** Benralizumab improved asthma and sinonasal outcomes up to 36 months. These findings support the potential of benralizumab to induce CR, emphasizing its role as a disease-modifying anti-asthmatic drug for the management of SEA. Further research is warranted to expand these findings by minimizing data loss and assessing benralizumab's long-term safety.

Keywords: severe eosinophilic asthma; benralizumab; effectiveness; long term; clinical remission

1. Introduction

Severe asthma (SA) is a debilitating chronic disorder that affects approximately 10% of asthma patients worldwide [1–3]. Due to its heterogeneous nature, distinct phenotypes and endotypes have been identified and prompted the sub-classification of the disease according to clinical characteristics and functional and inflammatory parameters [4]. Severe eosinophilic asthma (SEA) is one of the predominant subtypes of SA [5,6]; its pathophysiology is defined by an extensive type 2 (T2) inflammatory process mainly driven by the proliferation and activation of eosinophils. Accordingly, eosinophil number is increased in blood and sputum of SEA patients; other key characteristics are a scarce respiratory function that further deteriorates over time, and recurrent and/or life-threatening exacerbations [7–9]. Given the high burden of its manifestations and the poor prognosis, SEA has a devastating impact on patients' quality of life (QoL), which can be further aggravated by the presence of comorbidities, among which chronic rhinosinusitis with nasal polyposis (CRSwNP) is one of the most frequently observed [10,11].

The recommended background therapies, which include inhaled corticosteroids (ICS) and a second controller (usually a long-acting beta2-agonist [LABA]) [12] are not always effective in managing SEA symptoms. Based on their potent anti-inflammatory action, oral corticosteroids (OCS) have been traditionally added to background medications in cases of inadequate asthma control, to prevent exacerbations. However, given the cumulative risk of significant adverse effects and mortality associated with their usage, even moderate dosages of OCS should be avoided [12–16].

The development of several biological therapies has represented a giant step forward in the treatment of T2-high SA. Six biologics have thus far received approval (omalizumab, mepolizumab, reslizumab, benralizumab, dupilumab, tezepelumab); by targeting distinct pathways involved in the pathophysiology of the disease, they ensure superior efficacy and safety than OCS [17]. Based on their different mechanism of action (MoA), each one of these pharmacological agents is expected to be more successful in patients whose asthma is predominantly sustained by the corresponding inflammatory endotype. However, SA patients frequently show overlapping T2-high features [18]; as a result, precise pheno-endotypization is required to identify the driving pathway of the disease and anticipate the most effective biologic treatment.

Overall, the great clinical outcomes displayed by SA patients treated with biologic therapies have highlighted the potential of reaching a status of remission from the disease. To clarify this concept, a consensus on the criteria that define clinical remission (CR), both complete (cCR) and partial (pCR), was recently reached by a panel of experts from the Severe Asthma Network Italy (SANI) study group, allowing for the standardized assessment of patients regardless of the biological treatment received [19,20].

Benralizumab is a monoclonal antibody (mAb) approved for the treatment of SEA [21]. It is a humanized afucosilated immunoglobulin (Ig) Gk1 mAb that binds both interleukin 5 receptor alpha (IL-5Rα) and Fc gamma receptor IIIa (FcγRIIIa), expressed abundantly by eosinophils and natural killer (NK) cells, respectively. The simultaneous recognition of the two receptors allows benralizumab to activate antibody-dependent cell-mediated cytotoxicity (ADCC), a process through which NK cells induce the apoptosis of eosinophils [22,23]. The consequent nearly complete depletion of eosinophils differentiates benralizumab from the anti-IL-5 mAbs mepolizumab and reslizumab [24], and determines the well-established efficacy of benralizumab in SEA patients [25]. In a recent study, benralizumab has been shown to have profound immunological effects that are not limited to eosinophil apoptosis but include an increase in NK cell proliferation, maturation and cytotoxic activity, and the modulation of T cell subsets. Intriguingly, the number of circulating CD3 + T cells and activated NK cells significantly correlated with improvement in lung function parameters in benralizumab-treated SEA patients [26]. These results deepen our understanding of benralizumab MoA, which appears to be more complex than what was traditionally thought. These data suggest that the improvement in respiratory outcomes mediated by benralizumab may be due to a profound immunological modulation that takes place even in the absence of eosinophils.

To date, the 5-year-long MELTEMI trial represents the longest study evaluating the effects of benralizumab on SEA patients; the results indicated that benralizumab was safe and effective in eliminating exacerbations in up to 59% of patients during the entire extension period (BORA and MELTEMI studies, up to 4 years of treatment) [27]. Few real-life studies have investigated the benralizumab effectiveness over 20-month–4-year-long periods [25,28–33]. A marked and long-lasting reduction in exacerbations has been consistently shown across all studies, with impressive results obtained from the Italian ANANKE study, showing reductions of 94.9% and 96.9% in all and severe annual exacerbation rate (AER), respectively, after 96 weeks of treatment [25]. Positive outcomes have also been demonstrated in lung function and OCS reduction; however, the extent and the durability of benralizumab effectiveness on respiratory outcomes for periods longer than 2 years is still uncertain [31,33]. Recently published data from the phase IV randomized clinical trial (RCT) SHAMAL revealed that the benralizumab treatment was associated with a substantial reduction in the dose of background ICS, showcasing an additional clinical benefit of the anti-IL-5R therapy [34]. This Italian multicentric retrospective study includes a cohort of 108 SEA patients treated with benralizumab for up to 3 years. The data show changes in multiple clinical outcomes and provide a comprehensive analysis, as well as novel evidence, of the long-term effectiveness of benralizumab.

2. Materials and Methods

This is an observational retrospective study; data were collected from 9 Italian SANI centers specialized in the treatment of SA (Brescia, Catania, Modena, Montebelluna, Padova, Varese, Verona, Siena, Rome, Italy).

SA was diagnosed according to the European Respiratory Society (ERS) and the American Thoracic Society (ATS) guidelines [1]. Benralizumab was prescribed to adult patients as per Italian clinical practice, according to the eligibility and reimbursement criteria dictated by the therapeutic plan and previously established by the Italian regulatory drug agency (Agenzia Italiana del Farmaco, AIFA, Rome, Italy). To be eligible for benralizumab treatment, patients must have had any blood eosinophil count (BEC) $\geq$300 cells/μL in the absence of OCS treatment; such a BEC value may have been measured at any time before benralizumab initiation. In addition to this criterion, patients must meet one of the two following conditions: (1) at least two exacerbations in the previous 12 months despite maximum dose of inhaled therapy (steps 4–5 of the GINA document) and treated with systemic steroid or requiring hospitalization; (2) continuous OCS treatment received during the previous year in addition to maximal inhaled therapy [35]. Benralizumab was given subcutaneously at a dose of 30 mg; after the first three doses, which were administered every four weeks, benralizumab was administered every eight weeks.

A total of 108 patients were enrolled between January 2018 and February 2021; follow-up visits took place at 6, 12, 24, and 36 months after benralizumab initiation. Personal information including socio-demographic, clinical, functional and laboratory data were recorded as per clinical practice immediately before benralizumab initiation (i.e., at baseline) and during follow-up visits. Data were retrospectively collected from medical charts between April and June 2023. More specifically, the baseline characteristics included age, gender, body mass index (BMI), smoking habit, age at asthma diagnosis, age at benralizumab initiation, comorbidities, use and dose of asthma therapies (background inhaled medications, OCS, biologics received prior to benralizumab use), laboratory tests (BEC, IgE, fractioned exhaled nitric oxide [FeNO]), exacerbations (expressed as AER), as determined by treating physicians, and pre- and post-bronchodilator (BD) lung function parameters including forced expiratory volume in 1 second (FEV_1), and forced vital capacity (FVC). All respiratory measurements are pre-BD, unless otherwise specified.

Various patient reported outcomes (PROs) were also used to assess patients' asthma control (asthma control test, ACT, asthma control questionnaire-6, ACQ), and QoL (asthma quality of life questionnaire, AQLQ). The severity of sinonasal symptoms was specifically investigated in comorbid patients with CRSwNP using visual analogue scale (VAS) and sinonasal outcome test 22 (SNOT-22). The absolute differences in AER between 0 and 12 months and between 0 and 36 months were computed. Changes in laboratory parameters, AER, lung function parameters, PROs, background therapies, and OCS were evaluated over time. The number and percentages of patients reaching either pCR or cCR (defined according to the criteria detailed by Canonica et al. [19]) were determined at 12, 24 and 36 months; CR was calculated for each time point either from the corresponding previous time point (i.e., from baseline to 12 months; from 12 months to 24 months; and from 24 months to 36 months) or from baseline. pCR was defined by three criteria: (1) no use of OCS, accompanied by two of the following: either (1) good asthma control defined by ACT score ≥ 20; and/or (2) elimination of exacerbations; and/or (3) pulmonary stability. cCR was achieved by patients who met all four of the following criteria: (1) no use of OCS; (2) good asthma control defined by ACT score ≥ 20; (3) elimination of exacerbations; and (4) pulmonary stability [19].

Informed consent was obtained from all patients involved in the study. This was a SANI study; the study was conducted in conformity with the Declaration of Helsinki and was approved by the Central Ethics Committee for the SANI Network.

Statistical Analyses

For descriptive analyses, continuous variables were given as the mean with standard deviations (SD), or a median with range or interquartile range (IQR) and categorical variables were expressed as the number of subjects (n) and percentage values.

Possible over-dispersion for count values was assayed using a formal test based on the code from Gelman and Hill (2007) [36]. Linear, logistic, and Poisson mixed-effect regression models were performed on the continuous, dichotomy, and count values, respectively, to evaluate changes in AER, lung function, PROs scores, OCS, and use of asthma medication over time. Regression coefficients, odds ratios (ORs), and exponential regression coefficients associated with each outcome were calculated with 95% confidence intervals (CI) for each factor.

The center and subject variability were considered to be random effects in all mixed-effect regression models. The likelihood ratio test was used as a test of statistical significance and p-values were adjusted for multiple comparisons using the Holm correction method.

Differences, with a p-value less than 0.05, were selected as significant. Data were acquired and analyzed in R version v4.3.1 software environment [37].

3. Results
3.1. Patients' Characteristics at Baseline

The demographics, biochemical, and clinical characteristics of the study participants at baseline are summarized in Table 1. Briefly, a total of 108 patients (59.26% female, mean age 55.96 years) took part in this study; the population was highly comorbid, with 94 patients (87.04%) with at least one comorbidity. Chronic rhinosinusitis (CRS), and specifically CRSwNP, was the most common comorbidity, being present in 65 patients (60.19%). A total of 28 out of 104 patients (26.96%) had bronchiectasis and 4 out of 96 patients (4.71%) had eosinophilic granulomatosis with polyangiitis (EGPA). The mean age at asthma diagnosis was 35.68 years (15.95). All patients used ICS and LABA as background therapies, the mean ICS dose used by patients was high (1006.93 mcg/day (402.56)) and the majority of patients required additional asthma medications, including long-acting muscarinic antagonists (LAMA) (79 out of 107 patients, 73.83%), anti-leukotrienes (anti LT) (52 out of 107 patients, 48.60%), theophylline (6 out of 106 patients, 5.66%). OCS were taken by 67 patients (62.04%) at a mean dose of 7.95 mg/day (7.42); a total of 41 patients used the OCS dose higher than 5 mg/day (61.19%). Of note, benralizumab was the first biologic therapy used in 89 patients (82.41%), while 19 patients were switched to benralizumab after being treated with other biologics (either omalizumab or mepolizumab).

Table 1. Demographic, social, and clinical characteristics of patient population at baseline. Data refer to $n = 108$ patients, unless otherwise specified, and are expressed as the number of subjects (percentage), mean (SD), or median (range) as appropriate.

Characteristics at Baseline	Patient Population
Age (years)	55.96 (11.38)
Sex (female)	64 (59.26%)
BMI (kg/m^2)	
Underweight/normal weight	46 (42.59%)
Overweight	46 (42.59%)
Obese	16 (14.81%)
Smoking status	
Non-smokers	78 (72.22%)
Previous smokers	29 (26.85%)
Current smokers	1 (0.93%)
Comorbidities	94 (87.04%)
CRS	67 (62.62%)
CRSwNP	65 (60.19%)
Allergic rhinitis	57 (52.78%)
Gastroesophageal reflux disease (GERD)	39 (36.11%)
Bronchiectasis ($n = 104$)	28 (26.96%)
EGPA ($n = 96$)	4 (4.71%)
Eosinophilic esophagitis ($n = 93$)	1 (1.08%)
Age at asthma diagnosis (years) ($n = 106$)	35.68 (15.95)
ICS dose (mcg/day) ($n = 87$)	1006.93 (402.56)
<500	8 (9.20%)
$\geq$500 and <1000	44 (50.57%)
$\geq$1000	35 (40.23%)
LAMA ($n = 107$)	79 (73.83%)
Anti LT ($n = 107$)	52 (48.60%)
Theophylline ($n = 106$)	6 (5.66%)
SABA and/or ICS/LABA as needed (times per day) ($n = 88$)	3.10 (4.19)
OCS	67 (62.04%)
OCS dose (prednisone equivalent) (mg/day) ($n = 67$)	7.95 (7.42)
$\leq$5 mg/day	26 (38.81%)
>5 mg/day	41 (61.19%)
Biologic switch ($n = 98$)	
Naïve	89 (82.41%)
Switched	19 (17.59%)
BEC (cells/mm^3) ($n = 104$)	600 (28–3350)
FeNO (ppb) (N = 55)	61.95 (55.66)
Total serum IgE (IU/mL) ($n = 91$)	209 (4.9–1940)
AER ($n = 107$)	3.84 (3.18)
Exacerbation phenotype ($n = 45$)	
Bacterial	24 (53.33%)
Viral	7 (15.56%)
Non-infectious	14 (31.11%)
Lung function	
FEV$_1$ (L/min) ($n = 101$)	1.94 (0.83)
FVC (L) ($n = 90$)	3.30 (1.00)
FEV$_1$ (% pred.) ($n = 86$)	74.50 (20.68)
FVC (% pred.) ($n = 91$)	93.97 (20.73)
FEV$_1$/FVC ($n = 91$)	54.11 (24.87)
Asthma PROs	
ACT score ($n = 104$)	14.41 (5.08)
ACQ score ($n = 39$)	2.33 (1.25)
AQLQ score ($n = 31$)	3.76 (1.45)
CRSwNP PROs	
VAS ($n = 60$)	5.14 (3.13)
SNOT-22 score ($n = 57$)	47.21 (20.67)

Biochemical analyses revealed that patients had a median BEC of 600 cells/mm^3 (28–3350) ($n = 104$), a median total IgE level of 209 IU/mL (4.9–1940) ($n = 91$), and a mean FeNO of 61.95 ppb (55.66) ($n = 55$). The frequency of asthma exacerbations approached four events/year, with a mean AER of 3.84 (3.18) (n = 107); the phenotype of exacerbations was assessed in 45 patients, among which 14 (31.11%) had exacerbations of non-infectious nature, whereas the rest of patients experienced either viral (15.56%) or bacterial-induced (53.33%) exacerbations. Patients were also characterized by suboptimal lung function, showing a mean FEV_1/FVC ratio of 54.11 (24.87) (n = 91), a mean FEV_1 of 1.94 L (0.83) (n = 101), and a mean predicted FEV_1 of 74.50% (20.68) (n = 86).

Overall, asthma was uncontrolled despite the use of multiple medications, and patients' QoL was poor, as demonstrated by the low scores achieved in various PROs, including ACT (n = 104), ACQ (n = 39) and AQLQ (n = 31) (mean values of 14.41, 2.33 and 3.76, respectively). VAS (n = 60) and SNOT-22 (n = 57) were administered to comorbid patients with CRSwNP and showed a mean score of 5.14 (3.13) and 47.21 (20.67), respectively, indicative of moderate sinonasal symptom severity [38].

3.2. Benralizumab Reduced Exacerbations and Inflammatory Markers

Patients experienced a significant and remarkable reduction in AER throughout the three years of treatment with benralizumab ($p < 0.0001$, Figure 1A); baseline AER declined from a mean of 3.84 (3.18) to 0.26 (0.83) (0.07, 95% CI 0.05:0.10) already after 6 months of treatment and remained low at all time points, reaching 0.43 (0.93) (0.11, 95% CI 0.08:0.16) at 36 months. Compared with the baseline, the decline in AER amounted to 93%, 95%, 91%, and 89% at 6, 12, 24, and 36 months, respectively.

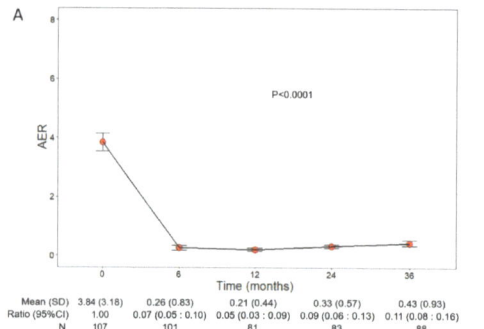 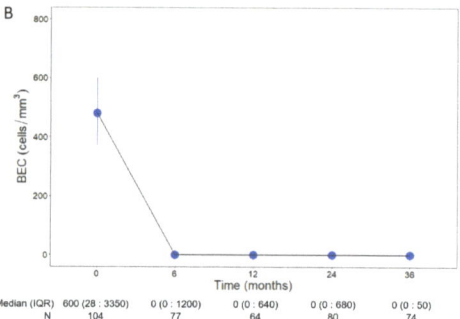

Figure 1. Change in AER (**A**) and BEC (**B**) during the treatment with benralizumab. Data were recorded at baseline and at 6, 12, 24, and 36 months. Mean (SD), *n* values and exponential beta regression coefficients (i.e., ratio) with 95% CI, or median (IQR) and *n* values are reported for each time point.

Consistent with its anti-eosinophilic effect, benralizumab treatment induced an almost complete depletion of BEC that was sustained over time, with a median BEC of 0 (0:50) displayed at all time points (Figure 1B). The drop in BEC was accompanied by a persistent reduction in FeNO, which decreased from a mean of 61.95 ppb (55.66) at baseline to 42.27 ppb (32.31) at 36 months ($p = 0.0001$, Table S1).

3.3. Benralizumab Improved Lung Function

Patients treated with benralizumab ameliorated their lung function throughout the 36-month period, with a significant increment observed in FEV_1 ($p < 0.0001$) (Figure 2). The mean volume of FEV_1 increased from 1.94 L (0.83) at baseline to 2.38 L (0.79) at 36 months (+440 mL), with the maximal value of 2.41 L (0.88) recorded at 12 months (Figure 2A), while percentage of predicted FEV_1 peaked at 36 months (87.62%, with a mean increase of 13.12% from baseline) (12.38, 95% CI 8.14:16.62) (Figure 2B). Variations in other respiratory measurements are reported in Table S1.

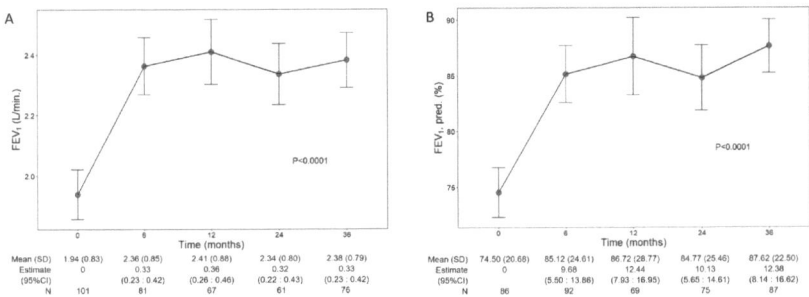

Figure 2. Change in FEV$_1$ volume (**A**) and percentage of predicted (**B**) during the treatment with benralizumab. Data were recorded at baseline and at 6, 12, 24, and 36 months. Mean (SD), n values and regression coefficients (i.e., estimate) with 95% CI are reported for each time point.

3.4. Benralizumab Increased Asthma Control and QoL

Asthma control and QoL significantly ameliorated during benralizumab treatment, with net improvements observed already at 6 months after the start of the treatment (Figure 3A). In detail, the mean ACT score was 14.41 (5.08) at baseline and increased to 21.66 points (4.50) at 6 months (7.18, 95% CI 6.35:8.01); the ACT score remained either stable or further increased throughout the treatment period, indicating a durable good control of asthma. In addition, benralizumab enhanced the patients' QoL as determined by the significant changes of both ACQ and AQLQ scores over time (mean ACQ: from 2.33 to 0.73, $p < 0.0001$; mean AQLQ: from 3.76 to 5.33, $p = 0.0001$) (Figure 3B,C).

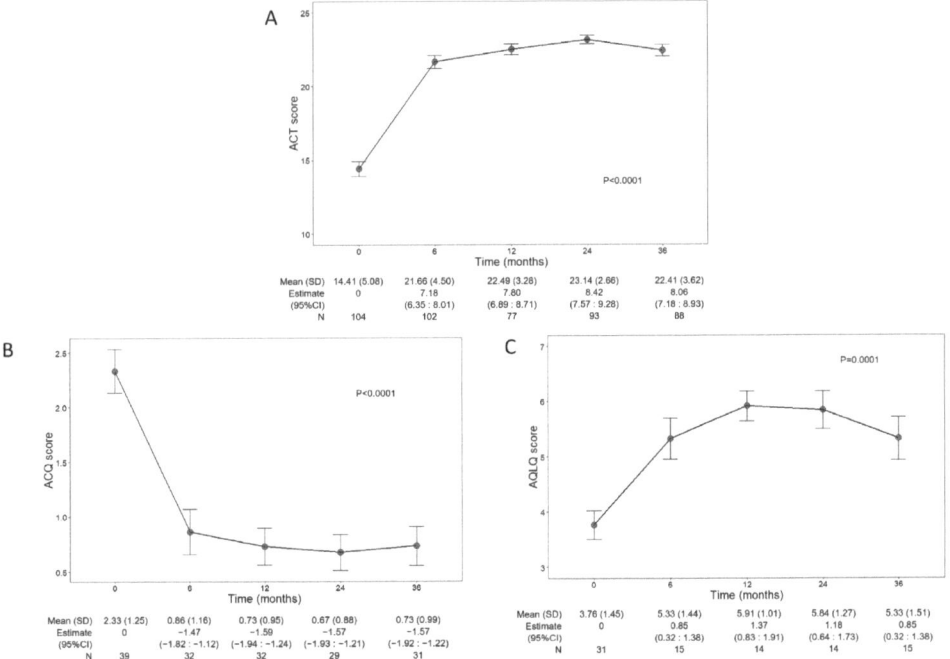

Figure 3. Change in ACT (**A**), ACQ (**B**), and AQLQ (**C**) scores during the treatment with benralizumab. Data were recorded at baseline and at 6, 12, 24, and 36 months. Mean (SD), n values and regression coefficients (i.e., estimate) with 95% CI are reported for each time point.

3.5. Benralizumab Alleviated Sinonasal Symptoms in Comorbid Patients

Beyond the asthma control improvement, benralizumab also decreased the severity of sinonasal symptoms in the subset of comorbid patients with CRSwNP. The mean VAS score significantly declined over the treatment period ($p = 0.0007$), decreasing from 5.14 (3.13) at baseline to 3.29 (3.20) at 36 months (-1.39, 95% CI $-2.11:-0.66$) (Figure 4A). In parallel, the mean SNOT-22 score also significantly dropped ($p < 0.0001$) from 47.21 (20.67) at baseline to 24.27 (16.69) at 36 months (-22.02, 95% CI $-27.55:-16.49$) (Figure 4B).

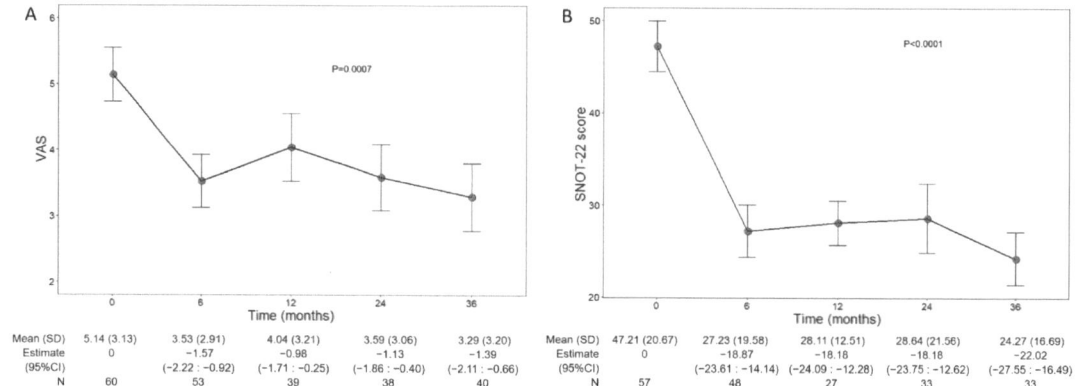

Figure 4. Change in VAS (**A**) and SNOT-22 (**B**) score during the treatment with benralizumab. Data were recorded at baseline and at 6, 12, 24, and 36 months. Mean values (SD), n and regression coefficients (i.e., estimate) with 95% CI are reported for each time point.

3.6. Benralizumab Decreased the Use of OCS

As shown in Figure 5, a significant reduction in OCS use was observed over time ($p < 0.0001$). The mean dose of OCS decreased to 3.18 mg/day (6.52) at 6 months (-6.73, 95% CI $-8.55:-4.91$) and continued to decline, reaching a mean dose of 1.80 mg/day (6.02) at 36 months (-8.35, 95% CI $-10.40:-6.29$). A total of 39 out of 64 (60.94%) eliminated the use of OCS already after 6 months from the start of benralizumab, and 38 out of 45 patients (84.44%) remained free from OCS at 36 months. Only three patients (6.67%) maintained (or increased) the baseline OCS dose, showing no reduction at 36 months (Table 2).

Table 2. Extent of OCS dose reduction achieved by patients during the treatment with benralizumab. Data are expressed as n (%).

Extent of OCS Reduction	Month 6 (n = 64)	Month 12 (n = 47)	Month 24 (n = 43)	Month 36 (n = 45)
Any reduction	52 (81.25%)	41 (87.23%)	39 (90.7%)	42 (93.33%)
≥90%	39 (60.94%)	34 (72.34%)	34 (79.07%)	38 (84.44%)
≥75%	42 (65.62%)	38 (80.85%)	37 (86.05%)	39 (86.67%)
≥50%	50 (78.12%)	41 (87.23%)	38 (88.37%)	42 (93.33%)
≥25%	51 (79.69%)	41 (87.23%)	39 (90.7%)	42 (93.33%)
No reduction	12 (18.75%)	6 (12.77%)	4 (9.3%)	3 (6.67%)
Elimination	39 (60.94%)	34 (72.34%)	33 (76.74%)	38 (84.44%)

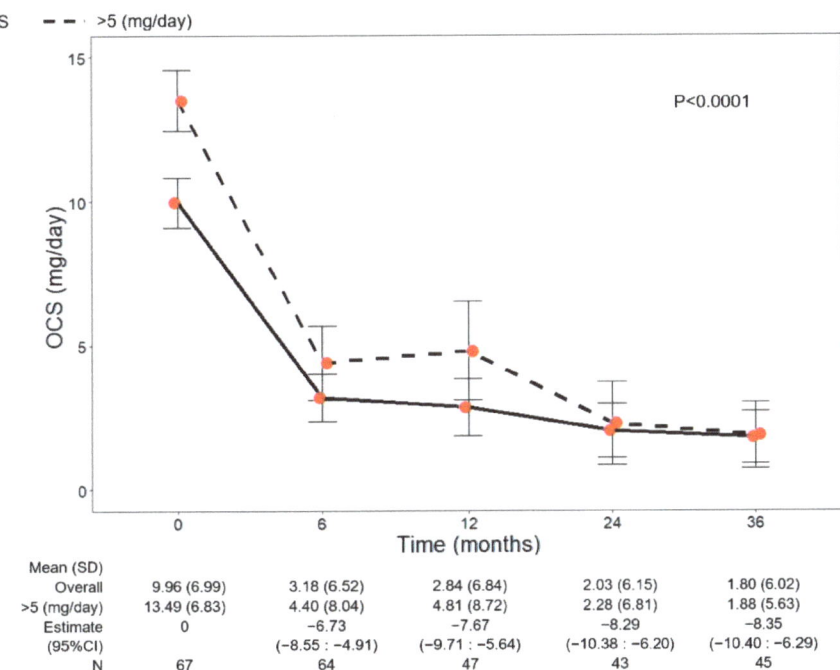

Figure 5. Change in OCS dose in the overall patient population and in patients with baseline OCS dose > 5 mg/day during the treatment with benralizumab. Data were recorded at baseline and at 6, 12, 24, and 36 months. Mean (SD), n values and regression coefficients (i.e., estimate) with 95% CI are reported for each time point.

The change in OCS use was also investigated in patients grouped according to their baseline OCS dose (≤5 mg/day or >5 mg/day) (Figure 5 and Table S2). The overall population and the subgroup of patients with a baseline OCS dose >5 mg/day showed a similar OCS reduction pattern, with mean OCS doses of 1.80 (6.02) and 1.88 (5.63) at 36 months, respectively (Figure 5). An almost identical percentage of patients discontinued OCS at 36 months regardless of the baseline OCS dose (85.71% of patients with OCS ≤ 5 mg/day and 83.33% of patients with OCS > 5 mg/day) (Table S2).

3.7. Benralizumab Reduced the Need for Asthma Background Medication

The daily ICS dose used by patients decreased progressively over time, from a mean of 1006.93 (402.56) at baseline (n = 87) to a mean of 800.04 (394.89) at 36 months (n = 70), with an overall reduction of 20.55%. Accordingly, the percentage of patients taking a low dose of ICS (<500 mcg/day) increased from 9.20% at baseline to 32.86% at 36 months, and a significant reduction in the required dose of ICS was observed over time (p = 0.0010, Table 3). In particular, the chances of patients requiring a medium ICS dose (≥500 and <1000 mcg/day) at 12, 24, and 36 months were reduced by 78%, 83%, and 89% compared with baseline (0.22 [0.07:0.71], 0.17 [0.06:0.55], and 0.11 [0.02:0.68], respectively), and the chances of requiring a high ICS dose (≥1000 mcg/day) at 6, 12, 24, and 36 months were reduced by 87%, 90%, 91%, and 85% compared with baseline (0.13, 95% CI 0.02:0.77; 0.10, 95% CI 0.02:0.57; 0.09, 95% CI 0.01:0.54), and 0.15 (95% CI 0.05:0.47), respectively) (Table 3). Benralizumab treatment not only lowered the ICS dose but also decreased the need for other asthma medications, such as the use of as-needed relievers SABA or ICS/LABA (p < 0.0001), LAMA (p = 0.0008), anti LT (p < 0.0001), and theophylline (p = 0.0070) (Table 3).

Table 3. Change in asthma medication use during the treatment with benralizumab. Descriptive statistics with a summary output of mixed-model on asthma medications other than OCS (ICS, SABA or ICS-LABA as needed, LAMA, anti LT, and theophylline) recorded at baseline and during the treatment with benralizumab. Mean (SD) and n values or n (percentage) and the beta regression coefficient (or OR where appropriate) with 95% CI are reported for each time point.

Parameter	Baseline	Month 6	Month 12	Month 24	Month 36	p-Value
ICS dose (mcg/day)	1006.93 (402.56) $n = 87$	895.09 (420.65) $n = 85$	853.93 (408.02) $n = 68$	841.47 (411.64) $n = 70$	800.04 (394.89) $n = 70$	
ICS dose (mcg/day)	1006.93 (402.56)	895.09 (420.65)	853.93 (408.02)	841.47 (411.64)	800.04 (394.89)	0.0010 †
<500	8 (9.20%)	17 (20.00%)	19 (27.94%)	21 (30.00%)	23 (32.86%)	
≥500 and <1000	44 (50.57%)	43 (50.59%)	32 (47.06%)	32 (45.71%)	31 (44.29%)	
≥1000	35 (40.23%)	25 (29.41%)	17 (25.00%)	17 (24.29%)	16 (22.86%)	
*	1	0.37 (0.12:1.13)	0.22 (0.07:0.71)	0.17 (0.06:0.55)	0.11 (0.02:0.68)	
#	1	0.13 (0.02:0.77)	0.10 (0.02:0.57)	0.09 (0.01:0.54)	0.15 (0.05:0.47)	
SABA or ICS-LABA as needed (times per day)	3.10 (4.19) 0 $n = 88$	0.35 (0.96) −2.72 (−3.37:−2.07) $n = 85$	0.2 (0.6) −2.78 (−3.51:−2.06) $n = 61$	0.43 (1.42) −2.59 (−3.3:−1.89) $n = 67$	0.38 (1.85) −2.73 (−3.43:−2.04) $n = 71$	<0.0001
LAMA						
No	28 (26.17%)	29 (28.16%)	28 (29.17%)	34 (40%)	38 (44.19%)	
Yes	79 (73.83%) 1 $n = 107$	74 (71.84%) 0.50 (0.13:1.85) $n = 103$	68 (70.83%) 0.29 (0.07:1.12) $n = 96$	51 (60%) 0.13 (0.03:0.53) $n = 85$	48 (55.81%) 0.04 (0.01:0.20) $n = 86$	0.0008
Anti LT						
No	55 (51.40%)	56 (54.9%)	55 (57.89%)	57 (67.06%)	59 (68.6%)	
Yes	52 (48.60%) 1 $n = 107$	46 (45.10%) 0.48 (0.16:1.40) $n = 102$	40 (42.11%) 0.22 (0.07:0.70) $n = 95$	28 (32.94%) 0.06 (0.02:0.23) $n = 85$	27 (31.4%) 0.06 (0.02:0.23) $n = 86$	<0.0001
Theophylline						
No	100 (94.34%)	100 (99.01%)	95 (98.96%)	82 (96.47%)	84 (100%)	
Yes	6 (5.66%) 1 $n = 106$	1 (0.99%) 0.01 (0:0.68) $n = 101$	1 (1.04%) 0.01 (0:0.38) $n = 96$	3 (3.53%) 0.08 (0.01:1.14) $n = 85$	0 (0%) 0 (0:Inf) $n = 84$	0.0070

† p value estimated by fitting a multinomial log-linear model corrected for center and patients variability * ICS dose contrast, ≥500 and <1000 mcg/day versus <500 mcg/day; # ICS dose contrast, ≥500 1000 and <1000 mcg/day versus <500 mcg/day.

3.8. Benralizumab Promoted the Achievement of CR

Figure 6 shows the number and percentage of patients who achieved any CR, including pCR and cCR, at 12, 24, and 36 months (from the corresponding previous time point). A total of 36 out of 46 patients (78.26%) reached CR (either pCR, 8.70% or cCR, 69.57%) after 12 months; the rate of CR further increased at the following time points, with 90.00% and 84.31% of patients in CR at 24 and 36 months, respectively. When pCR and cCR were considered separately, the percentage of patients in pCR steadily increased from 8.70% at 12 months to 15.69% at 36 months, while most patients were in cCR from 12 months onwards (69.57% at 12 months, 77.50% at 24 months, and 68.63% at 36 months). The percentage of patients who did not achieve any kind of CR dropped from 21.74% at 12 months to 10.00% and 15.69% at 24 and 36 months, respectively (Figure 6). We also considered the percentage of patients who reached CR from baseline to each time point; as shown in Figure S1, similar results were obtained (at 36 months, 85.71% of patients achieved any CR, with 12.50% patients in pCR and 73.21% patients in cCR).

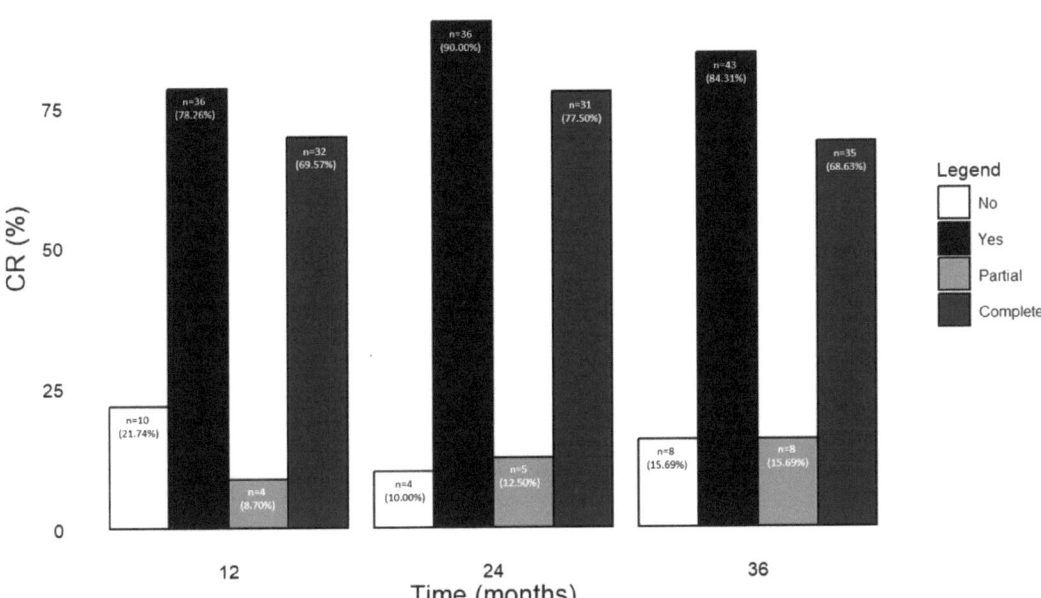

Figure 6. Number and percentage of patients who achieved and did not achieve CR (either pCR or cCR) at 12, 24, and 36 months during the treatment with benralizumab (from a previous time point).

4. Discussion

This study provides a comprehensive analysis of benralizumab effectiveness by retrospectively evaluating a total of 108 Italian patients with SEA treated for up to 36 months. Even though a high number of real-life studies have thus far evaluated the effectiveness of benralizumab on SEA patients, to our knowledge this is the first study conducted on more than 100 SEA patients treated over a period longer than 2 years. The longest real-life study (up to 48 months) was published by Numata and colleagues; however, only 23 SEA patients were initially included and fewer were followed for the entire period [33]. Similarly, Caminati and colleagues evaluated asthma outcomes in 68 mepolizumab-switched patients treated with benralizumab for a median period of 31 months [30]. In a more recent work, Fyles et al. considered a population of 81 SEA patients treated with either mepolizumab or benralizumab for up to 36 months; however, the majority of data were presented for the overall population, and thus, it is not possible to extrapolate the clinical improvements experienced by benralizumab-treated patients for each single outcome [31].

The baseline clinical characteristics reveal a severely compromised SEA patient population. The presence of circulating eosinophils (600 cells/mm^3), the high AER (3.84), the suboptimal FEV_1/FVC and FEV_1 (predicted: 74.50%), and the low scores of various PROs (with a mean ACT score: 14.41) confirm the poor control of the disease. In addition, the high percentages of patients taking OCS and experiencing comorbidities, including CRSwNP in 60.19% patients, bronchiectasis in almost 27% patients, and EGPA in 4.71% patients, further corroborate the high disease burden in our benralizumab-treated population. Nevertheless, the elevated number of comorbidities did not seem to impair the overall effectiveness of the anti-IL-5R. Additionally, benralizumab may also induce favorable outcomes in CRSwNP, bronchiectasis and EGPA; for these conditions, RCTs evaluating benralizumab efficacy are either currently ongoing (NCT04157335, NCT05006573) or terminated (NCT04157348), with positive effects demonstrated in EGPA patients [39].

The results from this long-term study reinforce the remarkable effectiveness of benralizumab in minimizing the number of exacerbations while maintaining minimal BEC throughout the study period. Benralizumab rapidly decreased the frequency of exacerbations, with a reduction in AER that persisted throughout the 36-month period (AER reduction ranging from 89% at 36 months to 95% at 12 months). Although the phenotype of exacerbations was determined in a small subgroup of patients at baseline only, we may speculate that benralizumab reduced all types of exacerbations, both infectious and non-infectious. This hypothesis is supported by (1) the extensive effect seen throughout the treatment period; (2) the high prevalence of bacterial-mediated exacerbations (more than 50%) observed at baseline; and (3) benralizumab novel MoA, which implies a broad modulation of the immune system, including the increased activation of NK cells [26]. Considering the antiviral and antibacterial role exerted by NK cells, it is plausible that their increased function contributed to prevent infections and infectious-related exacerbations in patients during benralizumab treatment. These data demonstrate that the effectiveness of benralizumab in preventing exacerbations is truly long-lasting, and the prominent extent of AER reduction is consistent with previous real-life studies [25,28–30].

Although benralizumab was anticipated to have a positive impact on AER over time, variable results have been published regarding its ability to enhance lung function over the long term. In our study, benralizumab significantly increased FEV_1 over time, with a remarkable +440 mL volume gain and predicted levels reaching normal values up to 36 months. This is the first time that benralizumab has been shown to induce a durable increase in respiratory function in real life up to 3 years; these results are in line with the recently published 96-week data from the ANANKE study, in which both pre-BD FEV_1 and FVC peaked after 96 weeks of treatment [25], and complement the data obtained from RCTs, where the initial improvement in lung function was stabilized over a two-year period [40]. As already mentioned, the novel MoA of benralizumab postulated by Bergantini et al., which involves the modulation of circulating CD3 + T subsets and increased activation of NK cells, even in the absence of eosinophils, may play a key role in the benralizumab-mediated long-term improvement in lung function [26].

Furthermore, McIntosh et al. found that benralizumab significantly reduced the mucus score in SEA patients treated up to 2.5 years; this result was accompanied by a parallel decrease in airway occlusion and improved ventilation, FEV_1, and ACQ-6 score [41]. As mucus accumulation has a profound impact on respiratory function in asthma patients, the benralizumab-mediated dissolution of mucus plugs may have contributed to the long-term favorable respiratory outcomes in our study. On the other hand, Numata and colleagues reported a decline in FEV_1 levels registered after 24 months [33]. In light of the data obtained from our study and other studies, it is possible that this result is biased due to the low number of patients considered in the study. The authors also speculated that the observed FEV_1 reduction may be caused by an airway obstruction mechanism induced by the long-term administration of a single biological, or a decrease adherence to inhaled therapies, or a physiological decline in pulmonary function [33]. Regardless of the reason justifying the different results, more studies with a greater number of patients are needed to ascertain benralizumab's long-term effectiveness on lung function and further elucidate the specific mechanism/s leading to increased lung function.

As measured by the ACT questionnaire, asthma control was significantly improved, with a mean ACT score greater than 21 at all timepoints. The significant results obtained in ACQ and AQLQ reinforced the achievement of good asthma control and demonstrated an overall improvement of QoL.

Benralizumab not only induced profound beneficial effects in terms of asthma symptoms but also improved sinonasal symptoms in comorbid patients with CRSwNP, as demonstrated by the significant and progressive changes recorded in VAS and SNOT-22. Although benralizumab currently lacks the indication for the treatment of CRSwNP, growing evidence indicates that the anti-IL-5R has a positive impact on nasal symptoms in comorbid patients [42–45]. Notably, a recent work by Santomasi and colleagues showed that benralizumab was not only effective in decreasing the SNOT-22 score, but it also significantly reduced the nasal polyps score (NPS), determined by nasal endoscopy, and the number of nasal eosinophils and neutrophils, assessed via nasal cytology, in SEA patients with CRSwNP [45]. Collectively, these data corroborate the theory of "united airway disease" [46], implying that SEA and CRSwNP share the same eosinophilic-driven pathophysiology in comorbid patients, and benralizumab could indeed represent the optimal therapeutic strategy to tackle both pathologies simultaneously.

The marked OCS-sparing effect of benralizumab is well recognized. In the pivotal PONENTE study, almost 63% of patients completely eliminated the use of OCS and more than 80% of patients either eliminated OCS or maintained a minimum dose due to adrenal insufficiency [47]. Similarly, the OCS dose has been either reduced or zeroed in real-life studies where patients were treated for periods longer than one year [25,29,30,33]. Our data indicate that benralizumab induced a durable OCS reduction, and this effect further increased over time. Indeed, the minimal mean dose of OCS was registered at 36 months; at this time point, almost the totality of patients (93.33%) successfully decreased their OCS dose by any extent, and 84.44% patients permanently discontinued OCS therapy. To our knowledge, these percentages are the highest ever recorded in the literature. The sub-analysis conducted on patients requiring a daily OCS dose of either $\leq$ or >5 mg substantiated the findings from the PONENTE trial, which showed that benralizumab OCS-sparing effect, was independent of the baseline dose [47].

Beyond the high rate of OCS reduction and elimination, benralizumab treatment was associated with a net and significant decrease in the dose of the maintenance ICS dose, with an overall reduction of 20.55% and a decreased probability of requiring medium and high ICS doses over time. Consistently, there were more than 20% patients transitioning from medium or high ICS doses to low ICS doses (<500 mcg/day) at 36 months. We also observed a progressive decline in the use of all other asthma therapies, including LAMA, anti-LT, theophylline, and as needed SABA and/or ICS/LABA. Notably, patients could reduce all these medications while maintaining good asthma control, as demonstrated by ACT and ACQ scores. To date, the effect of benralizumab on asthma medication other than OCS has not been extensively investigated. In the RCT SHAMAL, up to 92% of patients successfully reduced their high-dose ICS and 96% maintained such reductions up to 48 weeks without compromising asthma control (87% of patients were free from exacerbations by week 48) [34]. In real life, 66.3% of patients decreased the use of maintenance medications (ICS dose reduction and/or LABA, LAMA montelukast interruption) over a mean treatment period of 19.7 months. Similarly to our data, approximately 25% of patients reduced the ICS dose [29]. Given the extremely poor adherence to inhaled therapy in SA patients [48], benralizumab-mediated reduction in ICS and other background therapies may provide further beneficial effects by leading to (1) higher compliance to inhalers; (2) better asthma control in patients who do not strictly adhere to inhaled therapy regimen.

Since the advent of biological therapies for asthma and the compelling amelioration of patients' symptoms, the achievement of CR in SA patients has become possible. However, the criteria defining CR used in the various studies published so far have been somehow arbitrary. Recently, a Delphi consensus reached by members of the SANI study group agreed on the criteria to identify patients in pCR and cCR [19]. Based on these criteria, our results show that CR, and specifically cCR, was achieved by more than the half of the patients at all time points considered (up to 90.00% patients in CR at 24 months, of which 77.50% patients were in cCR). These data mean that benralizumab could permanently eradicate the disease in the vast majority of patients during the three-year study duration. CR was evaluated in previous studies, both RCT and in real life; the results show that benralizumab induced CR in percentages of SEA patients ranging from 14.5% (in the SIROCCO and CALIMA RCTs) [49] to 43% (in the real-world XALOC-1 study [50]). Compared to the latter studies, a slightly higher percentage of patients (54%) reached clinical remission at 48 weeks in the SHAMAL RCT despite the reduction in background ICS dose [34].

The percentage of patients achieving CR in our study seems to exceed the results previously reported; however, attention should be paid to the criteria employed to define CR, as they vary across the studies, and they differ from the criteria used herein. For instance, in the XALOC-1 study, the percentage of patients reaching CR (43%) was calculated without including any respiratory parameters and considering an ACT score ≥ 16 points [50]. Importantly, Campisi et al. found that SEA patients achieved CR more frequently in the absence of bronchiectasis [51], suggesting a negative impact of this comorbidity on benralizumab effectiveness [51]. The inclusion of a variable proportion of patients with this comorbidity, accompanied by the methodological differences used across the studies, may justify the variable results obtained so far. In our study, CR was evaluated in all patients, including those with bronchiectasis (which affected approximately a quarter of our patient population). The strict criteria employed in our study to define cCR and the inclusion of patients with bronchiectasis add further value to the rates of cCR reported here, which are unprecedented but justified by the striking effect of benralizumab observed in all the single outcomes (exacerbations, lung function, asthma control and OCS use). The long-term implications of achieving clinical remission through benralizumab treatment could encompass a better prognosis and extended life expectancy in SEA patients. These aspects are even more relevant considering the increasing prevalence and severity of late-onset asthma, and SEA in particular, as the global population ages [52].

Drawing upon the notion of "deep remission" related to rheumatoid arthritis, Oishi and colleagues also assessed deep remission in SA patients by considering the successful inhibition of T2 inflammation with BEC < 300 cells/mm^3 and FeNO < 35 ppb or < 50 ppb. [53,54]. While we did not formally assess the rate of patients achieving deep remission in our study, we anticipate a similar rate to those who achieved CR, owing to the extensive drop in BEC specifically induced by benralizumab MoA.

The retrospective design of this study represents its main limitation, as it is associated with a considerable loss of data during the 36-month treatment period. In general, a certain degree of missing data is anticipated in real-life, and retrospective multicentric studies can be attributed to several factors, including (1) variability in the collection of certain parameters across different centers, (2) loss of patients at follow-up due to various reasons (e.g., patient relocation, change in healthcare provider, etc.), and (3) data recording and collection from medical charts (not originally intended for research purposes) [55]. In our case, the extensive study duration and the monitoring of patients amid the COVID-19 pandemic also negatively affected patients' attendance at follow-up visits, further contributing to the loss of data during the observation period. Adverse events were not collected because the study's main purpose was to evaluate the effectiveness of benralizumab and this may represent another limitation. As already mentioned above, additional studies will be needed to validate our results over even longer treatment periods and by considering greater numbers of patients. Ideally, future studies will be conducted with a prospective design to limit the loss of data. A thorough evaluation of safety would also be valuable to confirm the long-term safety of benralizumab already observed in the MELTEMI study [27].

5. Conclusions

This study offers a comprehensive assessment of benralizumab long-term effectiveness on SEA by examining a meaningful sample population at various time points, up to 36 months of treatment. These impressive data not only comprehensively illustrate the long-lasting response to benralizumab in all the considered asthma clinical outcomes, but also reveal the simultaneous positive effects on CRSwNP symptoms. The large percentage of patients who reached either pCR or cCR is indicative of the long-term well-being induced by benralizumab and support its role as a disease-modifying anti-asthmatic therapy for the management of SEA. More research should corroborate these results, with a focus on minimizing data loss and exploring further facets of benralizumab MoA and effectiveness, including the impact on adherence to inhaled therapy, airway remodeling, and the achievement of deep remission.

Supplementary Materials: The following supporting information can be downloaded at: https://www.mdpi.com/article/10.3390/jcm13103013/s1, List of additional members of SANI. Table S1: Descriptive statistics with a summary output of a mixed model on FeNO and lung function parameters recorded at baseline and during the treatment with benralizumab (n = 108 unless otherwise specified). Mean (SD) and n values or n (percentage) and beta regression coefficients with 95% CI are reported for each time point. Table S2: Extent of OCS dose reduction during treatment with benralizumab in patients grouped according to OCS dose at baseline ($\leq$5 mg/day or >5 mg/day). Figure S1: Number and percentage of patients who achieved and did not achieve CR (either pCR or cCR) at 12, 24, and 36 months during the treatment with benralizumab (values calculated from baseline).

Author Contributions: Conceptualization, L.P.; Investigation, B.B. (Bianca Beghè), P.C., C.C. (Cristiano Caruso), C.C. (Claudia Crimi)., G.G., M.L., F.M., B.B. (Benedetta Bondi), Y.E.M., J.G., A.M., M.M., S.P. and M.Z.; Data curation, M.C., A.P. and D.V.; Validation, D.B., F.B. (Fulvio Braido), C.M. and A.V.; Writing—original draft, L.P.; Writing—review of the manuscript for intellectual content, G.S., A.S., P.P., F.B. (Francesco Blasi) and G.W.C.; Funding acquisition: SANI Study Group. All authors have read and agreed to the published version of the manuscript.

Funding: This project was supported by AstraZeneca.

Institutional Review Board Statement: The SANI registry was constructed according to the Declarations of Helsinki and Oviedo. The study was approved by the Central Ethics Committee for the SANI Network (Comitato Etico Area Vasta Nord-Ovest Toscana; protocol number: 1245/2016, protocol ID: 73714, 7 December 2016).

Informed Consent Statement: Informed consent was obtained from all subjects involved in the study.

Data Availability Statement: The data presented in this study are available upon reasonable request from the corresponding author (Laura Pini, laura.pini@unibs.it).

Acknowledgments: The authors would like to thank all the participants who took part in the study and their families. Statistical analyses were conducted by Fabio Gallo; writing and editorial assistance were provided by Alessandra Rossi, on behalf of EDRA S.p.A.

Conflicts of Interest: All authors reported no financial interests or potential conflicts of interest related to this study. L.P. received grants for educational events from AstraZeneca, Chiesi Farmaceutici, Glaxo Smith Kline and speaker fees from AstraZeneca, Chiesi Farmaceutici S.p.A, Glaxo Smith Kline, Guidotti, Grifols, Menarini, Novartis AG; D.B, B.Be, F.Br, D.V. received speaker fees from AstraZeneca, Chiesi Farmaceutici S.p.A, Glaxo Smith Kline, Guidotti, Grifols, Menarini, Novartis AG, Sanofi; P.C. received grants and speaker fees from AstraZeneca and GSK; M.C. received financial grants from AstraZeneca, GSK and Sanofi; C.Cr. received honoraria for lectures from AZ, GSK, Sanofi, Novartis, Resmed, F&P; C.M. received fees as a speaker in national and international congress from Astrazeneca, Sanofi, Novartis, GSK, Menarini, Guidotti, Firma, Roche, Berlin Chemie, Chiesi, Zambon; G.S. received financial grants from AstraZeneca, GSK, Novartis and Sanofi; P.P. received grants for educational events from AstraZeneca, Chiesi Farmaceutici, Glaxo Smith Kline, Guidotti and Sanofi and grants for participation to Advisory Board from Chiesi Farmaceutici, Glaxo Smith Kline, and Sanofi; F.Bl. received financial grants from AstraZeneca, Chiesi Farmaceutici S.p.A and Insmed Inc. and speaker fees from AstraZeneca, Chiesi Farmaceutici S.p.A, Glaxo Smith Kline, Guidotti, Grifols, Insmed Inc., Menarini, Novartis AG, Sanofi-Genzyme, Viatris Inc., Vertex Pharmaceuticals and Zambon; G.W.C. recceived research grants from A. Menarini, Allergy Therapeutics, AstraZeneca, Chiesi Farmaceutici, Faes, Firma, Glaxo Smith Kline, Guidotti-Malesci, Hal Allergy, Innovacaremd, Novartis, OmPharma, RedMaple, Sanofi-Aventis, Sanofi-Genzyme, Stallergenes-Greer, Uriach Pharma, ThermoFisher, Valeas.

References

1. Chung, K.F.; Wenzel, S.E.; Brozek, J.L.; Bush, A.; Castro, M.; Sterk, P.J.; Adcock, I.M.; Bateman, E.D.; Bel, E.H.; Bleecker, E.R.; et al. International ERS/ATS guidelines on definition, evaluation and treatment of severe asthma. *Eur. Respir. J.* **2014**, *43*, 343–373. [CrossRef] [PubMed]
2. Hekking, P.-P.W.; Wener, R.R.; Amelink, M.; Zwinderman, A.H.; Bouvy, M.L.; Bel, E.H. The prevalence of severe refractory asthma. *J. Allergy Clin. Immunol.* **2015**, *135*, 896–902. [CrossRef] [PubMed]

3. Bagnasco, D.; Paggiaro, P.; Latorre, M.; Folli, C.; Testino, E.; Bassi, A.; Milanese, M.; Heffler, E.; Manfredi, A.; Riccio, A.M.; et al. Severe asthma: One disease and multiple definitions. *World Allergy Organ. J.* **2021**, *14*, 100606. [CrossRef] [PubMed]
4. Buhl, R.; Humbert, M.; Bjermer, L.; Chanez, P.; Heaney, L.G.; Pavord, I.; Quirce, S.; Virchow, J.C.; Holgate, S. Severe eosinophilic asthma: A roadmap to consensus. *Eur. Respir. J.* **2017**, *49*, 1700634. [CrossRef] [PubMed]
5. Perez-de-Llano, L.; Tran, T.N.; Al-ahmad, M.; Alacqua, M.; Bulathsinhala, L.; Busby, J.; Canonica, G.W.; Carter, V.; Chaudhry, I.; Christoff, G.C.; et al. Characterization of Eosinophilic and Non-Eosinophilic Severe Asthma Phenotypes and Proportion of Patients with These Phenotypes in the International Severe Asthma Registry (ISAR). In *C21. Advances in Adult and Pediatric Asthma Phenotyping and Endotyping*; American Thoracic Society: New York, NY, USA, 2020; p. A4525.
6. Maio, S.; Baldacci, S.; Bresciani, M.; Simoni, M.; Latorre, M.; Murgia, N.; Spinozzi, F.; Braschi, M.; Antonicelli, L.; Brunetto, B.; et al. RItA: The Italian severe/uncontrolled asthma registry. *Allergy* **2018**, *73*, 683–695. [CrossRef] [PubMed]
7. Bakakos, A.; Loukides, S.; Bakakos, P. Severe Eosinophilic Asthma. *J. Clin. Med.* **2019**, *8*, 1375. [CrossRef] [PubMed]
8. de Groot, J.C.; Ten Brinke, A.; Bel, E.H.D. Management of the patient with eosinophilic asthma: A new era begins. *ERJ Open Res.* **2015**, *1*, 00024–02015. [CrossRef] [PubMed]
9. Heaney, L.G.; Perez de Llano, L.; Al-Ahmad, M.; Backer, V.; Busby, J.; Canonica, G.W.; Christoff, G.C.; Cosio, B.G.; FitzGerald, J.M.; Heffler, E.; et al. Eosinophilic and Noneosinophilic Asthma: An Expert Consensus Framework to Characterize Phenotypes in a Global Real-Life Severe Asthma Cohort. *Chest* **2021**, *160*, 814–830. [CrossRef]
10. Laidlaw, T.M.; Mullol, J.; Woessner, K.M.; Amin, N.; Mannent, L.P. Chronic Rhinosinusitis with Nasal Polyps and Asthma. *J. Allergy Clin. Immunol. Pract.* **2021**, *9*, 1133–1141. [CrossRef]
11. Massoth, L.; Anderson, C.; McKinney, K.A. Asthma and Chronic Rhinosinusitis: Diagnosis and Medical Management. *Med. Sci.* **2019**, *7*, 53. [CrossRef]
12. 2023 Gina Main Report. Available online: https://ginasthma.org/wp-content/uploads/2023/05/GINA-2023-Full-Report-2023-WMS.pdf (accessed on 8 May 2024).
13. Price, D.B.; Trudo, F.; Voorham, J.; Xu, X.; Kerkhof, M.; Ling Zhi Jie, J.; Tran, T.N. Adverse outcomes from initiation of systemic corticosteroids for asthma: Long-term observational study. *J. Asthma Allergy* **2018**, *11*, 193–204. [CrossRef] [PubMed]
14. Lee, H.; Ryu, J.; Nam, E.; Chung, S.J.; Yeo, Y.; Park, D.W.; Park, T.S.; Moon, J.-Y.; Kim, T.-H.; Sohn, J.W.; et al. Increased mortality in patients with corticosteroid-dependent asthma: A nationwide population-based study. *Eur. Respir. J.* **2019**, *54*, 1900804. [CrossRef] [PubMed]
15. Bourdin, A.; Molinari, N.; Vachier, I.; Pahus, L.; Suehs, C.; Chanez, P. Mortality: A neglected outcome in OCS-treated severe asthma. *Eur. Respir. J.* **2017**, *50*, 1701486. [CrossRef] [PubMed]
16. Lommatzsch, M.; Brusselle, G.G.; Levy, M.L.; Canonica, G.W.; Pavord, I.D.; Schatz, M.; Virchow, J.C. A2BCD: A concise guide for asthma management. *Lancet Respir. Med.* **2023**, *11*, 573–576. [CrossRef] [PubMed]
17. Chen, W.; Tran, T.N.; Sadatsafavi, M.; Murray, R.; Wong, N.C.B.; Ali, N.; Ariti, C.; Bulathsinhala, L.; Gil, E.G.; FitzGerald, J.M.; et al. Impact of Initiating Biologics in Patients With Severe Asthma on Long-Term Oral Corticosteroids or Frequent Rescue Steroids (GLITTER): Data From the International Severe Asthma Registry. *J. Allergy Clin. Immunol. Pract.* **2023**, *11*, 2732–2747. [CrossRef] [PubMed]
18. Chen, M.; Shepard, K., 2nd; Yang, M.; Raut, P.; Pazwash, H.; Holweg, C.T.J.; Choo, E. Overlap of allergic, eosinophilic and type 2 inflammatory subtypes in moderate-to-severe asthma. *Clin. Exp. Allergy J. Br. Soc. Allergy Clin. Immunol.* **2021**, *51*, 546–555. [CrossRef]
19. Canonica, G.W.; Blasi, F.; Carpagnano, G.E.; Guida, G.; Heffler, E.; Paggiaro, P.; Allegrini, C.; Antonelli, A.; Aruanno, A.; Bacci, E.; et al. Severe Asthma Network Italy Definition of Clinical Remission in Severe Asthma: A Delphi Consensus. *J. Allergy Clin. Immunol. Pract.* **2023**, *11*, 3629–3637. [CrossRef] [PubMed]
20. Lommatzsch, M.; Brusselle, G.G.; Canonica, G.W.; Jackson, D.J.; Nair, P.; Buhl, R.; Virchow, J.C. Disease-modifying anti-asthmatic drugs. *Lancet* **2022**, *399*, 1664–1668. [CrossRef] [PubMed]
21. Available online: https://www.ema.europa.eu/en/documents/product-information/fasenra-epar-product-information_en.pdf (accessed on 8 May 2024).
22. Dagher, R.; Kumar, V.; Copenhaver, A.M.; Gallagher, S.; Ghaedi, M.; Boyd, J.; Newbold, P.; Humbles, A.A.; Kolbeck, R. Novel mechanisms of action contributing to benralizumab's potent anti-eosinophilic activity. *Eur. Respir. J.* **2022**, *59*, 2004306. [CrossRef]
23. Caminati, M.; Bagnasco, D.; Vaia, R.; Senna, G. New horizons for the treatment of severe, eosinophilic asthma: Benralizumab, a novel precision biologic. *Biol. Targets Ther.* **2019**, *13*, 89–95. [CrossRef]
24. Menzella, F.; Biava, M.; Bagnasco, D.; Galeone, C.; Simonazzi, A.; Ruggiero, P.; Facciolongo, N. Efficacy and steroid-sparing effect of benralizumab: Has it an advantage over its competitors? *Drugs Context* **2019**, *8*, 212580. [CrossRef] [PubMed]
25. Vultaggio, A.; Aliani, M.; Altieri, E.; Bracciale, P.; Brussino, L.; Caiaffa, M.F.; Cameli, P.; Canonica, G.W.; Caruso, C.; Centanni, S.; et al. Long-term effectiveness of benralizumab in severe eosinophilic asthma patients treated for 96-weeks: Data from the ANANKE study. *Respir. Res.* **2023**, *24*, 135. [CrossRef] [PubMed]
26. Bergantini, L.; d'Alessandro, M.; Pianigiani, T.; Cekorja, B.; Bargagli, E.; Cameli, P. Benralizumab affects NK cell maturation and proliferation in severe asthmatic patients. *Clin. Immunol.* **2023**, *253*, 109680. [CrossRef] [PubMed]
27. Korn, S.; Bourdin, A.; Chupp, G.; Cosio, B.G.; Arbetter, D.; Shah, M.; Gil, E.G. Integrated Safety and Efficacy Among Patients Receiving Benralizumab for Up to 5 Years. *J. Allergy Clin. Immunol. Pract.* **2021**, *9*, 4381–4392.e4. [CrossRef] [PubMed]

28. Vitale, C.; Maglio, A.; Pelaia, C.; D'Amato, M.; Ciampo, L.; Pelaia, G.; Molino, A.; Vatrella, A. Effectiveness of Benralizumab in OCS-Dependent Severe Asthma: The Impact of 2 Years of Therapy in a Real-Life Setting. *J. Clin. Med.* **2023**, *12*, 985. [CrossRef] [PubMed]
29. Sposato, B.; Scalese, M.; Camiciottoli, G.; Carpagnano, G.E.; Pelaia, C.; Santus, P.; Pelaia, G.; Palmiero, G.; Di Tomassi, M.; Ronchi, M.C.; et al. Severe asthma and long-term Benralizumab effectiveness in real-life. *Eur. Rev. Med. Pharmacol. Sci.* **2022**, *26*, 7461–7473. [CrossRef] [PubMed]
30. Caminati, M.; Marcon, A.; Guarnieri, G.; Miotti, J.; Bagnasco, D.; Carpagnano, G.E.; Pelaia, G.; Vaia, R.; Maule, M.; Vianello, A.; et al. Benralizumab Efficacy in Late Non-Responders to Mepolizumab and Variables Associated with Occurrence of Switching: A Real-Word Perspective. *J. Clin. Med.* **2023**, *12*, 1836. [CrossRef] [PubMed]
31. Fyles, F.; Nuttall, A.; Joplin, H.; Burhan, H. Long-Term Real-World Outcomes of Mepolizumab and Benralizumab Among Biologic-Naive Patients With Severe Eosinophilic Asthma: Experience of 3 Years' Therapy. *J. Allergy Clin. Immunol. Pract.* **2023**, *11*, 2715–2723. [CrossRef] [PubMed]
32. Risco, M.; Sotomayor, J.; Alvarez-Sala, P.; Piorno, I.; Diaz-Campos, R.; Moya, B.; Crespo, J.F.; Fernandez, C.; GarcÃa Moguel, I. Long-term effectiveness and safety of benralizumab for uncontrolled eosinophilic asthma in real-word practice. *J. Allergy Clin. Immunol.* **2022**, *149*, AB16. [CrossRef]
33. Numata, T.; Araya, J.; Okuda, K.; Miyagawa, H.; Minagawa, S.; Ishikawa, T.; Hara, H.; Kuwano, K. Long-Term Efficacy and Clinical Remission After Benralizumab Treatment in Patients with Severe Eosinophilic Asthma: A Retrospective Study. *J. Asthma Allergy* **2022**, *15*, 1731–1741. [CrossRef]
34. Jackson, D.J.; Heaney, L.G.; Humbert, M.; Kent, B.D.; Shavit, A.; Hiljemark, L.; Olinger, L.; Cohen, D.; Menzies-Gow, A.; Korn, S.; et al. Reduction of daily maintenance inhaled corticosteroids in patients with severe eosinophilic asthma treated with benralizumab (SHAMAL): A randomised, multicentre, open-label, phase 4 study. *Lancet* **2024**, *403*, 271–281. [CrossRef] [PubMed]
35. Piano Terapeutico AIFA per la Prescrizione SSN di Fasenra (Benralizumab) Nell'asma Grave Eosinofilico Refrattario [Internet]. Gazzetta Ufficiale della Repubblica Italiana. Available online: https://www.gazzettaufficiale.it/atto/serie_generale/caricaDettaglioAtto/originario?atto.dataPubblicazioneGazzetta=2019-02-12&atto.codiceRedazionale=19A00829&elenco30giorni=false (accessed on 8 May 2024).
36. Gelman, A.; Hill, J. *Data Analysis Using Regression and Multilevel/Hierarchical Models*; Cambridge University Press: Cambridge, UK; New York, NY, USA, 2007.
37. Available online: https://www.r-project.org/ (accessed on 8 May 2024).
38. Toma, S.; Hopkins, C. Stratification of SNOT-22 scores into mild, moderate or severe and relationship with other subjective instruments. *Rhinol. J.* **2016**, *54*, 129–133. [CrossRef] [PubMed]
39. Wechsler, M.E.; Nair, P.; Terrier, B.; Walz, B.; Bourdin, A.; Jayne, D.R.W.; Jackson, D.J.; Roufosse, F.; Börjesson Sjö, L.; Fan, Y.; et al. Benralizumab versus Mepolizumab for Eosinophilic Granulomatosis with Polyangiitis. *N. Engl. J. Med.* **2024**, *390*, 911–921. [CrossRef] [PubMed]
40. FitzGerald, J.M.; Bleecker, E.R.; Bourdin, A.; Busse, W.W.; Ferguson, G.T.; Brooks, L.; Barker, P.; Martin, U.J. Two-Year Integrated Efficacy And Safety Analysis Of Benralizumab In Severe Asthma. *J. Asthma Allergy* **2019**, *12*, 401–413. [CrossRef] [PubMed]
41. McIntosh, M.J.; Kooner, H.K.; Eddy, R.L.; Wilson, A.; Serajeddini, H.; Bhalla, A.; Licskai, C.; Mackenzie, C.A.; Yamashita, C.; Parraga, G. CT Mucus Score and 129Xe MRI Ventilation Defects after 2.5 Years' Anti-IL-5Rα in Eosinophilic Asthma. *CHEST* **2023**, *164*, 27–38. [CrossRef]
42. Nolasco, S.; Crimi, C.; Pelaia, C.; Benfante, A.; Caiaffa, M.F.; Calabrese, C.; Carpagnano, G.E.; Ciotta, D.; D'Amato, M.; Macchia, L.; et al. Benralizumab Effectiveness in Severe Eosinophilic Asthma with and without Chronic Rhinosinusitis with Nasal Polyps: A Real-World Multicenter Study. *J. Allergy Clin. Immunol. Pract.* **2021**, *9*, 4371–4380.e4. [CrossRef] [PubMed]
43. Lombardo, N.; Pelaia, C.; Ciriolo, M.; Della Corte, M.; Piazzetta, G.; Lobello, N.; Viola, P.; Pelaia, G. Real-life effects of benralizumab on allergic chronic rhinosinusitis and nasal polyposis associated with severe asthma. *Int. J. Immunopathol. Pharmacol.* **2020**, *34*, 205873842095085. [CrossRef] [PubMed]
44. Bagnasco, D.; Brussino, L.; Bonavia, M.; Calzolari, E.; Caminati, M.; Caruso, C.; D'Amato, M.; De Ferrari, L.; Di Marco, F.; Imeri, G.; et al. Efficacy of Benralizumab in severe asthma in real life and focus on nasal polyposis. *Respir. Med.* **2020**, *171*, 106080. [CrossRef] [PubMed]
45. Santomasi, C.; Buonamico, E.; Dragonieri, S.; Iannuzzi, L.; Portacci, A.; Quaranta, N.; Carpagnano, G.E. Effects of benralizumab in a population of patients affected by severe eosinophilic asthma and chronic rhinosinusitis with nasal polyps: A real life study. *Acta Biomed. Atenei Parm.* **2023**, *94*, e2023028. [CrossRef]
46. Kanda, A.; Kobayashi, Y.; Asako, M.; Tomoda, K.; Kawauchi, H.; Iwai, H. Regulation of Interaction between the Upper and Lower Airways in United Airway Disease. *Med. Sci.* **2019**, *7*, 27. [CrossRef]
47. Menzies-Gow, A.; Gurnell, M.; Heaney, L.G.; Corren, J.; Bel, E.H.; Maspero, J.; Harrison, T.; Jackson, D.J.; Price, D.; Lugogo, N.; et al. Oral corticosteroid elimination via a personalised reduction algorithm in adults with severe, eosinophilic asthma treated with benralizumab (PONENTE): A multicentre, open-label, single-arm study. *Lancet Respir. Med.* **2022**, *10*, 47–58. [CrossRef] [PubMed]
48. Caminati, M.; Vianello, A.; Andretta, M.; Menti, A.M.; Tognella, S.; Esposti, L.D.; Gianenrico, S. Astonishing low adherence to inhaled therapy characterizes patients with severe asthma treated with biologics. *World Allergy Organ. J.* **2020**, *13*, 100377. [CrossRef]

49. Menzies-Gow, A.; Hoyte, F.L.; Price, D.B.; Cohen, D.; Barker, P.; Kreindler, J.; Jison, M.; Brooks, C.L.; Papeleu, P.; Katial, R. Clinical Remission in Severe Asthma: A Pooled Post Hoc Analysis of the Patient Journey with Benralizumab. *Adv. Ther.* **2022**, *39*, 2065–2084. [CrossRef] [PubMed]
50. Jackson, D.; Pelaia, G.; Padilla-Galo, A.; Watt, M.; Kayaniyil, S.; Boarino, S.; Tena, J.S.; Shih, V.; Tran, T.; Arbetter, D.; et al. Asthma Clinical Remission with Benralizumab in an Integrated Analysis of the Real-World XALOC-1 Study. *J. Allergy Clin. Immunol.* **2023**, *151*, AB13. [CrossRef]
51. Campisi, R.; Nolasco, S.; Pelaia, C.; Impellizzeri, P.; D'Amato, M.; Portacci, A.; Ricciardi, L.; Scioscia, G.; Crimi, N.; Scichilone, N.; et al. Benralizumab Effectiveness in Severe Eosinophilic Asthma with Co-Presence of Bronchiectasis: A Real-World Multicentre Observational Study. *J. Clin. Med.* **2023**, *12*, 3953. [CrossRef] [PubMed]
52. Hirano, T.; Matsunaga, K. Late-onset asthma: Current perspectives. *J. Asthma Allergy* **2018**, *11*, 19–27. [CrossRef] [PubMed]
53. Oishi, K.; Hamada, K.; Murata, Y.; Yamaji, Y.; Asami, M.; Edakuni, N.; Hirano, T.; Matsunaga, K. Achievement rate and predictive factors of the deep remission to biologics in severe asthma. *Eur. Respir. J.* **2022**, *60*, 4401. [CrossRef]
54. Oishi, K.; Hamada, K.; Murata, Y.; Matsuda, K.; Ohata, S.; Yamaji, Y.; Asami-Noyama, M.; Edakuni, N.; Kakugawa, T.; Hirano, T.; et al. A Real-World Study of Achievement Rate and Predictive Factors of Clinical and Deep Remission to Biologics in Patients with Severe Asthma. *J. Clin. Med.* **2023**, *12*, 2900. [CrossRef]
55. Talari, K.; Goyal, M. Retrospective Studies–Utility and Caveats. *J. R. Coll. Physicians Edinb.* **2020**, *50*, 398–402. [CrossRef]

Disclaimer/Publisher's Note: The statements, opinions and data contained in all publications are solely those of the individual author(s) and contributor(s) and not of MDPI and/or the editor(s). MDPI and/or the editor(s) disclaim responsibility for any injury to people or property resulting from any ideas, methods, instructions or products referred to in the content.

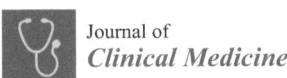

Article

Trends and Hospital Outcomes in HOSPITAL Admissions for Anaphylaxis in Children with and without Asthma in Spain (2016–2021)

Javier De Miguel-Díez [1], Ana Lopez-de-Andres [2,*], Francisco J. Caballero-Segura [1], Rodrigo Jimenez-Garcia [2], Valentin Hernández-Barrera [3], David Carabantes-Alarcon [2], Jose J. Zamorano-Leon [2], Ricardo Omaña-Palanco [2] and Natividad Cuadrado-Corrales [2]

[1] Respiratory Department, Hospital General Universitario Gregorio Marañón, Facultad de Medicina, Instituto de Investigación Sanitaria Gregorio Marañón (IiSGM), Universidad Complutense de Madrid, 28007 Madrid, Spain; javier.miguel@salud.madrid.org (J.D.M.-D.); fcabal01@ucm.es (F.J.C.-S.)
[2] Department of Public Health and Maternal & Child Health, Faculty of Medicine, Universidad Complutense de Madrid, 28040 Madrid, Spain; rodrijim@ucm.es (R.J.-G.); dcaraban@ucm.es (D.C.-A.); josejzam@ucm.es (J.J.Z.-L.); romana@ucm.es (R.O.-P.); mariancu@ucm.es (N.C.-C.)
[3] Preventive Medicine and Public Health Teaching and Research Unit, Health Sciences Faculty, Universidad Rey Juan Carlos, 28922 Alcorcón, Spain; valentin.hernandez@urjc.es
* Correspondence: anailo04@ucm.es; Tel.: +34-913941520

Abstract: (1) Background: To assess and compare the temporal trends in the incidence, characteristics and hospital outcomes among children with and without asthma who were hospitalized with anaphylaxis in Spain from 2016 to 2021, and identify the variables associated with severe anaphylaxis among children with asthma. (2) Methods: An observational, retrospective study was conducted using a population-based database. The study population included pediatric patients with anaphylaxis. This population was stratified based on whether they had asthma. (3) Results: The number of hospital admissions was stable from 2016 to 2019, dropping in 2020 and raising to the highest number in 2021. A total of 60.63% of hospitalizations occurred in boys and the most common anaphylactic reactions were due to food consumption (67.28%), increasing over time. The in-hospital mortality (IHM) remained stable and under 1% in all the years studied. The incidence of anaphylaxis was 2.14 times higher in children with asthma than in those without asthma (IRR 2.14; 95% CI 1.87–2.44). Furthermore, it was 1.79 times higher in boys with asthma than in those without asthma (IRR 1.79; 95% CI 1.06–2.45) and 2.68 times higher in girls with asthma than in those without asthma (IRR 2.68; 95% CI 2.23–3.12). Asthma was not associated with severe anaphylaxis (OR 1.31; 95% CI 0.88–1.96). (4) Conclusions: The number of hospitalizations for anaphylaxis in children remained stable from 2016 to 2019, dropping in 2020 and recovering in 2021. IHM was low and remained stable during the study period. The incidence of hospitalizations for anaphylaxis was higher in asthmatic children than in non-asthmatics, but there were no differences in the occurrence of severe anaphylaxis among them.

Keywords: anaphylaxis; children; hospitalizations; trends; asthma; sex-differences

1. Introduction

Anaphylaxis is a serious, potentially life threatening, allergic reaction that is triggered suddenly by exposure to specific allergen substances [1–4]. It may occur at any age and often results in hospital and/or emergency department admissions [5]. For this reason, healthcare professionals require training in how to recognize anaphylaxis and differentiate it from other diagnoses [6]. The lifetime prevalence of anaphylaxis is around 5% and appears to be rising [7]. In children, the estimated prevalence ranges from 0.04% to 1.8% and is also increasing, mostly at pre-school age [8].

Epidemiological factors associated with anaphylaxis vary with age, culture and lifestyle [9]. Food has been considered the predominating cause of anaphylaxis, particularly among children, and represents a significant health problem, as anaphylaxis caused by food can contribute to mortality [10].

Between 11% and 38% of children who experienced anaphylaxis have a history of asthma or recurrent wheezing [11]. Asthma has been identified as a risk factor for severe and potentially fatal anaphylaxis [12]. However, in a recent study, children hospitalized for anaphylaxis with a history of asthma did not have a higher chance of severe anaphylactic reactions compared with children without asthma [13].

Despite the substantial burden that this problem produces in the pediatric population, data concerning the characteristics of anaphylaxis in children in Spain are spare and they are not updated [14,15]. Studies on temporal trends based on large national admission databases could help to address this knowledge gap. The objectives of our study were as follows: (a) to assess the temporal trends in the incidence, anaphylactic reaction triggers, clinical characteristics, and hospital outcomes among children with and without asthma who were hospitalized with anaphylaxis in Spain from 2016 to 2021; (b) to compare study variables between children with and without asthma stratified by age and sex; (c) to identify variables associated with severe anaphylaxis, defined as causing admission to the intensive care unit (ICU) and/or mortality during hospitalization, among children with asthma, and to evaluate the effect of asthma on the occurrence of severe anaphylaxis.

2. Materials and Methods

An observational, retrospective study (from 1 January 2016 to 31 December 2021) was conducted using a population-based database, the Minimum Basic Data Set of Specialized Care Activity Registry (RAE-CMBD in Spanish). The RAE-CMBD, owned by the Spanish Ministry of Health (SMH), records individual information of all patients admitted to Spanish hospitals. The collected information includes sex, age, admission date, discharge date, diagnoses (up to 20), procedures (up to 20), and discharge destination (voluntary discharge, home, social institution, deceased) [16]. The RAE-CMBD uses the International Classification of Diseases, Tenth Revision (ICD-10) for coding. All diagnosis and procedure codes used in this study are detailed in Table S1.

The study population included pediatric patients (17 years old or younger) with an ICD-10 code for anaphylaxis in any diagnostic position within the RAE-CMBD. Subsequently, this population was stratified based on whether they had an asthma code in any diagnostic position within the RAE-CMBD. Hospitalized patients with lacking data for age, sex, dates of admission and/or discharge and discharge destination were excluded.

Different types of anaphylactic reaction triggers were recorded: food, drugs, serum, or unspecified, according to the ICD-10 coding methodology.

The use of mechanical ventilation (invasive and non-invasive), codified in any position in the RAE-CMBD procedure field, was also analyzed (Table S1).

Admission to the ICU refers to being admitted to the intensive care unit during hospitalization with anaphylaxis for at least 24 h. In-hospital mortality (IHM) was the proportion of deaths during hospitalization. A child with severe anaphylaxis was defined as someone who required admission to the ICU and/or died during hospitalization.

2.1. Statistical Analysis

The incidence of hospitalization with anaphylaxis per 100,000 children with and without asthma was calculated for each of the six years analyzed. Incidence rates were calculated based on the Spanish pediatric population with asthma, grouped by age and sex, according to the National Health Survey of 2016/2017 [17]. The pediatric populations with asthma for the missing years (2018, 2019, 2020, and 2021) were estimated assuming that the growth rate remained stable throughout the period. Poisson regression was used to calculate age- and sex-adjusted incidence rate ratios (IRR) with their 95% confidence intervals (CI).

A descriptive statistical analysis was conducted, categorical variables were expressed as frequencies and percentages, and for quantitative variables, mean and standard deviation were provided.

Temporal trends were analyzed using Cochran–Mantel–Haenszel statistics or the Cochran–Armitage test for categorical variables, and linear regression t-test or Jonckheere-Terpstra test for continuous variables.

Categorical variables were compared using Fisher's exact test, and continuous variables were compared using t-test or Mann–Whitney test, as necessary.

Multivariable logistic regression was used to identify variables associated with severe anaphylaxis among children with anaphylaxis according to asthma status. The models were constructed, including sex, age, year, reaction triggers and use of mechanical ventilation. The results of these models are presented as odds ratios (OR) with 95% CI.

Statistical analysis was performed using Stata version 14 software (Stata, College Station, TX, USA). A p-value of <0.05 (two-tailed) was considered significant.

2.2. Ethical Statement

According to Spanish legislation, written consent from patients or evaluation by an ethics committee is not required since the RAE-CMBD is an administrative, mandatory, ammonized registry, and its data can be requested online to the SMH [18]. The SMH will evaluate the ethical and methodological issues of the suggested study protocol and, if considered adequate, will provide the database.

3. Results

As can be seen in Table 1, during the study period, 2016–2021, there were 2573 hospital admissions with anaphylaxis in children under 18 years old in Spain.

Table 1. Characteristics of hospital admissions with a diagnosis of anaphylaxis among children in Spain, 2016–2021.

	2016	2017	2018	2019	2020	2021	Total	p Trend
N	431	421	439	432	346	504	2573	NA
Age, mean (SD)	6.9 (4.82)	7 (4.86)	6.35 (4.77)	6.94 (4.95)	6.78 (5.15)	6.68 (4.99)	6.77 (4.92)	0.396
0–5 years old, n (%)	189 (43.85)	189 (44.89)	214 (48.75)	189 (43.75)	159 (45.95)	238 (47.22)	1178 (45.78)	0.558
6–11 years old, n (%)	153 (35.5)	130 (30.88)	145 (33.03)	149 (34.49)	107 (30.92)	165 (32.74)	849 (33)	
12–17 years old, n (%)	89 (20.65)	102 (24.23)	80 (18.22)	94 (21.76)	80 (23.12)	101 (20.04)	546 (21.22)	
Boys, n (%)	280 (64.97)	245 (58.19)	255 (58.09)	250 (57.87)	225 (65.03)	305 (60.52)	1560 (60.63)	0.081
Anaphylactic reaction due to food, n (%)	292 (67.75)	260 (61.76)	282 (64.24)	270 (62.5)	244 (70.52)	383 (75.99)	1731 (67.28)	<0.001
Anaphylactic reaction due to serum, n (%)	15 (3.48)	14 (3.33)	17 (3.87)	8 (1.85)	10 (2.89)	14 (2.78)	78 (3.03)	0.600
Anaphylactic reaction due to drugs, n (%)	35 (8.12)	43 (10.21)	67 (15.26)	83 (19.21)	51 (14.74)	55 (10.91)	334 (12.98)	<0.001
Anaphylactic shock, unspecified, n (%)	91 (21.11)	105 (24.94)	72 (16.4)	73 (16.9)	42 (12.14)	53 (10.52)	436 (16.95)	<0.001
Invasive mechanical ventilation, n (%)	11 (2.55)	8 (1.9)	12 (2.73)	17 (3.94)	9 (2.6)	12 (2.38)	69 (2.68)	0.578
Noninvasive mechanical ventilation, n (%)	2 (0.46)	4 (0.95)	1 (0.23)	8 (1.85)	8 (2.31)	11 (2.18)	34 (1.32)	0.021
Admission to ICU, n (%)	29 (6.73)	55 (13.06)	49 (11.16)	59 (13.66)	44 (12.72)	36 (7.14)	272 (10.57)	0.001
IHM, n (%)	4 (0.93)	2 (0.48)	4 (0.91)	3 (0.69)	2 (0.58)	2 (0.4)	17 (0.66)	0.890
Admission to ICU or IHM, n (%)	31 (7.19)	55 (13.06)	49 (11.16)	60 (13.89)	45 (13.01)	37 (7.34)	277 (10.77)	0.001

ICU: Intensive Care Unit; IHM: In-hospital mortality; NA Not applicable.

Of all the hospital admissions, 60.63% occurred in boys, with a mean age of the study population of 6.77 years.

The most common anaphylactic reactions were due to food consumption (67.28%), followed by drug consumption (12.98%) and serum consumption (3.03%). Unspecified reactions were codified in 16.95% of the cases.

The need for mechanical ventilation was infrequent, with overall values of 2.68% for invasive and 1.32% for noninvasive, respectively.

Among the children diagnosed with anaphylaxis from 2016 to 2021, 10.57% were admitted to the ICU, and the IHM rate was 0.66%. Severe anaphylaxis, defined as either admission to the ICU or IHM, occurred in 10.77% of the children.

3.1. Temporal Trends in Hospital Admissions with Anaphylaxis in the Spanish Pediatric Population between 2016 and 2021

As indicated in Table 1, the number of hospital admissions was stable from 2016 to 2019 (around 430 per year) dropping to 346 in 2020 and rising to the highest number in 2021 (504).

Between 2016 and 2021, there was a significant increase in reactions associated with food consumption (67.75% vs. 75.99%; $p < 0.001$) and reactions associated with drug consumption (8.12% vs. 10.91%; $p < 0.001$). However, non-specific reactions decreased over the study period (21.11% vs. 10.52%; $p < 0.001$). Figure 1 shows the evolution over time according to the trigger type.

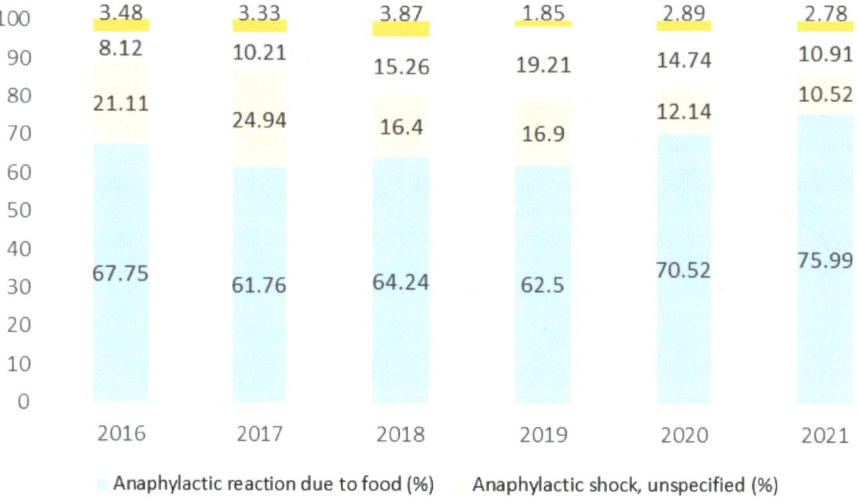

Figure 1. Triggers of anaphylaxis hospitalizations among Spanish children from 2016 to 2021.

The use of non-invasive mechanical ventilation increased in children with anaphylactic reactions between 2016 and 2021 (0.46% vs. 2.18%; $p = 0.021$), as observed in Table 1.

The IHM remained stable and under 1% in all the years studied. The ICU admissions and the prevalence of severe anaphylaxis showed significant variations over the study period. oscillating between 6.73% in 2016 and 13.66% in 2019.

3.2. Temporal Trends and Characteristics of Hospital Admissions with Anaphylaxis in the Spanish Pediatric Population Based on the Presence of Asthma

The presence of asthma among children admitted with anaphylaxis from 2016 to 2021 was codified in 12.59% (n = 324) of cases and remained stable overtime (Table 2).

Children with asthma had a higher mean age than children without asthma (9.85 years vs. 6.33 years; $p < 0.001$) and a similar sex distribution.

Anaphylactic reactions due to food consumption (73.46% vs. 66.39%; $p = 0.011$) were more frequent among children with asthma, but fewer reactions due to drug consumption (7.1% vs. 13.83%; $p < 0.001$) were found, as shown in Table 2.

Both in children with and without asthma, reactions associated with food consumption significantly increased over the study period (70% and 67.39% in 2016 vs. 87.32% and 74.13% in 2021; $p = 0.044$ and $p < 0.001$, respectively). Reactions associated with drug consumption increased in the group of non-asthmatic children (8.36% in 2016 vs. 12.01% in 2021). However, non-specific anaphylactic reactions decreased in both asthmatic children (23.33% in 2016 vs. 5.63% in 2021; $p = 0.037$) and non-asthmatic children (20.75% vs. 11.32%; $p < 0.001$). Figure 2 shows the triggers of anaphylaxis among Spanish children with and without asthma from 2016 to 2021

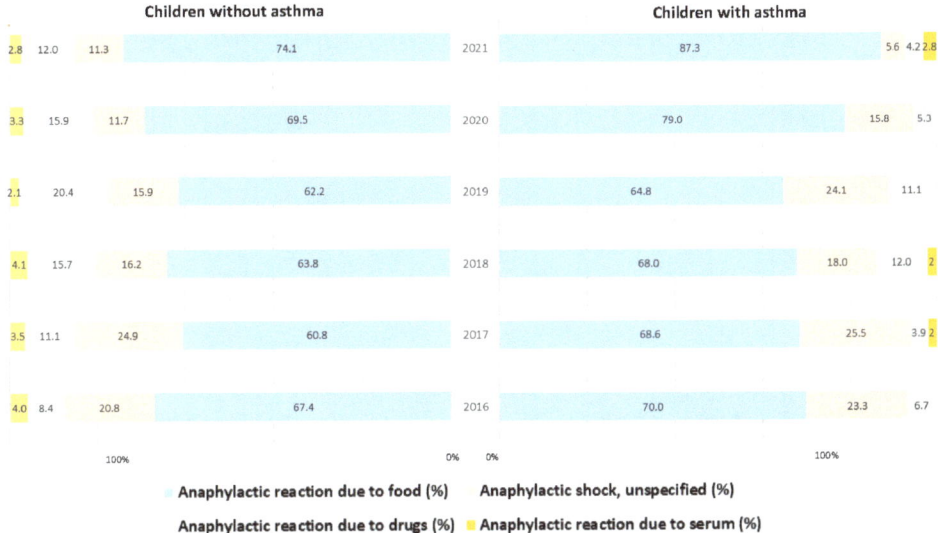

Figure 2. Triggers of anaphylaxis hospitalizations among Spanish children from 2016 to 2021, according to asthma status.

The use of non-invasive mechanical ventilation significantly increased ($p = 0.018$) in the group of non-asthmatic children between 2016 and 2021, as indicated in Table 2.

In non-asthmatic children, the frequency of ICU admissions increased over the study bperiod ($p = 0.004$). However, the frequency of severe anaphylaxis decreased ($p = 0.006$). In children with asthma, over the study period, ICU admissions, in-hospital mortality, and the frequency of severe anaphylaxis remained stable, as shown in Table 2.

Table 2. Characteristics of hospital admissions with a diagnosis of anaphylaxis among children with and without asthma in Spain, 2016–2021.

	Asthma	2016	2017	2018	2019	2020	2021	Total	p Trend	p "with Asthma" vs. "without Asthma"
N (%)	Yes	60 (13.92)	51 (12.11)	50 (11.39)	54 (12.5)	38 (10.98)	71 (14.09)	324 (12.59)	0.670	NA
	No	371 (86.08)	370 (87.89)	389 (88.61)	378 (87.5)	308 (89.02)	433 (85.91)	2249 (87.41)		
Age, mean (SD)	Yes	9.97 (4.04)	9.63 (3.39)	9.08 (4.45)	9.63 (3.81)	10.5 (3.87)	10.25 (3.5)	9.85 (3.84)	0.520	<0.001
	No	6.41 (4.76)	6.64 (4.92)	5.99 (4.7)	6.55 (4.98)	6.32 (5.1)	6.1 (4.95)	6.33 (4.9)	0.399	
0–5 years old, n (%)	Yes	10 (16.67)	6 (11.76)	13 (26)	6 (11.11)	5 (13.16)	6 (8.45)	46 (14.2)	0.194	<0.001
	No	179 (48.25)	183 (49.46)	201 (51.67)	183 (48.41)	154 (50)	232 (53.58)	1132 (50.33)	0.496	
6–11 years old, n (%)	Yes	27 (45)	25 (49.02)	20 (40)	31 (57.41)	15 (39.47)	42 (59.15)	160 (49.38)	0.194	<0.001
	No	126 (33.96)	105 (28.38)	125 (32.13)	118 (31.22)	92 (29.87)	123 (28.41)	689 (30.64)	0.496	
12–17 years old, n (%)	Yes	23 (38.33)	20 (39.22)	17 (34)	17 (31.48)	18 (47.37)	23 (32.39)	118 (36.42)	0.194	<0.001
	No	66 (17.79)	82 (22.16)	63 (16.2)	77 (20.37)	62 (20.13)	78 (18.01)	428 (19.03)	0.496	
Boys, n (%)	Yes	40 (66.67)	26 (50.98)	24 (48)	35 (64.81)	25 (65.79)	38 (53.52)	188 (58.02)	0.186	0.305
	No	240 (64.69)	219 (59.19)	231 (59.38)	215 (56.88)	200 (64.94)	267 (61.66)	1372 (61)	0.165	
Anaphylactic reaction due to food, n (%)	Yes	42 (70)	35 (68.63)	34 (68)	35 (64.81)	30 (78.95)	62 (87.32)	238 (73.46)	0.044	0.011
	No	250 (67.39)	225 (60.81)	248 (63.75)	235 (62.17)	214 (69.48)	321 (74.13)	1493 (66.39)	<0.001	
Anaphylactic reaction due to serum, n (%)	Yes	0 (0)	1 (1.96)	1 (2)	0 (0)	0 (0)	2 (2.82)	4 (1.23)	0.576	0.053
	No	15 (4.04)	13 (3.51)	16 (4.11)	8 (2.12)	10 (3.25)	12 (2.77)	74 (3.29)	0.616	
Anaphylactic reaction due to drugs, n (%)	Yes	4 (6.67)	2 (3.92)	6 (12)	6 (11.11)	2 (5.26)	3 (4.23)	23 (7.1)	0.413	0.001
	No	31 (8.36)	41 (11.08)	61 (15.68)	77 (20.37)	49 (15.91)	52 (12.01)	311 (13.83)	<0.001	
Anaphylactic shock, unspecified, n (%)	Yes	14 (23.33)	13 (25.49)	9 (18)	13 (24.07)	6 (15.79)	4 (5.63)	59 (18.21)	0.037	0.516
	No	77 (20.75)	92 (24.86)	63 (16.2)	60 (15.87)	36 (11.69)	49 (11.32)	377 (16.76)	<0.001	
Invasive mechanical ventilation, n (%)	Yes	2 (3.33)	2 (3.92)	0 (0)	5 (9.26)	1 (2.63)	0 (0)	10 (3.09)	0.054	0.630
	No	9 (2.43)	6 (1.62)	12 (3.08)	12 (3.17)	8 (2.6)	12 (2.77)	59 (2.62)	0.803	
Noninvasive mechanical ventilation, n (%)	Yes	0 (0)	2 (3.92)	0 (0)	2 (3.7)	2 (5.26)	0 (0)	6 (1.85)	0.152	0.374
	No	2 (0.54)	2 (0.54)	1 (0.26)	6 (1.59)	6 (1.95)	11 (2.54)	28 (1.24)	0.018	
Admission to ICU, n (%)	Yes	4 (6.67)	8 (15.69)	8 (16)	10 (18.52)	5 (13.16)	6 (8.45)	41 (12.65)	0.336	0.193
	No	25 (6.74)	47 (12.7)	41 (10.54)	49 (12.96)	39 (12.66)	30 (6.93)	231 (10.27)	0.004	
IHM, n (%)	Yes	1 (1.67)	0 (0)	1 (2)	0 (0)	0 (0)	0 (0)	2 (0.62)	0.555	0.918
	No	3 (0.81)	2 (0.54)	3 (0.77)	3 (0.79)	2 (0.65)	2 (0.46)	15 (0.67)	0.986	
Admission to ICU or IHM, n (%)	Yes	4 (6.67)	8 (15.69)	8 (16)	10 (18.52)	5 (13.16)	6 (8.45)	41 (12.65)	0.336	0.241
	No	27 (7.28)	47 (12.7)	41 (10.54)	50 (13.23)	40 (12.99)	31 (7.16)	236 (10.49)	0.006	

ICU: Intensive Care Unit; IHM: In-hospital mortality; NA Not applicable.

3.3. Incidence of Hospital Admission Due to Anaphylactic Reaction According to the Presence of Asthma and Characteristics of Admission According to Age and Sex

Table 3 presents the characteristics of hospital admissions with anaphylaxis by age groups and according to the asthma status.

Table 3. Characteristics of hospital admissions with a diagnosis of anaphylaxis among children with and without asthma according to age groups in Spain, 2016–2021.

	Asthma	0–5 Years Old	6–11 Years Old	12–17 Years Old	p
Rate per 100,000 children per year	Yes	49.72	82.56	46.10	<0.001
	No	45.48	24.56	15.60	<0.001
Age, mean (SD)	Yes	3.67 (1.25)	8.63 (1.65)	13.91 (1.63)	<0.001
	No	2.22 (1.79)	8.3 (1.76)	14.02 (1.58)	<0.001
Boys, n (%)	Yes	30 (65.22)	97 (60.63)	61 (51.69)	0.186
	No	709 (62.63)	437 (63.43)	226 (52.8)	0.001
Anaphylactic reaction due to food, n (%)	Yes	39 (84.78)	119 (74.38)	80 (67.8)	0.081
	No	852 (75.27)	459 (66.62)	182 (42.52)	<0.001
Anaphylactic reaction due to serum, n (%)	Yes	0 (0)	1 (0.63)	3 (2.54)	0.257
	No	38 (3.36)	19 (2.76)	17 (3.97)	0.534
Anaphylactic reaction due to drugs, n (%)	Yes	0 (0)	12 (7.5)	11 (9.32)	0.109
	No	104 (9.19)	97 (14.08)	110 (25.7)	<0.001
Anaphylactic shock, unspecified, n (%)	Yes	7 (15.22)	28 (17.5)	24 (20.34)	0.708
	No	142 (12.54)	115 (16.69)	120 (28.04)	<0.001
Invasive mechanical ventilation, n (%)	Yes	0 (0)	5 (3.13)	5 (4.24)	0.370
	No	34 (3)	13 (1.89)	12 (2.8)	0.340
Noninvasive mechanical ventilation, n (%)	Yes	1 (2.17)	3 (1.88)	2 (1.69)	0.979
	No	16 (1.41)	6 (0.87)	6 (1.4)	0.568
Admission to ICU, n (%)	Yes	4 (8.7)	21 (13.13)	16 (13.56)	0.680
	No	105 (9.28)	61 (8.85)	65 (15.19)	0.001
IHM, n (%)	Yes	0 (0)	2 (1.25)	0 (0)	0.357
	No	8 (0.71)	5 (0.73)	2 (0.47)	0.852
Admission to ICU or IHM, n (%)	Yes	4 (8.7)	21 (13.13)	16 (13.56)	0.680
	No	109 (9.63)	62 (9)	65 (15.19)	0.002

p values for comparison by age groups. ICU: Intensive Care Unit; IHM: In-hospital mortality.

The crude incidence of hospital admission with anaphylaxis in patients with asthma was 59.75 cases per 100,000 subjects with asthma per year, while in patients without asthma, it was 27.98 cases. Among patients with asthma, the highest incidence was observed in the age group of 6–11 years (82.56), whereas in patients without asthma, it was in the age group between 0 and 5 years (45.48). After using the Poisson regression model, adjusted for age and sex, it was found that the incidence of anaphylaxis for the period 2016–2021 was 2.14 times higher among children with asthma than among those without asthma (IRR 2.14; 95% CI 1.87–2.44).

When comparing the characteristics of anaphylaxis admission based on age groups, patients without asthma, aged between 12 and 17 years, had fewer reactions associated with food consumption and more reactions associated with drug consumption and non-specific reactions (all $p < 0.001$) compared to the other age groups (0–5 years old and 6–11 years old). Additionally, they had more admissions to the ICU ($p = 0.001$) and more severe anaphylactic reactions ($p = 0.002$), as indicated in Table 3.

Table 4 presents the characteristics of hospital admissions with anaphylaxis by sex and according to the asthma status.

The incidence of hospital admission with anaphylaxis in boys with asthma was 60.19 cases per 100,000 subjects with asthma, while in boys without asthma, it was 33.37. In girls, the incidence was 59.14 in those with asthma and 22.33 in those without asthma. After conducting the Poisson regression model, the incidence of anaphylaxis was 1.79 times higher in boys with asthma than in those without asthma (IRR 1.79; 95% CI 1.06–2.45) and

2.68 times higher in girls with asthma than in those without asthma (IRR 2.68; 95% CI 2.23–3.12).

Table 4. Characteristics of hospital admissions with a diagnosis of anaphylaxis among children with and without asthma according to sex in Spain, 2016–2021.

	Asthma	Boys	Girls	p
Rate per 100,000 subjects per year	Yes	60.19	59.14	NA
	No	33.37	22.33	NA
Age, mean (SD)	Yes	9.51 (3.84)	10.32 (3.8)	0.060
	No	6.09 (4.74)	6.7 (5.11)	0.004
0–5 years old, n (%)	Yes	30 (15.96)	16 (11.76)	0.186
	No	709 (51.68)	423 (48.23)	0.001
6–11 years old, n (%)	Yes	97 (51.6)	63 (46.32)	0.186
	No	437 (31.85)	252 (28.73)	0.001
12–17 years old, n (%)	Yes	61 (32.45)	57 (41.91)	0.186
	No	226 (16.47)	202 (23.03)	0.001
Anaphylactic reaction due to food, n (%)	Yes	134 (71.28)	104 (76.47)	0.296
	No	938 (68.37)	555 (63.28)	0.013
Anaphylactic reaction due to serum, n (%)	Yes	4 (2.13)	0 (0)	0.087
	No	38 (2.77)	36 (4.1)	0.083
Anaphylactic reaction due to drugs, n (%)	Yes	13 (6.91)	10 (7.35)	0.880
	No	181 (13.19)	130 (14.82)	0.274
Anaphylactic shock, unspecified, n (%)	Yes	37 (19.68)	22 (16.18)	0.420
	No	221 (16.11)	156 (17.79)	0.298
Invasive mechanical ventilation, n (%)	Yes	5 (2.66)	5 (3.68)	0.601
	No	35 (2.55)	24 (2.74)	0.788
Noninvasive mechanical ventilation, n (%)	Yes	6 (3.19)	0 (0)	0.035
	No	16 (1.17)	12 (1.37)	0.673
Admission to ICU, n (%)	Yes	20 (10.64)	21 (15.44)	0.199
	No	138 (10.06)	93 (10.6)	0.677
IHM, n (%)	Yes	0 (0)	2 (1.47)	0.095
	No	8 (0.58)	7 (0.8)	0.541
Admission to ICU or IHM, n (%)	Yes	20 (10.64)	21 (15.44)	0.199
	No	141 (10.28)	95 (10.83)	0.675

p values for comparison by sex. ICU: Intensive Care Unit; IHM: In-hospital mortality; NA Not applicable.

When comparing admission characteristics by sex, it was observed that in those without asthma, the mean age of girls was higher than that of boys (6.7 years vs. 6.09 years; $p = 0.004$). Additionally, girls had significantly fewer reactions associated with food consumption (63.28% vs. 68.37%; $p = 0.013$). In patients with asthma, only the use of non-invasive mechanical ventilation was higher in boys than in girls ($p = 0.035$). The rest of the study variables presented similar values between boys and girls, as indicated in Table 4.

3.4. Multivariable Analysis of Factors Associated with Severe Anaphylaxis during Hospital Admission with Anaphylaxis in the Pediatric Population with and without Asthma

As indicated in Table 5, older age (12–17 years) was a risk factor for severe anaphylaxis in children without asthma (OR 1.48; 95% CI 1.02–2.15).

The presence of reactions associated with drug consumption was associated with severe anaphylaxis in children without asthma and in the total study population.

Additionally, in the total study population, undergoing invasive and non-invasive mechanical ventilation (OR 17.54; 95% CI 9.87–31.15 and OR 4.9; 95% CI 2.07–11.6, respectively) were risk factors associated tor severe anaphylaxis.

After adjustment, severe anaphylaxis was significantly higher in the study population in years 2017, 2018, 2019, and 2020 compared to the year 2016.

Finally, when using the non-asthma status as the reference category, the analysis of the entire database revealed that the presence of asthma was not associated with severe anaphylaxis (OR 1.31; 95%CI 0.88–1.96).

Table 5. Multivariable analysis of the factors associated with in hospital mortality or admission to intensive care unit during hospital admission among children with a diagnosis of anaphylaxis in Spain, 2016–2021 according to asthma status.

	No Asthma	Asthma	Both
	OR (95% CI)	OR (95% CI)	OR (95% CI)
0–5 years old	1	1	1
6–11 years old	0.97 (0.68–1.38)	1.48 (0.43–5.16)	1.03 (0.74–1.43)
12–17 years old	1.48 (1.02–2.15)	1.22 (0.34–4.45)	1.39 (0.98–1.99)
Girls	0.97 (0.72–1.32)	1.87 (0.87–4.03)	1.05 (0.8–1.39)
Anaphylactic reaction due to drugs	2.03 (1.33–3.11)	1.77 (069–3.99)	1.95 (1.3–2.91)
Invasive mechanical ventilation	17.63 (9.5–32.73)	27.59 (4.77–159.64)	17.54 (9.87–31.15)
Noninvasive mechanical ventilation	3.59 (1.34–9.64)	42.5 (3.76–481.1)	4.9 (2.07–11.6)
2016	1	1	1
2017	2.17 (1.26–3.74)	2.2 (0.5–9.56)	2.25 (1.36–3.74)
2018	1.58(0.9–2.77)	3.64 (0.88–15.06)	1.79 (1.06–3)
2019	1.88 (1.09–3.25)	2.41 (0.58–10.09)	1.96 (1.18–3.26)
2020	1.97 (1.11–3.48)	2.26 (0.44–11.63)	2.03 (1.19–3.47)
2021	0.91 (0.5–1.67)	1.97 (0.45–8.58)	1.02 (0.58–1.78)
Asthma	NA	NA	1.31 (0.88–1.96)

OR: Odds Ratio; CI: Confidence Interval; NA: Not applicable.

4. Discussion

Our study provides new data regarding anaphylaxis among children. We reported that the number of hospital admissions for anaphylaxis in children remained stable from 2016 to 2021. Previous studies investigating trends in anaphylaxis hospitalization among children have reported conflicting results. Agreeing with us, Robinson et al. [19] found that anaphylaxis hospitalizations among infants and toddlers in the United States were stable from 2006 to 2015, in contrast to rising trends in older children. Similarly, Shrestha et al. [20] reported a stable rate of anaphylaxis hospitalizations among children and adults in the United States from 2001 to 2014, finding only an increase in children aged 5 to 14 years with food-related reactions.

Declining trends have been reported by Motosue et al. [21] who showed a significant decline in hospitalizations for United States children presenting with food-induced anaphylaxis from 2005 to 2014, despite a rise in emergency department visits.

Finally, increments in hospitalizations have been published by Dyer et al. [22], who described rising rates of food-induced anaphylaxis hospitalizations and emergency department visits in children in Illinois from 2008 to 2012. Also, Tejedor–Alonso et al. [14] reported an increase in the frequency of admission due to anaphylaxis in Spanish hospitals from 1998 to 2011, particularly in patients aged 0–14 years and in food anaphylaxis. More recently, Baseggio Conrado et al. [23] evidenced a threefold increase in hospital admissions for food anaphylaxis between 1998 and 2018 in the United Kingdom, with cow's milk being the most common single cause of fatal anaphylaxis.

The underlying reasons for the stable trends in anaphylaxis hospitalizations in children obtained in our study are not known. We do not believe that our findings are due to a decline in prevalence of anaphylaxis. In fact, recent studies on the trends in prevalence of anaphylaxis and food allergy support a rising prevalence [5]. It is likely that our findings are the results of several factors, including changes in disease recognition, severity, management, and health care utilization, as already described by other authors [19,24,25].

We also found a drop in the number of hospital admissions for anaphylaxis in 2020, coinciding with the start of the COVID pandemic, which was recovered in 2021. The decrease in the frequency of anaphylaxis at the start of the pandemic has been described by other authors [26], as well as the subsequent recovery [27]. It may reflect decreased accidental exposures due to reduced social gatherings and closed schools. The reluctance to present to the emergency department for fear of contagion may also contribute [26,27].

Our data showed that anaphylaxis hospitalization was more likely in male than in female children. These results are consistent with those reported by the majority of previous studies [28,29]. Regardless of gender, we also found that food was the most common cause of anaphylaxis in children, as previously described [30,31], representing more than two thirds of the cases. Furthermore, unspecified causes decreased, while reactions caused by food and drugs increased over time, possibly influenced, at least in part, by improved coding.

Severe anaphylaxis requiring ICU admission is a rare event and difficult to study since the number of affected patients is usually small [32]. We identified that 10.57% of children with anaphylaxis required admission to the ICU. Sundquist et al. [33] also found a lower ICU admission rate in children with anaphylaxis, which is clearly less than in adults.

Consistent with other studies [34], we found that IHM was low and remained stable over time. So, the vast majority hospital admissions with anaphylaxis did not result in death, reflecting in part the quality-of-care provided [35]. In fact, mortality appears similar in those regions where data are available [24]. An exception is Australia, where all-cause fatal anaphylaxis rates increased by 6.2% per annum from 1997 to 2013, primarily due to food triggers [36]. However, when these data are analyzed by case-fatality rate (proportion of cases admitted to hospital that result in a fatal outcome), mortality has decreased, including with respect to fatal food-related anaphylaxis in Australia [24].

Asthma seems to be associated with the risk of anaphylaxis. In the current study, the incidence of hospitalizations for anaphylaxis was higher in asthmatic children than in non-asthmatic children. González–Pérez et al. [37] also demonstrated that patients with asthma have a greater risk of anaphylaxis than those without asthma, with the risk greater in severe than no severe asthma. Like us, they also found that women are at higher risk of anaphylaxis than men, especially if they have severe asthma.

The relationship between asthma and severe anaphylaxis is controversial. Despite asthma having been identified as a risk factor for severe anaphylaxis [38–41], our study did not find that children with asthma had more severe anaphylaxis compared with those without asthma. Similar results have been described by other authors [11,13,42]. Furthermore, Motosue et al. [43] reported that asthma was less likely to be a predictor of hospitalizations, admissions to the ICU, and endotracheal intubation. However, other authors have indicated that suboptimal asthma control, rather than the presence of asthma, may increase the likelihood of having severe anaphylaxis [44,45]. In fact, good asthma control may prevent life-threatening acute bronchospasm after ingestion of nuts, although there may be little effect on the severity of other symptoms of anaphylaxis such as pharyngeal edema [46].

This study has several potential limitations. First, we used administrative data, which are susceptible to coding errors and diagnostic misclassification. Therefore, we lack detailed information on the clinical criteria for diagnosing anaphylaxis. However, in Spain the medical societies recommend using the Guidelines of the European Academy of Allergy and Clinical Immunology [6]. Second, due to the nature of the national database, we did not have information that could be relevant such as complete information on etiology and risk factors/co-factors for anaphylaxis, detailed clinical presentation, serum (or plasma) tryptase, or pharmacologic treatments such as epinephrin injection. Third, our study did not include patients who were judged not to require hospitalization after an emergency department visit. Forth, in our study, we stratified by asthma and not by other atopic disease and clinical manifestation allergic rhinitis or/and eczema. We have chosen asthma because in Spain it is an important public health problem and has greater severity than other atopic diseases and clinical manifestations of allergic rhinitis and/or eczema. Furthermore, as commented before, there are few studies in our country and elsewhere that assess the association of anaphylaxis and asthma and the results have been contradictory. However, future investigations should focus on the relationship of anaphylaxis with other atopic disease and clinical manifestation allergic rhinitis or/and eczema. Fifth, in our investigation we have not included anaphylaxis triggered by a "toxic effect of contact with venomous animals and plants" (ICD10 codes T63.xxx). The reason for this is that from 2016 to 2021, only four children in the entire database (0.16%) had a T63.xxx code in their diagnosis fields. Sixth, we also could not identify those children that suffered anaphylaxis triggered by allergen immunotherapy or latex, as no ICD10 codes were available to identify a patient with anaphylaxis triggered by these allergens. Regarding allergen immunotherapy, the incidence rates of severe systemic reactions are estimated to be probably <1% [47].

The strengths of this study include the use of a large, nationally representative database, with a 6-year study period, which provides the ability to study trends of anaphylaxis in Spain over time. In addition, we used rigorous methods to select the study population and meticulous data analysis to measure outcomes.

5. Conclusions

In summary, using nationally representative data, we found that the number of hospitalizations for anaphylaxis in children remained stable from 2016 to 2019, with a drop in 2020 and recovery in 2021. Anaphylaxis hospitalization was more likely in male children, and food was the most common cause, increasing over time. IHM was low and remained stable during the study period. On the other hand, the incidence of hospitalizations for anaphylaxis was higher in asthmatic children than in non-asthmatics, but there were no differences in the occurrence of severe anaphylaxis among them. Increased knowledge regarding the epidemiology of pediatric anaphylaxis in children may contribute to improve its management.

Supplementary Materials: The following supporting information can be downloaded at: https://www.mdpi.com/article/10.3390/jcm12196387/s1, Table S1: ICD-10 diagnosis and procedures codes used in this investigation.

Author Contributions: Conceptualization, J.D.M.-D., R.J.-G. and N.C.-C.; Methodology: A.L.-d.-A., F.J.C.-S. and J.J.Z.-L.; Validation: D.C.-A. and R.O.-P.; Data curation: V.H.-B.; Formal analysis: V.H.-B.; Funding: A.L.-d.-A. and R.J.-G.; Writing—original draft; J.D.M.-D., F.J.C.-S., R.J.-G. and N.C.-C.; Writing—review and editing: A.L.-d.-A., J.J.Z.-L., D.C.-A. and R.O.-P. All authors have read and agreed to the published version of the manuscript.

Funding: This work has been supported by the Madrid Government (Comunidad de Madrid-Spain) under the Multiannual Agreement with Universidad Complutense de Madrid in the line Excellence Programme for university teaching staff, in the context of the V PRICIT (Regional Programme of Research and Technological Innovation). And by Universidad Complutense de Madrid. Grupo de Investigación en Epidemiología de las Enfermedades Crónicas de Alta Prevalencia en España-GEPIECAP-(970970).

Institutional Review Board Statement: Not applicable.

Informed Consent Statement: Not applicable.

Data Availability Statement: According to the contract signed with the Spanish Ministry of Health and Social Services, which provided access to the databases from the Spanish National Hospital Database (*Registro de Actividad de Atención Especializada. Conjunto Mínimo Básico de Datos*, Registry of Specialized Health Care Activities. Minimum Basic Data Set), we cannot share the databases with any other investigator, and we have to destroy the databases once the investigation has concluded. Consequently, we cannot upload the databases to any public repository. However, any investigator can apply for access to the databases by filling out the questionnaire available at https://www.sanidad.gob.es/estadEstudios/estadisticas/estadisticas/estMinisterio/SolicitudCMBD.htm (accessed on 20 May 2023). All other relevant data are included in the paper.

Conflicts of Interest: The authors declare no conflict of interest.

References

1. Sampson, H.A.; Muñoz-Furlong, A.; Campbell, R.L.; Adkinson, N.F.; Bock, S.A.; Branum, A.; Brown, S.G.; Camargo, C.A.; Cydulka, R.; Galli, S.J.; et al. Second Symposium on the Definition and Management of Anaphylaxis: Summary Report—Second National Institute of Allergy and Infectious Disease/Food Allergy and Anaphylaxis Network Symposium. *Ann. Emerg. Med.* **2006**, *47*, 373–380. [CrossRef] [PubMed]
2. Jares, E.J.; Cardona, V.; Gómez, R.M.; Bernstein, J.A.; Filho, N.A.R.; Cherrez-Ojeda, I.; Ensina, L.F.; De Falco, A.; Díaz, M.C.; Vereau, P.A.C.; et al. Latin American anaphylaxis registry. *World Allergy Organ. J.* **2023**, *16*, 100748. [CrossRef] [PubMed]
3. Yao, T.-C.; Wu, A.C.; Huang, Y.-W.; Wang, J.-Y.; Tsai, H.-J. Increasing trends of anaphylaxis-related events: An analysis of anaphylaxis using nationwide data in Taiwan, 2001–2013. *World Allergy Organ. J.* **2018**, *11*, 23. [CrossRef]
4. Lin, R.Y.; Anderson, A.S.; Shah, S.N.; Nurruzzaman, F. Increasing anaphylaxis hospitalizations in the first 2 decades of life: New York State, 1990–2006. *Ann. Allergy Asthma Immunol.* **2008**, *101*, 387–393. [CrossRef] [PubMed]
5. Gurkha, D.; Podolsky, R.; Sethuraman, U.; Levasseur, K. Comparison of anaphylaxis epidemiology between urban and suburban pediatric emergency departments. *BMC Pediatr.* **2023**, *23*, 85. [CrossRef] [PubMed]
6. Muraro, A.; Worm, M.; Alviani, C.; Cardona, V.; DunnGalvin, A.; Garvey, L.H.; Riggioni, C.; de Silva, D.; Angier, E.; Arasi, S.; et al. EAACI guidelines: Anaphylaxis (2021 update). *Allergy* **2022**, *77*, 357–377. [CrossRef]
7. Wood, R.A.; Camargo, C.A.; Lieberman, P.; Sampson, H.A.; Schwartz, L.B.; Zitt, M.; Collins, C.; Tringale, M.; Wilkinson, M.; Boyle, J.; et al. Anaphylaxis in America: The prevalence and characteristics of anaphylaxis in the United States. *J. Allergy Clin. Immunol.* **2014**, *133*, 461–467. [CrossRef]
8. Gaspar, Â.; Santos, N.; Faria, E.; Pereira, A.M.; Gomes, E.; Câmara, R.; Rodrigues-Alves, R.; Borrego, L.; Carrapatoso, I.; Carneiro-Leão, L.; et al. Anaphylaxis in children and adolescents: The Portuguese Anaphylaxis Registry. *Pediatr. Allergy Immunol.* **2021**, *32*, 1278–1286. [CrossRef]
9. Anagnostou, K. Anaphylaxis in Children: Epidemiology, Risk Factors and Management. *Curr. Pediatr. Rev.* **2018**, *14*, 180–186. [CrossRef]
10. Vetander, M.; Helander, D.; Flodström, C.; Östblom, E.; Alfvén, T.; Ly, D.H.; Hedlin, G.; Lilja, G.; Nilsson, C.; Wickman, M. Anaphylaxis and reactions to foods in children—A population-based case study of emergency department visits. *Clin. Exp. Allergy* **2012**, *42*, 568–577. [CrossRef]
11. Jiang, N.; Xu, W.; Huang, H.; Hou, X.; Xiang, L. Anaphylaxis in Chinese Children: Different Clinical Profile Between Children with and without a History of Asthma/Recurrent Wheezing. *J. Asthma Allergy* **2022**, *15*, 1093–1104. [CrossRef] [PubMed]
12. Campbell, R.L.; Li, J.T.; Nicklas, R.A.; Sadosty, A.T.; Members of the Joint Task Force; Practice Parameter Workgroup. Emergency department diagnosis and treatment of anaphylaxis: A practice parameter. *Ann. Allergy Asthma Immunol.* **2014**, *113*, 599–608. [CrossRef] [PubMed]
13. Dribin, T.E.; Michelson, K.A.; Zhang, Y.; Schnadower, D.; Neuman, M.I. Are Children with a History of Asthma More Likely to Have Severe Anaphylactic Reactions? A Retrospective Cohort Study. *J. Pediatr.* **2020**, *220*, 159–164.e2. [CrossRef] [PubMed]
14. Tejedor-Alonso, M.A.; Moro-Moro, M.; González, M.M.; Rodriguez-Alvarez, M.; Fernández, E.P.; Zamalloa, P.L.; Aquino, E.F.; Gil Prieto, R.; Gil De Miguel, A. Increased incidence of admissions for anaphylaxis in Spain 1998–2011. *Allergy* **2015**, *70*, 880–883. [CrossRef]
15. Nieto-Nieto, A.; Tejedor-Alonso, M.; Farias-Aquino, E.; Moro-Moro, M.; Ingelmo, A.R.; Gonzalez-Moreno, A.; Gil de Miguel, A. Clinical profile of patients with severe anaphylaxis hospitalized in the spanish hospital system: 1997–2011. *J. Investig. Allergol. Clin. Immunol.* **2017**, *27*, 111–126. [CrossRef]
16. Ministerio de Sanidad, Servicios Sociales e Igualdad. Real Decreto 69/2015, de 6 de Febrero, por el Que Se Regula el Registro de Actividad de Atención Sanitaria Especializada. (Spanish National Hospital Discharge Database). *BOE* **2015**, *35*, 10789–10809. Available online: https://www.mscbs.gob.es/estadEstudios/estadisticas/docs/BOE_RD_69_2015_RAE_CMBD.pdf (accessed on 19 January 2023).
17. Ministerio de Sanidad. National Health Survey in Spain 2020 [Encuesta Nacional de Salud de España 2017]. Available online: https://www.sanidad.gob.es/estadEstudios/estadisticas/encuestaNacional/encuesta2017.htm (accessed on 28 July 2023).
18. Ministerio de Sanidad, Consumo y Bienestar Social, Solicitud de Extracción de Datos—Extraction Request. (Spanish National Hospital Discharge Database). Available online: https://www.mscbs.gob.es/estadEstudios/estadisticas/estMinisterio/SolicitudCMBDdocs/2018_Formulario_Peticion_Datos_RAE_CMBD.pdf (accessed on 28 July 2023).
19. Robinson, L.B.; Arroyo, A.C.; Faridi, M.K.; Rudders, S.A.; Camargo, C.A., Jr. Trends in US hospitalizations for anaphylaxis among infants and toddlers: 2006 to 2015. *Ann. Allergy Asthma Immunol.* **2021**, *126*, 168–174.e3. [CrossRef]
20. Shrestha, P.; Dhital, R.; Poudel, D.; Donato, A.; Karmacharya, P.; Craig, T. Trends in hospitalizations related to anaphylaxis, angioedema, and urticaria in the United States. *Ann. Allergy Asthma Immunol.* **2019**, *122*, 401–406.e2. [CrossRef]
21. Motosue, M.S.; Bellolio, M.F.; Van Houten, H.K.; Shah, N.D.; Campbell, R.L. National trends in emergency department visits and hospitalizations for food-induced anaphylaxis in US children. *Pediatr. Allergy Immunol.* **2018**, *29*, 538–544. [CrossRef]
22. Dyer, A.A.; Lau, C.H.; Smith, T.L.; Smith, B.M.; Gupta, R.S. Pediatric emergency department visits and hospitalizations due to food-induced anaphylaxis in Illinois. *Ann. Allergy Asthma Immunol.* **2015**, *115*, 56–62. [CrossRef]
23. Conrado, A.B.; Ierodiakonou, D.; Gowland, M.H.; Boyle, R.J.; Turner, P.J. Food anaphylaxis in the United Kingdom: Analysis of national data, 1998-2018. *BMJ* **2021**, *372*, n251. [CrossRef]

24. Turner, P.J.; Campbell, D.E.; Motosue, M.S.; Campbell, R.L. Global Trends in Anaphylaxis Epidemiology and Clinical Implications. *J. Allergy Clin. Immunol. Pract.* **2020**, *8*, 1169–1176. [CrossRef]
25. Gaffney, L.K.; Porter, J.; Gerling, M.; Schneider, L.C.; Stack, A.M.; Shah, D.; Michelson, K.A. Safely Reducing Hospitalizations for Anaphylaxis in Children Through an Evidence-Based Guideline. *Pediatrics.* **2022**, *149*, e2020045831. [CrossRef] [PubMed]
26. Dribin, T.E.; Neuman, M.I.; Schnadower, D.; Sampson, H.A.; Porter, J.J.; Michelson, K.A. Trends and Variation in Pediatric Anaphylaxis Care From 2016 to 2022. *J. Allergy Clin. Immunol. Pract.* **2023**, *11*, 1184–1189. [CrossRef] [PubMed]
27. Al Ali, A.; Gabrielli, S.; Colli, L.D.; Colli, M.D.; McCusker, C.; Clarke, A.E.; Morris, J.; Gravel, J.; Lim, R.; Chan, E.S.; et al. Temporal trends in anaphylaxis ED visits over the last decade and the effect of COVID-19 pandemic on these trends. *Expert Rev. Clin. Immunol.* **2023**, *19*, 341–348. [CrossRef] [PubMed]
28. Abunada, T.; Al-Nesf, M.A.; Thalib, L.; Kurdi, R.; Khalil, S.; ElKassem, W.; Mobayed, H.M.; Zayed, H. Anaphylaxis triggers in a large tertiary care hospital in Qatar: A retrospective study. *World Allergy Organ. J.* **2018**, *11*, 20. [CrossRef] [PubMed]
29. Okubo, Y.; Nochioka, K.; Testa, M.A. Nationwide Survey of Hospitalization Due to Pediatric Food-Induced Anaphylaxis in the United States. *Pediatr. Emerg. Care* **2019**, *35*, 769–773. [CrossRef]
30. Dinakar, C. Anaphylaxis in Children: Current Understanding and Key Issues in Diagnosis and Treatment. *Curr. Allergy Asthma Rep.* **2012**, *12*, 641–649. [CrossRef]
31. Ramsey, N.B.; Guffey, D.; Anagnostou, K.; Coleman, N.E.; Davis, C.M. Epidemiology of Anaphylaxis in Critically Ill Children in the United States and Canada. *J. Allergy Clin. Immunol. Pract.* **2019**, *7*, 2241–2249. [CrossRef]
32. Krmpotic, K.; Weisser, C.; O'Hanley, A.; Soder, C. Incidence and Outcomes of Severe Anaphylaxis in Paediatric Patients in Atlantic Canada. *J. Pediatr. Intensive Care* **2019**, *8*, 113–116. [CrossRef]
33. Sundquist, B.K.; Jose, J.; Pauze, D.; Pauze, D.; Wang, H.; Järvinen, K.M. Anaphylaxis risk factors for hospitalization and intensive care: A comparison between adults and children in an upstate New York emergency department. *Allergy Asthma Proc.* **2019**, *40*, 41–47. [CrossRef] [PubMed]
34. Turner, P.J.; Gowland, M.H.; Sharma, V.; Ierodiakonou, D.; Harper, N.; Garcez, T.; Pumphrey, R.; Boyle, R.J. Increase in anaphylaxis-related hospitalizations but no increase in fatalities: An analysis of United Kingdom national anaphylaxis data, 1992–2012. *J. Allergy Clin. Immunol.* **2015**, *135*, 956–963.e1. [CrossRef] [PubMed]
35. Ma, L.; Danoff, T.M.; Borish, L. Case fatality and population mortality associated with anaphylaxis in the United States. *J. Allergy Clin. Immunol.* **2014**, *133*, 1075–1083. [CrossRef] [PubMed]
36. Mullins, R.J.; Wainstein, B.K.; Barnes, E.H.; Liew, W.K.; Campbell, D.E. Increases in anaphylaxis fatalities in Australia from 1997 to 2013. *Clin. Exp. Allergy* **2016**, *46*, 1099–1110. [CrossRef] [PubMed]
37. González-Pérez, A.; Aponte, Z.; Vidaurre, C.F.; Rodríguez, L.A.G. Anaphylaxis epidemiology in patients with and patients without asthma: A United Kingdom database review. *J. Allergy Clin. Immunol.* **2010**, *125*, 1098–1104.e1. [CrossRef] [PubMed]
38. Simons, F.E.R.; Ardusso, L.R.; Bilò, M.B.; El-Gamal, Y.M.; Ledford, D.K.; Ring, J.; Sanchez-Borges, M.; Senna, G.E.; Sheikh, A.; Thong, B.Y.; et al. World Allergy Organization Guidelines for the Assessment and Management of Anaphylaxis. *World Allergy Organ. J.* **2011**, *4*, 13–37. [CrossRef]
39. Muraro, A.; Roberts, G.; Worm, M.; Bilò, M.B.; Brockow, K.; Fernández Rivas, M.; Santos, A.F.; Zolkipli, Z.Q.; Bellou, A.; Beyer, K.; et al. Anaphylaxis: Guidelines from the European Academy of Allergy and Clinical Immunology. *Allergy* **2014**, *69*, 1026–1045. [CrossRef]
40. Simons, F.E.R.; Ardusso, L.R.; Bilò, M.B.; Cardona, V.; Ebisawa, M.; El-Gamal, Y.M.; Lieberman, P.; Lockey, R.F.; Muraro, A.; Roberts, G.; et al. International consensus on (ICON) anaphylaxis. *World Allergy Organ. J.* **2014**, *7*, 9. [CrossRef]
41. Greenhawt, M.; Gupta, R.S.; Meadows, J.A.; Pistiner, M.; Spergel, J.M.; Camargo, C.A.; Simons, F.E.R.; Lieberman, P.L. Guiding Principles for the Recognition, Diagnosis, and Management of Infants with Anaphylaxis: An Expert Panel Consensus. *J. Allergy Clin. Immunol. Pract.* **2019**, *7*, 1148–1156.e5. [CrossRef]
42. Clark, S.; Wei, W.; Rudders, S.A.; Camargo, C.A., Jr. Risk factors for severe anaphylaxis in patients receiving anaphylaxis treatment in US emergency departments and hospitals. *J. Allergy Clin. Immunol.* **2014**, *134*, 1125–1130. [CrossRef]
43. Motosue, M.S.; Bellolio, M.F.; Van Houten, H.K.; Shah, N.D.; Campbell, R.L. Risk factors for severe anaphylaxis in the United States. *Ann. Allergy Asthma Immunol.* **2017**, *119*, 356–361.e2. [CrossRef] [PubMed]
44. Bock, S.A.; Muñoz-Furlong, A.; Sampson, H.A. Further fatalities caused by anaphylactic reactions to food, 2001–2006. *J. Allergy Clin. Immunol.* **2007**, *119*, 1016–1018. [CrossRef]
45. Bock, S.; Muñoz-Furlong, A.; Sampson, H.A. Fatalities due to anaphylactic reactions to foods. *J. Allergy Clin. Immunol.* **2001**, *107*, 191–193. [CrossRef] [PubMed]
46. Summers, C.W.; Pumphrey, R.S.; Woods, C.N.; McDowell, G.; Pemberton, P.W.; Arkwright, P.D. Factors predicting anaphylaxis to peanuts and tree nuts in patients referred to a specialist center. *J. Allergy Clin. Immunol.* **2008**, *121*, 632–638.e2. [CrossRef] [PubMed]
47. Lieberman, P. The Risk and Management of Anaphylaxis in the Setting of Immunotherapy. *Am. J. Rhinol. Allergy* **2012**, *26*, 469–474. [CrossRef]

Disclaimer/Publisher's Note: The statements, opinions and data contained in all publications are solely those of the individual author(s) and contributor(s) and not of MDPI and/or the editor(s). MDPI and/or the editor(s) disclaim responsibility for any injury to people or property resulting from any ideas, methods, instructions or products referred to in the content.

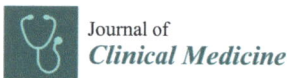

Article

Switching to Dupilumab from Other Biologics without a Treatment Interval in Patients with Severe Asthma: A Multi-Center Retrospective Study

Hisao Higo [1,2,3], Hirohisa Ichikawa [4], Yukako Arakawa [4], Yoshihiro Mori [4], Junko Itano [5], Akihiko Taniguchi [2], Satoru Senoo [2], Goro Kimura [5], Yasushi Tanimoto [5], Kohei Miyake [6], Tomoya Katsuta [7], Mikio Kataoka [8], Yoshinobu Maeda [2], Katsuyuki Kiura [1], Nobuaki Miyahara [1,9,*] and Okayama Respiratory Disease Study Group (ORDSG)

[1] Department of Allergy and Respiratory Medicine, Okayama University Hospital, Okayama 700-8558, Japan; prea4jsb@s.okayama-u.ac.jp (H.H.)
[2] Department of Hematology, Oncology, and Respiratory Medicine, Okayama University Graduate School of Medicine, Dentistry, and Pharmaceutical Sciences, Okayama 700-8558, Japan
[3] Department of Internal Medicine, Kagawa Rosai Hospital, Marugame 763-8502, Japan
[4] Department of Respiratory Medicine, KKR Takamatsu Hospital, Takamatsu 760-0018, Japan
[5] Department of Allergy and Respiratory Medicine, National Hospital Organization Minami-Okayama Medical Center, Okayama 701-0304, Japan
[6] Department of Respiratory Medicine, National Hospital Organization Himeji Medical Center, Himeji 670-8520, Japan
[7] Department of Respiratory Medicine, Ehime Prefectural Central Hospital, Matsuyama 790-0024, Japan
[8] Department of Respiratory Medicine, Onomichi Municipal Hospital, Onomichi 722-8503, Japan
[9] Department of Medical Technology, Okayama University Graduate School of Health Sciences, Okayama 700-8558, Japan
* Correspondence: miyahara@md.okayama-u.ac.jp

Abstract: Background: Dupilumab is a fully humanized monoclonal antibody that blocks interleukin-4 and interleukin-13 signals. Several large clinical trials have demonstrated the efficacy of dupilumab in patients with severe asthma. However, few studies have examined a switch to dupilumab from other biologics. Methods: This retrospective, multi-center observational study was conducted by the Okayama Respiratory Disease Study Group. Consecutive patients with severe asthma who were switched to dupilumab from other biologics without a treatment interval between May 2019 and September 2021 were enrolled. Patients with a treatment interval of more than twice the standard dosing interval for the previous biologic prior to dupilumab administration were excluded. Results: The median patient age of the 27 patients enrolled in this study was 57 years (IQR, 45–68 years). Eosinophilic chronic rhinosinusitis (ECRS)/chronic rhinosinusitis with nasal polyp (CRSwNP) was confirmed in 23 patients. Previous biologics consisted of omalizumab (n = 3), mepolizumab (n = 3), and benralizumab (n = 21). Dupilumab significantly improved FEV_1 (median improvement: +145 mL) and the asthma control test score (median improvement: +2). The overall response rate in patients receiving dupilumab for asthma as determined using the Global Evaluations of Treatment Effectiveness (GETE) was 77.8%. There were no significant differences in the baseline characteristics of the GETE-improved group vs. the non-GETE-improved group. ECRS/CRSwNP improved in 20 of the 23 patients (87.0%). Overall, 8 of the 27 patients (29.6%) developed transient hypereosinophilia (>1500/μL), but all were asymptomatic and able to continue dupilumab therapy. Conclusions: Dupilumab was highly effective for the treatment of severe asthma and ECRS/CRSwNP, even in patients switched from other biologics without a treatment interval.

Keywords: dupilumab; severe asthma; treatment interval; eosinophilic chronic rhinosinusitis

1. Introduction

Asthma is a common disease that affects 300 million people worldwide [1]. The estimated prevalence of severe asthma is 3–10% of the total asthmatic population [2]. As the molecular mechanisms involved in the pathogenesis of asthma have been gradually elucidated, new biological therapies have been developed to treat severe asthma. The first biologic for severe asthma was the anti-IgE monoclonal antibody omalizumab, which suppresses allergic reactions by inhibiting IgE binding to high-affinity receptors on mast cells and basophils [3]. Omalizumab has been shown to reduce the rate of asthma exacerbation significantly [4]. The anti-interleukin-5 (IL-5) monoclonal antibody mepolizumab and the anti-IL-5 receptor α (IL-5Rα) monoclonal antibody benralizumab, both available in Japan, deplete eosinophils by binding to IL-5 or IL-5Rα, thus ameliorating eosinophilic inflammation of the airways in asthma patients [5].

Dupilumab (Dupixent®) is the fourth biologic to become available in Japan since 2018. It is a fully humanized monoclonal antibody of the IgG4 type, and it recognizes the alpha subunit of the IL-4 receptor α (IL-4Rα), blocking both IL-4 and IL-13 signals [6]. IL-4 induces the differentiation of type-2 helper T (Th2) cells and group 2 innate lymphoid cells (ILC2), and IgE production from B cells. Th2 cells and ILC2 produce IL-5 and activate eosinophils. IL-4 and IL-13 enhance the expression of adhesion molecules on endothelial cells and induce the production of chemokines such as eotaxin by airway epithelial cells, thereby recruiting eosinophils from the blood circulation to the airway mucosa. As a result of these mechanisms, IL-4 and IL-13 induce type-2 inflammation [7]. Several large clinical trials in patients with severe asthma have shown that dupilumab reduces asthma exacerbations, improves scores in obstructive pulmonary impairment and asthma control tests, and decreases the oral corticosteroid dose [8–11]. As the fourth biologic for asthma approved in Japan, dupilumab is likely to be administered to patients previously treated with other biologics. However, few studies have examined the effect of a switch to dupilumab from those biologics [12–14], and no study has focused on patients who were switched without a treatment interval. A long interval before a switch to dupilumab complicates comparisons of efficacy vs. previous biologics. Therefore, we conducted a retrospective study to examine the efficacy of dupilumab in patients who were switched from other biologics without a treatment interval.

2. Materials and Methods

2.1. Study Design

This retrospective, multi-center observational study was conducted by the Okayama Respiratory Disease Study Group. Participating institutions included Okayama University Hospital, KKR Takamatsu Hospital, National Hospital Organization Minami-Okayama Medical Center, National Hospital Organization Himeji Medical Center, Ehime Prefectural Central Hospital, Kagawa Rosai Hospital, and Onomichi Municipal Hospital. The study was approved by the institutional review boards of Okayama University Hospital (no. 2112–034) and all other participating hospitals. The requirement for written informed consent was waived because of the retrospective nature of the study. Consecutive patients with severe asthma who were switched to dupilumab at a dose of 300 mg (loading dose, 600 mg) every 2 weeks from other biologics between May 2019 and September 2021 were enrolled. Asthma was diagnosed based on the Japanese guidelines and the Global Initiative of Asthma guidelines [15,16]. ECRS/CRSwNP was diagnosed using the Japanese Epidemiological Survey of Refractory Eosinophilic Chronic Rhinosinusitis scoring system [17]. To compare the effects of previous biologics and dupilumab, patients with a treatment interval of more than twice the standard dosing interval for the previous biologic prior to dupilumab administration were excluded. Patients treated with the respective biologic for <3 months were also excluded. A high dose of inhaled corticosteroid (ICS) was defined as a total daily dose of fluticasone propionate of 1000 µg or equivalent. A medium dose of ICS was defined as a total daily dose of fluticasone propionate of 500 µg or equivalent. The clinical data of patients, including disease duration, body mass index, smoking history, allergies, comorbidities, treatment, blood eosinophil count, exhaled nitric oxide (FeNO), serum IgE level, and pulmonary function test, were collected from their medical records. Because biologics affect the levels of several biomarkers (blood eosinophil count, FeNO, and serum IgE), data prior to their administration were used to evaluate the characteristics of the study patients.

2.2. Study Assessments

The FeNO level was measured using a NIOX VERO™ device (Aerocrine AB, Stockholm, Sweden). The primary efficacy outcomes included the physician-reported Global Evaluation of Treatment Effectiveness (GETE) [4,18,19], in which the outcome is ranked as excellent (complete control of asthma), good (marked improvement), moderate (discernible but limited improvement), poor (no appreciable change), or worse. A GETE responder is defined as a patient with an excellent/good response to treatment with biologic agents. The GETE score determined after the introduction of the previous biologic was used if the overall evaluation did not change after the switch to dupilumab. Asthmatic symptoms were evaluated using the asthma control test (ACT), a clinically useful scoring system. This test contains five questions related to the frequency of asthma symptoms and rescue medication use during the previous 4 weeks [20]. Patients with ACT scores of 20–25 are considered to have well-controlled asthma, with a minimal clinically important difference in the ACT score of 3 points [21]. Dupilumab efficacy was evaluated between 3 months and 1 year in most cases.

2.3. Statistical Analysis

Statistical analyses were performed using EZR software version 1.36 (Saitama Medical Center, Jichi Medical University, Saitama, Japan) [22]. Patient characteristics were compared using Fisher's exact test for binary variables. Continuous variables were evaluated using the Mann–Whitney U test or the Wilcoxon signed-rank test. A p-value < 0.05 was considered to indicate statistical significance.

3. Results

3.1. Clinical Characteristics

Table 1 shows the clinical characteristics of the 27 patients with severe asthma who were enrolled in this study. Comorbidities included allergic bronchopulmonary aspergillosis (n = 3), eosinophilic chronic rhinosinusitis (ECRS)/chronic rhinosinusitis with nasal polyp (CRSwNP) (n = 23), and eosinophilic otitis media (EOM) (n = 11). All patients were treated with ICS, and nine patients (33.3%) received maintenance OCS, including five for the treatment of asthma. Previous biologics treatments consisted of omalizumab (n = 3), mepolizumab (n = 3), and benralizumab (n = 21). The median period of treatment with these previous biologics was 421 days (interquartile range (IQR), 301–673 days). Dupilumab was administered as a second-line biologic to 19 patients, as a third-line biologic to 7 patients, and as a fourth-line biologic to 1 patient.

Levels of three biomarkers of type-2 inflammation (blood eosinophil count, serum IgE, and FeNO) before the use of any biologics are shown in Table 1. Although analysis was not performed for all cases due to missing data, the percentages of patients with a blood eosinophil count >150/µL, a serum IgE level of >167 IU/mL, and an FeNO value of >25 ppb were 80.8% (21 of 26 patients), 80.0% (16 of 20 patients), and 85.7% (18 of 21 patients), respectively. In 6 of the 27 patients, the blood eosinophil count was >1500/µL. All but one case, in which the values of all biomarkers were not obtained, were positive for at least one biomarker. Despite the previous treatment with biologics, 18 of 19 patients had FeNO values greater than 25 ppb (94.7%).

The reasons for switching biologics included persistent asthmatic symptoms, persistent ECRS/CRSwNP symptoms, persistent EOM symptoms, and self-administration (Table 2). Asthma symptoms were among the reasons for switching in only 44% of cases, while ECRS was the reason for switching in 67% of cases.

Table 1. Clinical characteristics of the 27 study patients.

Characteristics	n = 27
Age, years—median (IQR)	57 (45–68)
Male sex—n (%)	15 (55.6)
Disease duration, years—median (IQR)	12 (8–26)
Body mass index—median (IQR)	24.3 (20.0–27.4)
Smoking history	
Never—n (%)	16 (59.3)
Former or current—n (%)	11 (40.7)
ACT—median (IQR)	20.5 (16–23) *
Allergies—n (%)	16 (59.3)
Comorbidity	
ABPA—n (%)	3 (11.1)
ECRS—n (%)	23 (85.2)
EOM—n (%)	11 (40.7)
AD—n (%)	2 (7.4)
AR—n (%)	10 (37.0)
Treatment	
High dose ICS—n (%)	18 (66.7)
Medium dose ICS—n (%)	9 (33.3)
LABA—n (%)	26 (96.3)
LAMA—n (%)	14 (51.9)
LTRA—n (%)	18 (66.7)
Xanthine—n (%)	8 (29.6)
Maintenance OCS—n (%)	9 (33.3)
Previous biologics	
Omalizumab—n (%)	3 (11.1)
Mepolizumab—n (%)	3 (11.1)
Benralizumab—n (%)	21 (77.8)
Treatment period—median (IQR)	421 (301–673)
Biomarkers (before the use of any biologics)	
Blood eosinophil count (/µL)—median (IQR)	690 (352–1407) *
Serum IgE (IU/mL)—median (IQR)	436 (188–881) †
FeNO (ppb)—median (IQR)	82 (56–116) ‡
FeNO before dupilumab use (ppb)—median (IQR)	60 (37–77) ‡
Pulmonary function	
FEV_1 (L)—median (IQR)	1.84 (1.50–2.39) ‡
%FEV_1 (%)—median (IQR)	80.0% (60.1–84.9) ‡
FEV_1/FVC (%)—median (IQR)	63.5 (54.0–75.3) ‡

* Data available for 26 patients. † Data available for 20 patients. ‡ Data available for 21 patients. Abbreviations: ACT, asthma control test; ABPA, allergic bronchopulmonary aspergillosis; ECRS, eosinophilic chronic rhinosinusitis; EOM, eosinophilic otitis media; AD, atopic dermatitis; AR, allergic rhinitis; ICS, inhaled corticosteroid; LABA, long-acting beta-2 agonist; LAMA, long-acting muscarinic antagonist; LTRA, leukotriene receptor antagonist; OCS, oral corticosteroids; FeNO, fractional exhaled nitric oxide; FEV_1, forced expiratory volume in one second; FVC, forced vital capacity; IQR, interquartile range.

Table 2. Reasons for switching biologics.

Reasons (n = 27)	n (%)
Asthmatic symptoms	5 (18.5)
Asthmatic and ECRS symptoms	7 (25.9)
ECRS symptoms	10 (37.0)
EOM symptoms	3 (11.1)
ECRS and EOM symptoms	1 (3.7)
Self-administration	1 (3.7)

Abbreviations: ECRS, eosinophilic chronic rhinosinusitis; EOM, eosinophilic otitis media.

3.2. Efficacy of Dupilumab

Figure 1a,b show the changes in FEV_1 and %FEV_1 values before and after dupilumab administration. Dupilumab significantly improved FEV_1 in the 20 patients for whom data were available (median improvement in FEV_1 of +145 mL; IQR, +88–358 mL; $p < 0.01$). FEV_1 decreased slightly in 2 patients (−20 mL and −70 mL) but increased in the remaining 18 patients, especially in 7 patients (35.0%) who had an improvement of >200 mL. The %FEV_1 improved by >5% in 55% of the patients; the median improvement was +5.4% (IQR, +3.0–15.9%; $p < 0.01$). It also significantly improved the ACT scores of 20 patients for whom data were available (Figure 1c). Only one patient had a one-point drop in the ACT score, whereas eight patients had a score improvement of ≥3 points. The median improvement in the ACT score was +2 (IQR, +1–5; $p < 0.01$).

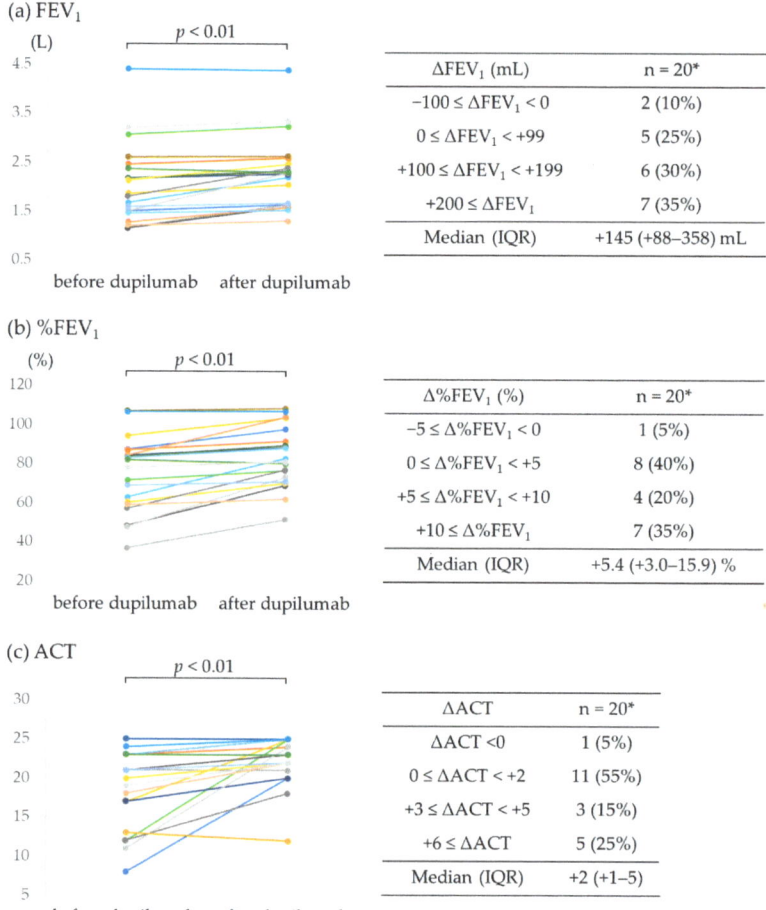

Figure 1. Effect of dupilumab on FEV_1 and ACT score. (**a**) FEV_1, (**b**) %FEV_1, and (**c**) ACT score before and after dupilumab administration. * Data available for 20 patients.

Table 3 shows the efficacy of dupilumab and previous biologics for the treatment of severe asthma based on the GETE. The overall responder rate (excellent/good) following dupilumab treatment was 77.8%. After switching, scores improved in 14 patients (51.9%) but deteriorated in 1 patient. Among the 15 patients for whom an improvement in asthma symptoms was not the reason for the switch to dupilumab, an improved GETE was recorded in 5 patients (33.3%). A decrease in the OCS dose was possible in four of the nine OCS-treated patients.

Table 3. GETE score of dupilumab-treated patients (n = 27).

GETE Score	Previous Biologics: n (%)	Dupilumab: n (%)
Excellent	3 (11.1)	6 (22.2)
Good	8 (29.6)	15 (55.6)
Moderate	12 (44.4)	4 (14.8)
Poor	4 (14.8)	1 (3.7)
Worsening	0 (0)	1 (3.7)
Excellent/Good	11 (40.7)	21 (77.8)

Abbreviations: GETE, global evaluations of treatment effectiveness.

The trends in FeNO levels from before treatment with any biologics to after dupilumab administration are shown in Figure 2. In all 16 patients for whom FeNO levels were available before and after dupilumab administration, dupilumab reduced levels, with a reduction >100 ppb achieved in 4 patients.

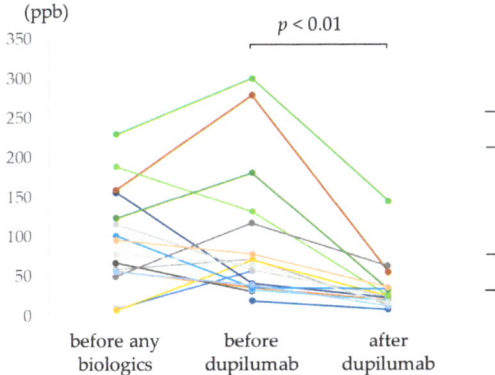

Figure 2. Trends in FeNO levels from before treatment with any biologics to after dupilumab administration. * Data available for 16 patients.

Our study included six patients with blood eosinophil counts >1500/µL before treatment with biologics, all of whom were switched from mepolizumab (n = 1) or benralizumab (n = 5). In four, the FEV_1 increased by >100 mL. In this group, according to the GETE, the overall responder rate (excellent/good) among dupilumab-treated patients was 66.7%.

The GETE-improved and non-improved groups were compared to detect predictors of the efficacy of dupilumab in asthma patients (Table 4). There were no significant differences between the two groups, and no predictors of response based on the GETE in patients switched to dupilumab from other biologics could be identified.

Although our analysis was limited to the 20 patients for whom data were available, the ACT-improved group (+3 ≤ ACT) was compared to the non-improved group (ACT < +3). Both blood eosinophil count before the use of any biologics and FeNO level before the use of dupilumab were significantly higher in the ACT-improved group than in the non-ACT-improved group (Table 5). A comparison of the FEV_1-improved group (100 mL ≤ ΔFEV_1) with the non-improved group (ΔFEV_1 < 100 mL) for the 20 patients for whom data were available did not reveal a significant difference between the two groups (Table 6).

Table 7 shows the efficacy of dupilumab for the treatment of ECRS/CRSwNP as evaluated based on physician assessment. ECRS/CRSwNP improved in 20 of the 23 patients (87.0%) with ECRS/CRSwNP.

Table 4. Comparison between the GETE-improved group and the non-GETE-improved group.

	GETE-Improved (n = 14)	Non-GETE-Improved (n = 13)	p-Value
Age, years—median (IQR)	62 (52–72)	55 (41–60)	0.14
Male sex—n (%)	10 (71.4)	5 (38.5)	0.13
Body mass index—median (IQR)	24.6 (22.8–27.8)	20.8 (18.5–26.4)	0.26
Never smoker—n (%)	6 (42.9)	10 (76.9)	0.12
ABPA—n (%)	3 (21.4)	0 (0)	0.22
ECRS—n (%)	11 (78.6)	12 (92.3)	0.60
EOM—n (%)	7 (50.0)	4 (30.8)	0.44
Maintenance OCS—n (%)	4 (28.6)	5 (38.5)	0.70
Biomarkers (before the use of any biologics)			
Blood eosinophil count (/μL)—median (IQR)	601 (270–1144)	703 (498–1695)	0.53
Serum IgE (IU/mL)—median (IQR)	395 (296–710)	272 (135–584)	0.43
FeNO (ppb)—median (IQR)	82 (50–124)	87 (57–103)	0.97
FeNO before dupilumab use (ppb)—median (IQR)	71 (49–125)	51 (36–68)	0.39

Abbreviations: GETE, global evaluations of treatment effectiveness; ABPA, allergic bronchopulmonary aspergillosis; ECRS, eosinophilic chronic rhinosinusitis; EOM, eosinophilic otitis media; OCS, oral corticosteroids; FeNO, fractional exhaled nitric oxide; IQR, interquartile range.

Table 5. Comparison between the ACT-improved group and the non-improved group.

	ACT-Improved (n = 8)	Non-ACT-Improved (n = 12)	p-Value
Age, years—median (IQR)	56 (43–64)	60 (46–73)	0.33
Male sex—n (%)	4 (50.0)	8 (66.7)	0.65
Body mass index—median (IQR)	25.5 (23.0–27.7)	21.2 (19.4–25.0)	0.22
Never smoker—n (%)	5 (62.5)	7 (58.3)	1.00
ABPA—n (%)	2 (25.0)	0 (0)	0.15
ECRS—n (%)	7 (87.5)	9 (75.0)	0.62
EOM—n (%)	3 (37.5)	5 (41.7)	1.00
Maintenance OCS—n (%)	3 (37.5)	2 (16.7)	0.35
Biomarkers (before the use of any biologics)			
Blood eosinophil count (/μL)—median (IQR)	1045 (699–1682)	439 (95–516) *	<0.01
Serum IgE (IU/mL)—median (IQR)	388 (183–710) †	272 (150–433) ‡	0.54
FeNO (ppb)—median (IQR)	87 (40–126)	67 (57–101) §	0.89
FeNO before dupilumab use (ppb)—median (IQR)	68 (58–88)	36 (33–47) ‡	0.04

* Data available for 11 patients. † Data available for 7 patients. ‡ Data available for 8 patients. § Data available for 9 patients. Abbreviations: ACT, asthma control test; ABPA, allergic bronchopulmonary aspergillosis; ECRS, eosinophilic chronic rhinosinusitis; EOM, eosinophilic otitis media; OCS, oral corticosteroids; FeNO, fractional exhaled nitric oxide; IQR, interquartile range.

3.3. Adverse Events

Figure 3a shows blood eosinophil counts before the use of any biologics, before the use of dupilumab, and after the use of dupilumab. Transient hypereosinophilia >1500/μL occurred in 8 of the 27 study patients (29.6%), and a value >3000/μL was observed in 3 patients (11.1%). The highest blood eosinophil count value was 5546/μL. The median time for the blood eosinophil count to reach its highest value was 182 days (IQR, 113–283 days). All patients with dupilumab-induced hypereosinophilia were asymptomatic. Dupilumab was interrupted due to hypereosinophilia in one patient but was later resumed. One patient had an adverse event of diarrhea, but dupilumab was continued. Figure 3b shows the changes in the eosinophil counts of the six patients with blood eosinophil counts >1500/μL before the use of any biologics. In four of the patients (66.7%), blood eosinophil counts increased to >1500/μL after dupilumab administration. All patients were asymptomatic and were able to continue dupilumab therapy.

Table 6. Comparison between the FEV$_1$-improved group and the non-improved group.

	FEV$_1$-Improved (n = 14)	Non-FEV$_1$-Improved (n = 6)	p-Value
Age, years—median (IQR)	62 (57–69)	46 (44–67)	0.54
Male sex—n (%)	10 (71.4)	3 (50.0)	0.61
Body mass index—median (IQR)	23.2 (20.5–25.8)	27.2 (22.6–32.0)	0.19
Never smoker—n (%)	6 (42.9)	5 (83.3)	0.16
ABPA—n (%)	1 (7.1)	1 (16.7)	0.52
ECRS—n (%)	12 (85.7)	5 (83.3)	1.00
EOM—n (%)	6 (42.9)	2 (33.3)	1.00
Maintenance OCS—n (%)	4 (28.6)	1 (16.7)	1.00
Biomarkers (before the use of any biologics)			
Blood eosinophil count (/μL)—median (IQR)	692 (460–1848)	488 (359–1059)	0.44
Serum IgE (IU/mL)—median (IQR)	395 (157–710) *	188 (150–206) †	0.28
FeNO (ppb)—median (IQR)	73 (55–100) ‡	101 (56–124) §	0.57
FeNO before dupilumab use (ppb)—median (IQR)	68 (57–77) ¶	39 (36–41) §	0.27

* Data available for 11 patients. † Data available for 4 patients. ‡ Data available for 12 patients. § Data available for 5 patients. ¶ Data available for 10 patients. Abbreviations: FEV$_1$, forced expiratory volume in one second; ABPA, allergic bronchopulmonary aspergillosis; ECRS, eosinophilic chronic rhinosinusitis; EOM, eosinophilic otitis media; OCS, oral corticosteroids; FeNO, fractional exhaled nitric oxide; IQR, interquartile range.

Table 7. Efficacy of dupilumab for ECRS based on assessment of each physician.

ECRS Symptoms (n = 23)	no. (%)
Improved	20 (87.0)
No change	3 (13.0)
Worsening	0 (0)

Abbreviations: ECRS, eosinophilic chronic rhinosinusitis.

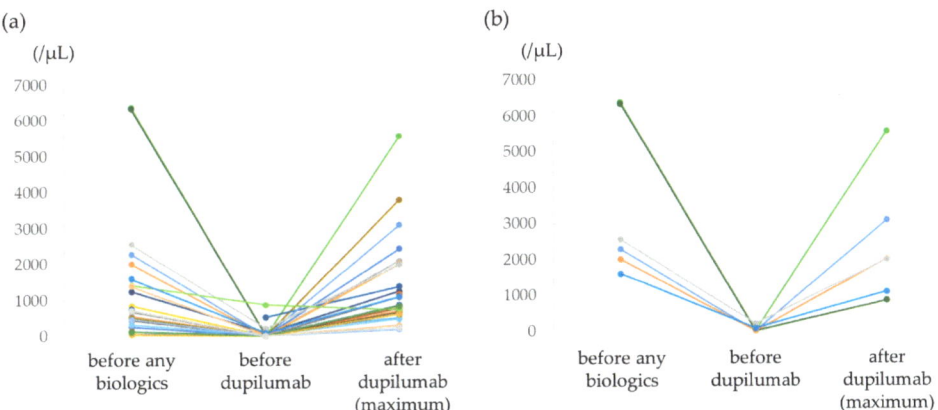

Figure 3. Trends in blood eosinophil counts from before treatment with any biologics to after dupilumab therapy. (**a**) All patients, (**b**) the six patients with blood eosinophil counts >1500/μL.

4. Discussion

A switch to dupilumab therapy has been examined in a few studies. Dupin et al. reported the efficacy of dupilumab in patients with severe asthma, nearly all (97%) with a history of biologics treatment [12]. The study showed significant improvements in ACT scores and FEV$_1$ values after dupilumab administration. Another study of 16 patients with a history of biologics treatment found that dupilumab was effective for preventing exacerbations and reducing the steroid dose [13]. However, those studies did not specify the period between discontinuation of the previous biologic and dupilumab administration.

Mümmler et al. reported the efficacy of a switch to dupilumab therapy. After the switch, patients had better asthma control, improved lung function, and decreased FeNO, total IgE, OCS dosage, and exacerbation rate [14]. The study allowed up to 6 months between the switch to dupilumab and the discontinuation of a previous biologic.

Despite the demonstrated efficacy of dupilumab in patients with a history of biologics treatment reported in previous studies, it is difficult to compare the efficacy of dupilumab with that of previous biologics due to differences in the interval before dupilumab initiation. The present study, however, was limited to a short switching interval and thus allowed a clear comparison between previous biologics and dupilumab. Our results show that dupilumab improved lung function and symptoms in the absence of a treatment interval following the discontinuation of previous biologics. The switch to dupilumab also led to a reduction in FeNO. In the QUEST study, dupilumab treatment significantly reduced FeNO levels [8], as is also reported for other biologics [23–25]. Our results similarly imply that dupilumab is more effective than other biologics in decreasing FeNO levels.

While some patients with severe asthma clearly responded better to dupilumab than to other biologics, we were unable to identify the predictors of a better response. GETE-improved and non-improved groups were compared to identify the predictors of dupilumab efficacy for the treatment of asthma. Blood eosinophil counts and FeNO were promising candidates, as their predictive ability was previously reported [8,9]. Dupilumab resulted in a greater benefit with respect to the prevention of severe asthma exacerbation, an improved FEV_1, and reduced glucocorticoid use among patients with relatively high blood eosinophil counts and FeNO levels. However, neither blood eosinophil count nor FeNO level could be confirmed as predictive of a response to dupilumab as defined by the GETE. Patients with a high blood eosinophil count or a high FeNO level are more likely to respond to other biologics, as well as to dupilumab [26–31]. Therefore, it may be difficult to predict whether dupilumab is more likely to be effective based on these biomarkers. In addition, ECRS/CRSwNP patients have elevated FeNO levels [32]. In the present study, 85.2% of patients had concomitant ECRS/CRSwNP, which may have influenced their FeNO levels, reducing the predictability of efficacy. Nonetheless, a previous study reported that FeNO levels were predictive of efficacy, even in patients who had switched biologics [14]. Our analysis based on the ACT also indicated higher FeNO levels before the use of dupilumab and higher blood eosinophil counts before the use of any biologics in the ACT-improved group than in the non-ACT-improved group. Therefore, while these biomarkers may be candidates, larger studies are needed to identify clear predictors of efficacy in patients who have switched to dupilumab from other biologics.

The efficacy of dupilumab in asthma patients with blood eosinophil counts >1500/μL was not established in the QUEST trial because it excluded these patients at screening [8]. In our study, the six patients with blood eosinophil counts >1500/μL were switched from anti-IL-5/IL-5 receptor antibody to dupilumab, resulting in an improved FEV_1 and a high response rate (66.7%) based on the GETE. These results imply that dupilumab is a worthwhile treatment option, even in patients with blood eosinophil counts >1500/μL, a condition under which anti-IL-5/IL-5 receptor antibody treatment is preferred.

The high efficacy of dupilumab determined in this study may have been influenced by patient selection. Among our patients, the proportion with ECRS/CRSwNP was very high (85.2%) and was higher than the proportion in severe asthma cohorts enrolled in recent randomized controlled trials (~20%) [8,33]. A post hoc analysis of the QUEST trial data implied higher dupilumab efficacy in patients with complicated chronic sinusitis [33]. Further studies are needed to determine whether dupilumab is equally effective for patients without ECRS/CRSwNP.

We observed that dupilumab improved ECRS/CRSwNP in 20 of the 23 patients (87.0%). Although other biologics (omalizumab, mepolizumab, benralizumab) have also been reported to be effective against ECRS/CRSwNP [34–36], the high efficacy of dupilumab in our switched cases implies that it is more effective against ECRS/CRSwNP than the other biologics.

Previous analyses of dupilumab-related adverse events among patients in clinical trials have reported that hypereosinophilia (>3000/μL) developed in 1–13% of them [7,8,37,38]. Most of these events occurred in patients with high baseline eosinophil levels (>500/μL) and were not associated with symptoms or discontinuation of therapy [38]. In our study, 11.1% of patients had eosinophilia >3000/μL, but all were asymptomatic and were able to continue dupilumab therapy. Although hypereosinophilia should be monitored, dupilumab was safe in patients switched from other biologics, even for those with baseline blood eosinophil counts >1500/μL.

Our study had several limitations. First, it was retrospective, was non-randomized, and had a small sample size. Second, some data were missing due to the retrospective nature of the study. Third, because of the high proportion of patients with ECRS/CRSwNP complications, it could not be determined whether our results can be generalized to all patients with severe asthma. Fourth, as 77.8% of patients switched from benralizumab, the efficacy of dupilumab in patients switching from omalizumab or mepolizumab could not be adequately studied. To address these limitations, larger prospective observational studies are needed that stratify patients according to ECRS/CRSwNP status and previous biologics. Despite these limitations, the real-world data provided by our study support the efficacy and safety of a therapeutic switch to dupilumab, particularly for patients with ECRS/CRSwNP.

5. Conclusions

Dupilumab is expected to be highly effective for the treatment of severe asthma and ECRS/CRSwNP, even in patients who are switched from other biologics without a treatment interval.

Author Contributions: Conceptualization, H.H, A.T, S.S., N.M. and ORDSG; methodology, H.H, A.T, S.S., N.M. and ORDSG; formal analysis, H.H., H.I., J.I., A.T., S.S. and N.M.; investigation, H.H., H.I., Y.A., Y.M. (Yoshihiro Mori), J.I., A.T., S.S., G.K., Y.T., K.M., T.K., M.K., N.M. and ORDSG; resources, H.H., H.I., Y.A., Y.M. (Yoshihiro Mori), J.I., A.T., S.S., G.K., Y.T., K.M., T.K., M.K., Y.M. (Yoshinobu Maeda), K.K. and N.M.; data curation, H.H., H.I., Y.M. (Yoshihiro Mori), J.I., K.M., T.K., N.M. and ORDSG; writing—original draft preparation, H.H., H.I. and N.M.; writing—review and editing, H.H., H.I., Y.A., Y.M. (Yoshihiro Mori), J.I., A.T., S.S., G.K., Y.T., K.M., T.K., M.K., Y.M. (Yoshinobu Maeda), K.K. and N.M.; visualization, H.H., Y.M. (Yoshinobu Maeda), K.K. and N.M.; supervision, Y.M. (Yoshinobu Maeda), K.K. and N.M. All authors have read and agreed to the published version of the manuscript.

Funding: This research received no external funding.

Institutional Review Board Statement: This study was carried out according to the principles of the Declaration of Helsinki for human investigations and approved by the local Ethics Committee (no. 2112-034).

Informed Consent Statement: The requirement for written informed consent was waived because of the retrospective nature of the study.

Data Availability Statement: The data presented in this study are available on request from the corresponding author.

Conflicts of Interest: The authors declare no conflict of interest.

References

1. Brusselle, G.G.; Koppelman, G.H. Biologic therapies for severe asthma. *N. Engl. J. Med.* **2022**, *386*, 157–171. [CrossRef] [PubMed]
2. Hekking, P.W.; Wener, R.R.; Amelink, M.; Zwinderman, A.H.; Bouvy, M.L.; Bel, E.H. The prevalence of severe refractory asthma. *J. Allergy Clin. Immunol.* **2015**, *135*, 896–902. [CrossRef] [PubMed]
3. Pelaia, G.; Gallelli, L.; Renda, T.; Romeo, P.; Busceti, M.T.; Grembiale, R.D.; Maselli, R.; Marsico, S.A.; Vatrella, A. Update on optimal use of omalizumab in management of asthma. *J. Asthma Allergy* **2011**, *4*, 49–59. [CrossRef]
4. Humbert, M.; Beasley, R.; Ayres, J.; Slavin, R.; Hébert, J.; Bousquet, J.; Beeh, K.M.; Ramos, S.; Canonica, G.W.; Hedgecock, S.; et al. Benefits of omalizumab as add-on therapy in patients with severe persistent asthma who are inadequately controlled despite best available therapy (GINA 2002 step 4 treatment): INNOVATE. *Allergy* **2005**, *60*, 309–316. [CrossRef] [PubMed]

5. Farne, H.A.; Wilson, A.; Powell, C.; Bax, L.; Milan, S.J. Anti-IL5 therapies for asthma. *Cochrane Database Syst. Rev.* **2017**, *9*, CD010834. [CrossRef]
6. Gandhi, N.A.; Pirozzi, G.; Graham, N.M.H. Commonality of the IL-4/IL-13 pathway in atopic diseases. *Expert. Rev. Clin. Immunol.* **2017**, *13*, 425–437. [CrossRef]
7. Maspero, J.; Adir, Y.; Al-Ahmad, M.; Celis-Preciado, C.A.; Colodenco, F.D.; Giavina-Bianchi, P.; Lababidi, H.; Ledanois, O.; Mahoub, B.; Perng, D.-W.; et al. Type 2 inflammation in asthma and other airway diseases. *ERJ Open Res.* **2022**, *8*, 00576–2021. [CrossRef]
8. Castro, M.; Corren, J.; Pavord, I.D.; Maspero, J.; Wenzel, S.; Rabe, K.F.; Busse, W.W.; Ford, L.; Sher, L.; Fitzgerald, J.M.; et al. Dupilumab Efficacy and Safety in Moderate-to-Severe Uncontrolled Asthma. *N. Engl. J. Med.* **2018**, *378*, 2486–2496. [CrossRef]
9. Rabe, K.F.; Nair, P.; Brusselle, G.; Maspero, J.F.; Castro, M.; Sher, L.; Zhu, H.; Hamilton, J.D.; Swanson, B.N.; Khan, A.; et al. Efficacy and safety of dupilumab in glucocorticoid-dependent severe asthma. *N. Engl. J. Med.* **2018**, *378*, 2475–2485. [CrossRef]
10. Wenzel, S.; Ford, L.; Pearlman, D.; Spector, S.; Sher, L.; Skobieranda, F.; Wang, L.; Kirkesseli, S.; Rocklin, R.; Bock, B.; et al. Dupilumab in persistent asthma with elevated eosinophil levels. *N. Engl. J. Med.* **2013**, *368*, 2455–2466. [CrossRef]
11. Wenzel, S.; Castro, M.; Corren, J.; Maspero, J.; Wang, L.; Zhang, B.; Pirozzi, G.; Sutherland, E.R.; Evans, R.R.; Joish, V.N.; et al. Dupilumab efficacy and safety in adults with uncontrolled persistent asthma despite use of medium-to-high-dose inhaled corticosteroids plus a long-acting beta2 agonist: A randomised double-blind placebo-controlled pivotal phase 2b dose-ranging trial. *Lancet* **2016**, *388*, 31–44. [CrossRef] [PubMed]
12. Dupin, C.; Belhadi, D.; Guilleminault, L.; Gamez, A.; Berger, P.; De Blay, F.; Bonniaud, P.; Leroyer, C.; Mahay, G.; Girodet, P.O.; et al. Effectiveness and safety of dupilumab for the treatment of severe asthma in a real-life French multi-centre adult cohort. *Clin. Exp. Allergy* **2020**, *50*, 789–798. [CrossRef] [PubMed]
13. Numata, T.; Araya, J.; Miyagawa, H.; Okuda, K.; Takekoshi, D.; Hashimoto, M.; Minagawa, S.; Ishikawa, T.; Hara, H.; Kuwano, K. Real-World Effectiveness of Dupilumab for Patients with Severe Asthma: A Retrospective Study. *J. Asthma Allergy* **2022**, *15*, 395–405. [CrossRef] [PubMed]
14. Mümmler, C.; Munker, D.; Barnikel, M.; Veit, T.; Kayser, M.Z.; Welte, T.; Behr, J.; Kneidinger, N.; Suhling, H.; Milger, K. Dupilumab improves asthma control and lung function in patients with insufficient outcome during previous antibody therapy. *J. Allergy Clin. Immunol. Pract.* **2021**, *9*, 1177–1185.e4. [CrossRef] [PubMed]
15. Ichinose, M.; Sugiura, H.; Nagase, H.; Yamaguchi, M.; Inoue, H.; Sagara, H.; Tamaoki, J.; Tohda, Y.; Munakata, M.; Yamauchi, K.; et al. Japanese guidelines for adult asthma 2017. *Allergol. Int.* **2017**, *66*, 163–189. [CrossRef] [PubMed]
16. Global Initiative for Asthma. *Asthma Management and Prevention*; Global Initiative for Asthma: Fontana, WI, USA, 2019; Volume 49.
17. Tokunaga, T.; Sakashita, M.; Haruna, T.; Asaka, D.; Takeno, S.; Ikeda, H.; Nakayama, T.; Seki, N.; Ito, S.; Murata, J.; et al. Novel scoring system and algorithm for classifying chronic rhinosinusitis: The JESREC Study. *Allergy* **2015**, *70*, 995–1003. [CrossRef]
18. Humbert, M.; Taille, C.; Mala, L.; Le Gros, V.; Just, J.; Molimard, M. Investigators S: Omalizumab effectiveness in patients with severe allergic asthma according to blood eosinophil count: The STELLAIR study. *Eur. Respir. J.* **2018**, *51*, 1702523. [CrossRef]
19. Lloyd, A.; Turk, F.; Leighton, T.; Walter Canonica, G. Psychometric evaluation of Global Evaluation of Treatment Effectiveness: A tool to assess patients with moderate-to-severe allergic asthma. *J. Med. Econ.* **2007**, *10*, 285–296. [CrossRef]
20. Nathan, R.A.; Sorkness, C.A.; Kosinski, M.; Schatz, M.; Li, J.T.; Marcus, P.; Murray, J.J.; Pendergraft, T.B. Development of the asthma control test: A survey for assessing asthma control. *J. Allergy Clin. Immunol.* **2004**, *113*, 59–65. [CrossRef]
21. Schatz, M.; Kosinski, M.; Yarlas, A.S.; Hanlon, J.; Watson, M.E.; Jhingran, P. The minimally important difference of the Asthma Control Test. *J. Allergy Clin. Immunol.* **2009**, *124*, 719–723.e711. [CrossRef]
22. Kanda, Y. Investigation of the freely available easy-to-use software 'EZR' for medical statistics. *Bone Marrow Transplant.* **2013**, *48*, 452–458. [CrossRef]
23. Kayser, M.Z.; Drick, N.; Milger, K.; Fuge, J.; Kneidinger, N.; Korn, S.; Buhl, R.; Behr, J.; Welte, T.; Suhling, H. Real-world multicenter experience with mepolizumab and benralizumab in the treatment of uncontrolled severe eosinophilic asthma over 12 months. *J. Asthma Allergy* **2021**, *14*, 863–871. [CrossRef] [PubMed]
24. Pelaia, C.; Crimi, C.; Benfante, A.; Caiaffa, M.F.; Calabrese, C.; Carpagnano, G.E.; Ciotta, D.; D'Amato, M.; Macchia, L.; Nolasco, S.; et al. Therapeutic effects of benralizumab assessed in patients with severe eosinophilic asthma: Real-life evaluation correlated with allergic and non-allergic phenotype expression. *J. Asthma Allergy* **2021**, *14*, 163–173. [CrossRef] [PubMed]
25. Pianigiani, T.; Alderighi, L.; Meocci, M.; Messina, M.; Perea, B.; Luzzi, S.; Bergantini, L.; D'Alessandro, M.; Refini, R.M.; Bargagli, E.; et al. Exploring the interaction between fractional exhaled nitric oxide and biologic treatment in severe asthma: A systematic review. *Antioxidants* **2023**, *12*, 400. [CrossRef]
26. FitzGerald, J.M.; Bleecker, E.R.; Menzies-Gow, A.; Zangrilli, J.G.; Hirsch, I.; Metcalfe, P.; Newbold, P.; Goldman, M. Predictors of enhanced response with benralizumab for patients with severe asthma: Pooled analysis of the SIROCCO and CALIMA studies. *Lancet Respir. Med.* **2018**, *6*, 51–64. [CrossRef] [PubMed]
27. Kavanagh, J.E.; Hearn, A.P.; Dhariwal, J.; d'Ancona, G.; Douiri, A.; Roxas, C.; Fernandes, M.; Green, L.; Thomson, L.; Nanzer, A.M.; et al. Real-world effectiveness of benralizumab in severe eosinophilic asthma. *Chest* **2020**, *159*, 496–506. [CrossRef]
28. Sandhu, Y.; Harada, N.; Sasano, H.; Harada, S.; Ueda, S.; Takeshige, T.; Tanabe, Y.; Ishimori, A.; Matsuno, K.; Abe, S.; et al. Pretreatment frequency of circulating th17 cells and feno levels predicted the real-world response after 1 year of benralizumab treatment in patients with severe asthma. *Biomolecules* **2023**, *13*, 538. [CrossRef]

29. Watanabe, H.; Shirai, T.; Hirai, K.; Akamatsu, T.; Nakayasu, H.; Tamura, K.; Masuda, T.; Takahashi, S.; Tanaka, Y.; Kishimoto, Y.; et al. Blood eosinophil count and FeNO to predict benralizumab effectiveness in real-life severe asthma patients. *J. Asthma* **2021**, *59*, 1796–1804. [CrossRef]
30. Menigoz, C.; Dirou, S.; Chambellan, A.; Hassoun, D.; Moui, A.; Magnan, A.; Blanc, F.X. Use of FeNO to predict anti-IL-5 and IL-5R biologics efficacy in a real-world cohort of adults with severe eosinophilic asthma. *J. Asthma* **2023**, *60*, 1162–1170. [CrossRef]
31. Hanania, N.A.; Wenzel, S.; Rosen, K.; Hsieh, H.J.; Mosesova, S.; Choy, D.F.; Lal, P.; Arron, J.R.; Harris, J.M.; Busse, W. Exploring the effects of omalizumab in allergic asthma: An analysis of biomarkers in the EXTRA study. *Am. J. Respir. Crit. Care Med.* **2013**, *187*, 804–811. [CrossRef]
32. Takeno, S.; Taruya, T.; Ueda, T.; Noda, N.; Hirakawa, K. Increased exhaled nitric oxide and its oxidation metabolism in eosinophilic chronic rhinosinusitis. *Auris Nasus Larynx* **2013**, *40*, 458–464. [CrossRef] [PubMed]
33. Maspero, J.F.; Katelaris, C.H.; Busse, W.W.; Castro, M.; Corren, J.; Chipps, B.E.; Peters, A.T.; Pavord, I.D.; Ford, L.B.; Sher, L.; et al. Dupilumab efficacy in uncontrolled, moderate-to-severe asthma with self-reported chronic rhinosinusitis. *J. Allergy Clin. Immunol. Pract.* **2020**, *8*, 527–539.e9. [CrossRef] [PubMed]
34. Gevaert, P.; Omachi, T.A.; Corren, J.; Mullol, J.; Han, J.; Lee, S.E.; Kaufman, D.; Ligueros-Saylan, M.; Howard, M.; Zhu, R.; et al. Efficacy and safety of omalizumab in nasal polyposis: 2 randomized phase 3 trials. *J. Allergy Clin. Immunol.* **2020**, *146*, 595–605. [CrossRef] [PubMed]
35. Han, J.K.; Bachert, C.; Fokkens, W.; Desrosiers, M.; Wagenmann, M.; Lee, S.E.; Smith, S.G.; Martin, N.; Mayer, B.; Yancey, S.W.; et al. Mepolizumab for chronic rhinosinusitis with nasal polyps (SYNAPSE): A randomised, double-blind, placebo-controlled, phase 3 trial. *Lancet Respir. Med.* **2021**, *9*, 1141–1153. [CrossRef]
36. Bachert, C.; Han, J.K.; Desrosiers, M.Y.; Gevaert, P.; Heffler, E.; Hopkins, C.; Tversky, J.R.; Barker, P.; Cohen, D.; Emson, C.; et al. Efficacy and safety of benralizumab in chronic rhinosinusitis with nasal polyps: A randomized, placebo-controlled trial. *J. Allergy Clin. Immunol.* **2022**, *149*, 1309–1317.e1312. [CrossRef]
37. Bachert, C.; Han, J.K.; Desrosiers, M.; Hellings, P.W.; Amin, N.; Lee, S.E.; Mullol, J.; Greos, L.S.; Bosso, J.V.; Laidlaw, T.M.; et al. Efficacy and safety of dupilumab in patients with severe chronic rhinosinusitis with nasal polyps (LIBERTY NP SINUS-24 and LIBERTY NP SINUS-52): Results from two multicentre, randomised, double-blind, placebo-controlled, parallel-group phase 3 trials. *Lancet* **2019**, *394*, 1638–1650. [CrossRef]
38. Wechsler, M.E.; Klion, A.D.; Paggiaro, P.; Nair, P.; Staumont-Salle, D.; Radwan, A.; Johnson, R.R.; Kapoor, U.; Khokhar, F.A.; Daizadeh, N.; et al. Effect of dupilumab on blood eosinophil counts in patients with asthma, chronic rhinosinusitis with nasal polyps, atopic dermatitis, or eosinophilic esophagitis. *J. Allergy Clin. Immunol. Pract.* **2022**, *10*, 2695–2709. [CrossRef]

Disclaimer/Publisher's Note: The statements, opinions and data contained in all publications are solely those of the individual author(s) and contributor(s) and not of MDPI and/or the editor(s). MDPI and/or the editor(s) disclaim responsibility for any injury to people or property resulting from any ideas, methods, instructions or products referred to in the content.

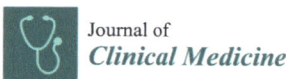 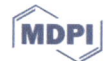

Article

Etiologies of Acute Bronchiolitis in Children at Risk for Asthma, with Emphasis on the Human Rhinovirus Genotyping Protocol

Ahmad R. Alsayed [1,*], Anas Abed [2], Mahmoud Abu-Samak [1], Farhan Alshammari [3] and Bushra Alshammari [4]

[1] Department of Clinical Pharmacy and Therapeutics, Applied Science Private University, Amman 11931, Jordan
[2] Pharmacological and Diagnostic Research Centre, Faculty of Pharmacy, Al-Ahliyya Amman University, Amman 11931, Jordan
[3] Department of Pharmaceutics, College of Pharmacy, University of Hail, Hail 2440, Saudi Arabia
[4] Department of Medical Surgical Nursing, College of Nursing, University of Hail, Hail 2440, Saudi Arabia
* Correspondence: a_alsayed@asu.edu.jo or a.alsayed.phd@gmail.com; Tel.: +962-786770778

Abstract: This research aims to determine acute bronchiolitis' causative virus(es) and establish a viable protocol to classify the Human Rhinovirus (HRV) species. During 2021–2022, we included children 1–24 months of age with acute bronchiolitis at risk for asthma. The nasopharyngeal samples were taken and subjected to a quantitative polymerase chain reaction (qPCR) in a viral panel. For HRV-positive samples, a high-throughput assay was applied, directing the VP4/VP2 and VP3/VP1 regions to confirm species. BLAST searching, phylogenetic analysis, and sequence divergence took place to identify the degree to which these regions were appropriate for identifying and differentiating HRV. HRV ranked second, following RSV, as the etiology of acute bronchiolitis in children. The conclusion of the investigation of all available data in this study distributed sequences into 7 HRV-A, 1 HRV-B, and 7 HRV-C types based on the VP4/VP2 and VP3/VP1 sequences. The nucleotide divergence between the clinical samples and the corresponding reference strains was lower in the VP4/VP2 region than in the VP3/VP1 region. The results demonstrated the potential utility of the VP4/VP2 region and the VP3/VP1 region for differentiating HRV genotypes. Confirmatory outcomes were yielded, indicating how nested and semi-nested PCR can establish practical ways to facilitate HRV sequencing and genotyping.

Keywords: acute bronchiolitis; asthma; genotyping; human rhinovirus; sequencing; virus; bioinformatics

1. Introduction

Due to wheezing, viral respiratory infections are the leading cause of hospitalization among newborns and young children [1]. The most common cause is thought to be respiratory syncytial virus (RSV). Other infections, in addition to *Mycoplasma pneumoniae*, cause wheezing in children, including human metapneumovirus (hMPV), influenza virus, parainfluenza virus, and adenovirus [2–5]. However, human rhinovirus (HRV) has been identified equally frequently as RSV in children hospitalized with wheezing disorders [6–11]. Several studies indicate that HRV is a substantial risk factor for later wheeze or asthma development [12–16].

The family "Picornaviridae", genus "Enterovirus" (EV), has three HRV species: HRV-A, -B, and -C. Over 160 rhinovirus types have been identified, which include 99 classic HRV-A and HRV-B types [17], in addition to six novel HRV-A genotypes, five novel HRV-B genotypes, and fifty-one novel HRV-C genotypes.

Screening methods based on polymerase chain reaction (PCR) are less complicated and more objective [18]. A classification system based on sequence data was optimal because PCR is a ubiquitous technique in laboratories and online databases contain a wealth of nucleotide sequence data. Such a system was devised for EV in 1999 [19]. Owing to their sensitive nature, it is possible to facilitate the diagnosis of previously unencountered HRV variants [20–23] and prototypic strains [24–26]. Noteworthy, sequence motifs of this kind constitute the aim of almost all primers and probes that have undergone publication, but it is important to recognize that they each reflect a distinct placement, length, and assay type (the standard, quantitative, nested, and one-step PCR approaches are employed).

The application of the HRV's 5′ untranslated region (UTR) for genotyping purposes does reflect a variety of limitations. As a case in point, the 5′ UTR is linked to the non-specific amplification of RNA large regulator non-coding RNA B2 or human genomic DNA chromosome 6 sequences, both of which give rise to a 424 bp non-specific product (similar in size to the virus-specific amplicon, 390 bp) [23,27,28]. It is expected for non-specific results of this kind to arise in the context of clinical samples reflecting high human RNA concentrations or clinical samples that have been contaminated with genomic DNA. Owing to the suggested recombination between species, aspects of the 5′ UTR sequences for the HRV-A and C types are characterized by a certain degree of genetic similarity [29,30]. Furthermore, structural genes, as a result of considerable sequence variance, cannot be viably employed as a universal diagnostic primer. Nevertheless, as identified with a phylogenetic analysis of the capsid-coding regions, the A, B, and C HRV species are clearly delineated, and the disparities that exist between each mean that the regions can be distinguished from one another [31–34].

It was necessary to consider the probable molecular genotype determinants to classify EV based on sequence data. Studies of the viral-capsid protein 1 (VP 1) sequence divergence led to the proposal of a 25% nucleotide and 12% amino acid divergence threshold for classifying EV types [19]. Numerous new varieties of EVs have been classified based on these thresholds [35–39]. As some EV isolates have documented evidence of recombination within the capsid region [40,41], it is recommended that only VP1 be used for typing in EV. Previous efforts to classify EV by VP2 sequences have been unsuccessful [42,43].

In standard practice, neutralization assays have been superseded by molecular methods for classifying EV isolates. It has been determined that these methods consistently outperform serotyping in terms of accuracy, efficiency, and classification of new types [44].

It is no longer practicable or desirable to consider all HRV types as a single biological and clinical entity, as their genetic diversity and range of distinct clinical manifestations are so extensive. There are currently no conclusive links between any HRV type and a specific disease. As the spectrum of severe clinical illnesses attributed to HRV infection becomes better understood, it will likely become necessary to routinely screen for HRV in diagnostic settings and initiate large-scale epidemiological studies to determine circulation patterns and strain associations. A simple and practical system of classifying HRV into types, analogous to the system currently used for EV [45], will facilitate the investigation of potential outbreaks and nosocomial transmission as well as type-specific biological properties, such as the identification of types with potentially increased virulence.

The immediate aim of this research has been to establish a viable protocol by which it is possible to classify HRV species and types and to ensure that this protocol is characterized by high sensitivity, specificity, and cost-effectiveness. There are no epidemiologic investigations in Jordan on the prevalence of the causative pathogens in young children with acute bronchiolitis, focusing on HRV genotypes. Therefore, we used reverse-transcriptase polymerase chain reaction (RT-PCR) testing on the nasopharyngeal secretion of young children brought to the emergency room (ER) for the first time for acute wheezing to identify the related pathogen(s).

2. Materials and Methods

2.1. Study Design and Population

The approval of the study was received from the Research Ethics Committee of the Al-Rayhan Medical Center, Amman, Jordan (ARMC-2021-IRB-7-1), with informed, written consent from the parents of the children.

Between August 2021 and August 2022, we invited the participation of children between 1 and 24 months of age admitted to the ER with the first episode of acute wheezing associated with a viral upper respiratory infection.

We excluded children with (1) symptoms for longer than seven days, (2) previous endotracheal intubation, (3) a history of asthma or atopy with an excellent response to the first dose of β2-agonist nebulization, (4) a contraindication to corticosteroid, (5) premature birth, or (6) current or a history of COVID-19.

2.2. Data and Specimens' Collection and Follow-Up

A sample of nasopharyngeal secretion was collected from each child upon admission to the ER by inserting a disposable suction catheter connected to a mucus extractor and applying gentle suction without inserting any solution into the nostrils. The obtained secretion was promptly placed in a tube containing viral transport media and sent to a laboratory, where samples for pathogen detection were aliquoted and frozen at −80 degrees Celsius until processing. The specimens were deposited in 2 mL cryo-safe-labeled tubes containing the laboratory's identification and the date.

Each child's demographic characteristics, medical history, treatments, and clinical course were thoroughly recorded. All children were offered optional follow-up consultations one month after discharge, then every three to six months for three years. Children diagnosed with respiratory disease or asthma were welcome to return for longer-term, routine follow-ups. All medical records will be examined at the end of the third year. Any child who misses a follow-up appointment will be contacted by phone to inquire about any respiratory diseases and treatments they may have received.

2.3. Nucleic Acid Extraction from Samples

The samples were thawed in a water bath at 37 °C before nucleic acid extraction. The automated total nucleic acid extraction was performed by the BIOBASE Kit from 200 µL samples using the magnetic beads method (Biobase Biodustry (Shandong) Co. Ltd., Shandong, China) [46,47]. After extraction, the 100 µL eluted nucleic acid samples were used for virus detection. Then, the remaining volume of samples was transferred to 1.5 mL conical tubes and deeply frozen at −80 °C for HRV retrospective investigation at the end of the study.

2.4. Respiratory Viral Detection

The respiratory samples were subjected to real-time qPCR testing (amplification mix preparation) in a respiratory viral panel, including Adenovirus (ADV), Bocavirus (BOV); Coronavirus (COV); Generic influenza (FLU); Human rhinovirus (HRV); Metapneumovirus (MPV); Parainfluenza (PF); and Respiratory syncytial virus (RSV), covering several subtypes as detailed in a recent study [48]. The TIANLONG: Real-Time PCR System with 48-well block equipment was used using the appropriate kits and primers, according to a recent publication [48]. HRV detection in those clinical specimens was carried out using specific primers that targeted the HRV genome's highly conserved 5′-NCR. According to a recent study, the absolute quantification approach was utilized to analyze the samples [49]. SARS-CoV-2 detection was performed using real-time PCR, as outlined in previous studies [49,50].

2.5. PCR Protocol for HRV-Positive Samples Targeting VP4/VP2 and VP3/VP1 Regions
2.5.1. PCR Primers for HRV VP Regions

Different PCR primers were used to cover various genome regions in the viral-capsid protein (VP) of HRV. All PCR primers were designed in previous studies (Table 1) and synthesized by Sigma-Aldrich, Gillingham, UK, using DST purification (the "stage A" of PCR optimization in this study, as shown in Figure S1) and HPLC purification (stage B of this study). These primers target VP1, VP3/VP1, the VP4 region, and a section of the VP2 genome region (VP4/VP2). As recommended by Sigma, the primers were reconstituted in the corresponding volumes of nuclease-free water to obtain a concentration of 100 µM. After 30 min, the tubes were vortexed for a few seconds. A quantity of 10 µM is prepared for each primer by diluting 20 µL of the original primers' tubes with 180 µL nuclease-free water. All primers were stored in a −20° freezer.

Table 1. Summary of master mixes used for nested and semi-nested PCR.

1st-Round PCR Assay	OS Primer	OAS Primer	2nd-Round PCR Assay	IS Primer	IAS Primer	PCR Product Length (bp)
			Nested PCR			
B	92,580 = F187	R 92383	E	F VP1F	R VP1R	665
W	W:F	W:R	X	X:F	X:R	929
Y	Y:F	Y:R	Z	Z:F	Z:R	563
			Semi-nested PCR			
A	F 92378	R 92379 [a]	D	F92580 = F187	R 92379 [a]	355
C	F 92380 [b]	R 92383	E	F VP1F [b]	R VP1R	455

[a] The reverse primer is the same in master mixes A and D. [b] The forward primer is the same in master mixes C and E. Throughout this study, the single letter, for example, A, B, C, and so forth, refers to assays (master mixes) used in a single-round PCR. Whereas a combination of 2 letters separated by a colon ":", for example, A:D, Y:Z., and so forth, is used to refer to nested or semi-nested PCR assays, the first letter (the assay, the master mix) means that its first-round PCR product was used as a template with the second master mix (the second letter). These master mixes (assays) target various regions in the HRV genome; assay A targets VP3/VP1, whereas assays B, C, A:D, B:E, and C:E target VP1. Assays W, Y, W:X, and Y:Z are directing the VP4/VP2 region in HRV. Abbreviations: OS: outer sense, OAS: outer antisense, IS: inner sense, IAS: inner antisense.

The term "serotype" indicates identification and classification by directly investigating antigenic properties. Therefore, we have used the term "genotype" or simply "type" to represent HRV types identified and classified by sequence data alone. The highly conserved "5′ untranslated region" (5′-UTR), and "5′ non-coding region" (5′-NCR) are used interchangeably throughout the paper.

2.5.2. Pre-PCR and PCR Protocol

Different master mixes were used with different primer combinations, as shown in Table S2. The second-round PCR used the D, E, X, and Z master mixes to increase the specificity of detection.

This study was divided into two main stages: "stage A" which is limited in the flow chart (Figure S1), briefly included ten steps of PCR optimization using DST-purified primers. Whereas "stage B" represents the second period and most of this method development study.

Regarding stage B, initially, the first-round PCR' master mix, which contained reverse transcriptase (RT) reagents from SuperScript™ III Platinum™ One-Step RT-PCR Kit (Invitrogen, Thermo Fisher, Oxford, UK), was processed following the manufacturer's instructions, and 20 µL aliquots were placed into the reaction tubes (Table S3). Following this, 5 µL of the RNA extraction eluate from the clinical samples was added to the reaction tubes containing the first-round PCR master mix to create a final volume of 25 µL before transferring the reaction mixture to the PCR machine.

The LightCycler® Multiplex DNA master (Roche, Burgess Hill, UK, cat. no. 07 339 577 001) and the Platinum® SYBR® Green qPCR SuperMix-UDG (Thermo Fisher, UK, cat. no. 11733038) were both used in the second-round PCR with the D, E, X, and Z master mixes (Tables S4 and S5, respectively). A master mix comparison was performed using the four highest HRV-load samples.

For HRV screening, DNA fragments were amplified via PCR. The PCR protocol involves a series of temperature-dependent stages performed cyclically. The reaction mixture was reverse-transcribed into cDNA. Then the mixture was subjected to denaturation of the target DNA (either cDNA or first-round PCR product), followed by primer annealing, nucleotide extension, and a final extension step. Table S6 represents the thermal cycles applied to all stage B's first and second-round PCR reactions in this study.

The DNA polymerase is rendered unreactive at room temperature by complexing the Platinum Taq with an activity-blocking antibody, thereby increasing sensitivity by halting non-specific annealing. Polymerase activity resumes at higher temperatures during thermal cycling (Table S6) as the complexed antibody is denatured.

The first-round product attained from the Superscript III reaction was used directly in the second round of PCR, as previously described by mixing 1 µL of this product with 24 µL of the second-round PCR' master mix.

2.5.3. Variations of the Standard PCR Technique (Nested and Semi-Nested PCR)

The study also adopted other PCR cycling profiles in addition to the standard PCR described. These were nested and semi-nested PCR. Table 1 shows the master mixes summary detailing the PCR products' length and the primers used for semi-nested and nested PCR.

2.5.4. Agarose Gel Electrophoresis

The gel electrophoresis used for stage B in this study is 1% agarose (ABgene Multi ABgarose, Thermo Fisher Scientific, UK). The agarose gels were dissolved in 1X Tris-Borate-EDTA (TBE) buffer (made from ×10 Gibco Ultra-Pure TBE buffer) (Thermo Fisher Scientific, UK) containing 1× pegGREEN. GeneRuler 1 kb or 100 bp DNA Ladder (Thermo Scientific, UK) was used. All PCR products were run at a constant voltage of 100 V for 1 h and 30 min. The resultant gels were observed under UV light and photographed using a BioSpectrumAC Imaging System V2.

2.5.5. PCR Product Clean-Up Procedure

All PCR products underwent a PCR clean-up step to remove unincorporated primers and deoxyribonucleotide triphosphates (dNTPs) and improve sequencing reaction fidelity. The spin column PCR purification step was performed using the QIAquick PCR Purification Kit (Qiagen, Manchester, UK), combining three main phases: binding, washing, and eluting the DNA. The resulting mixture was then used directly for sequencing reactions.

2.6. Sanger Sequencing Workflow

All HRV sequencing was performed using the Sanger method, in which the reaction mixture comprises all four-chain terminating dideoxynucleotides labeled with distinct fluorescent dyes, allowing the DNA sequence to be determined sequentially [18]. This was accomplished using the ABI BigDye Terminator kit (Applied Biosystems, Cheshire, UK), with the reagents and cycling conditions described in the supplementary data (Tables S7 and S8). Using appropriate PCR primers, PCR products were sequenced in both sense and antisense orientations to enable dual coverage (Figure 1). The quantity of BigDye used in each reaction was modified based on the fragment size.

A pGem and NTC were included as controls for each set of sequence reactions. The plate was sealed with an adhesive PCR seal (ABGene, AB-0558) and spun briefly (1500× g for 30 s) in a centrifuge to ensure the reaction mix was at the bottom of the well. The results of Sanger sequencing were returned in the form of FASTA and corresponding ABI files.

2.7. Bioinformatic Methods
2.7.1. Sequence Alignment and Database Searching

All phylogenetic and evolutionary analyses depend on correctly identifying and aligning homologous sequences in a sequence alignment. The alignment process is fundamental to all subsequent analyses and prevents erroneous conclusions regarding phylogeny, genetic diversity, and recombination.

Sequences were imported into Lasergene SeqMan Pro version 15 (DNASTAR Inc., Madison, WI, USA) and initially aligned with the Pro Assembler algorithm implemented within the software. Any gaps and mismatches between the sense and antisense sequences were resolved by inspecting the associated chromatograms. Amino acid sequences were obtained by translating nucleotide sequences in the DNASTAR V15 software package using a standard genetic code.

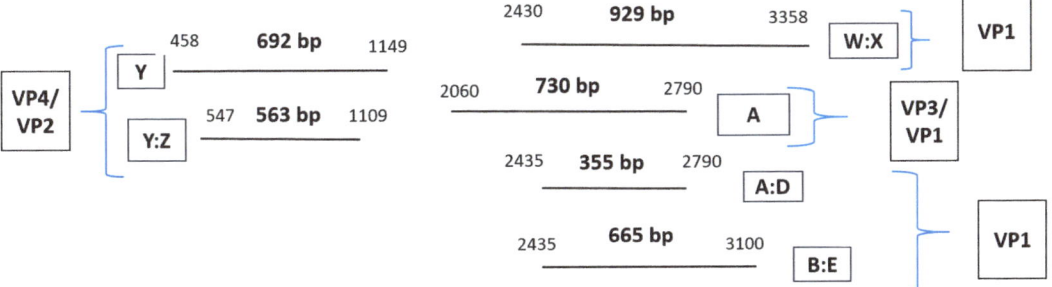

Figure 1. Illustration of polymerase chain reaction (PCR) products for the six optimal assays (with HRV genome targets' regions). Above are given the first- and second-round PCR products (i.e., the horizontal lines) for the six optimal assays in the research, including the lengths, placements (in relation to one another), and the VP target regions in the HRV genome. Product length (bp) is indicated, and the PCR product numbers give the positional number of the nucleotides inside the HRV genome (i.e., the 5′ and the 3′, on the left and right, respectively). Abbreviations: viral-capsid protein (VP).

Sequences of HRV PCR products were analyzed using nucleotide and protein BLAST (BLASTN and BLASTX, http://blast.ncbi.nlm.nih.gov/Blast.cgi, accessed on 1 November 2022) to obtain the maximum number of matching and potentially homologous sequences for analysis.

BLAST is a heuristic that, despite being rapid and relatively accurate, sacrifices some accuracy for speed and cannot guarantee that all homologous sequences will be returned. Consequently, optimizing particular parameters is essential for the endeavor's accuracy.

An input query sequence in FASTA format is separated into "words" of a particular length. The entire database is then searched for occurrences of every possible word derived from the query sequence. These are 11 nucleotides in length by default. As a precise match of the entire word length is required for the algorithm to advance, the word length can be specified to modify the sensitivity and specificity of the protocol. When a match is found in a database sequence, the hit is extended by adding bases from the query sequence to both the 5′ and 3′ ends and searching for additional matches. The alignment is scored sequentially according to a specified match/mismatch penalty. The match/mismatch score's default value is $1/-2$. This was reduced to $1/-1$ when searching for sequences with a greater dissimilarity. The alignment extension is continuously scored until its score falls below a predetermined threshold (20 for nucleotide sequences). The extension phase permits the distinction between meaningful and random matches. The returned sequences were allocated an expectation value (E-value), which estimates the probability that a hit is a false positive.

2.7.2. Assembly of VP Region Sequences

Sequence reads were downloaded, end-trimmed (to remove the primer sequence as well as low-quality sequences and base pairs), and assembled with the program SeqMan Pro version 15 (DNASTAR Inc., Madison, WI, USA). Pro Assembly algorithm parameters used for contigs assembly using SeqMan Pro are as follows: match size = 25, minimum match percentage = 70, minimum sequence length = 50, gap penalty = 0.00, gap length penalty = 0.00, match spacing = 150, and maximum mismatch end bases = 15. Additional manual inspections identified ambiguities or potential single nucleotide variants that were interrogated by further RT-PCRs and sequencing. To close gaps between assembled contigs, additional primer design and sequencing were investigated using SeqMan Pro and SeqBuilder version 15 (DNASTAR Inc., Madison, WI, USA) to enhance the sequence coverage. Figure 2 illustrates the analysis steps of HRV genotyping.

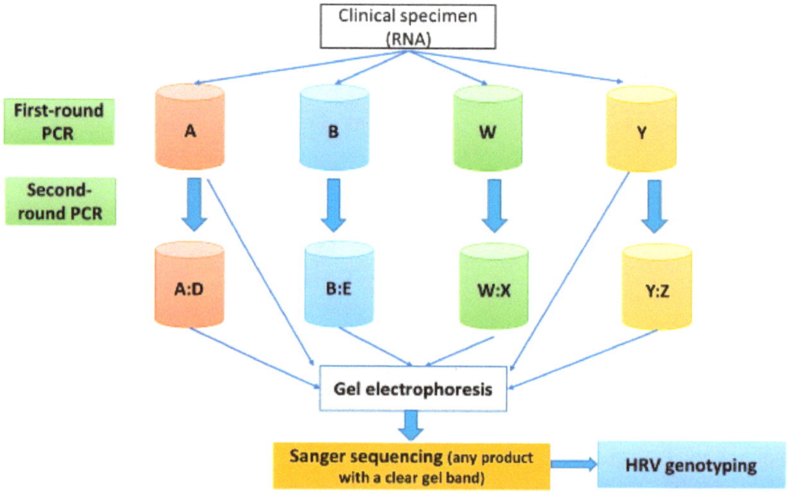

Figure 2. The workflow of HRV genotype analysis. A, B, W, and Y represent the first-round PCR assays (master mixes); A:D, B:E, W:X, and Y:Z are the second-round PCR assays (master mixes). Abbreviations: PCR: polymerase chain reaction; RNA: ribonucleic acid.

2.7.3. Multiple Sequence Alignment, Nucleotide p-Distances, and Phylogenetic Analysis

The regions of the HRV genome analyzed in this study included the VP4/VP2 and VP3/VP1 of HRV-A, HRV-B, and HRV-C that are commonly used in studies of HRV molecular epidemiology [51–55] and downloaded from GenBank. Any highly diverse sequences from the particular multiple sequence alignments (MSA) were excluded. Pairwise sequence alignment and multiple sequence alignment (MSA) were performed using the software MegAlign version 15 (DNASTAR Inc., Madison, WI, USA).

Phylogenetic trees illustrate the relationships among the HRV genotypes of the study's samples and the related references in the VP4/VP2 and VP3/VP1 regions. The input sequences were initially processed to produce the MSA and matrixes of identity and distances (divergences) between all sequence pairs. The unrooted phylogenetic trees were created using the Neighbor-Joining method [56] according to the distances (divergences) between all pairs of sequences in the MSA, with branch length proportional to the sequences' divergence. The evolutionary distances were calculated using the Maximum Composite Likelihood method [57] in units of the number of base substitutions per site. The confidence of associated sequence (taxa) clustering was assessed by bootstrapping calculated from 500 replicates [58]. Bootstrap values of >70% indicate highly significant clustering, whereas values < 50% indicate that the clustering is statistically insignificant. Phylogenetic analyses were performed using MEGA7 [59]. Pairwise nucleotide p-distances were computed using the "Sequence Distances" program within the MEGA7 package. Divergence values were calculated as distance values × 100%.

2.7.4. Recombination Analysis within the VP4/VP2 and VP3/VP1 Regions

The recombination predictions of the genomic sequences, aligned as described above, were conducted with a suite of programs within the RDP4 package version 3.2 [60]. The individual programs: RDP4 v3.2, Bootscan, Maximum X2, Chimaera, SiScan, and 3Seq were applied for the analysis.

Since no single program provides optimal performance under all conditions, any event supported by evidence from two or more analyses with p-values < 1.00×10^{-5} was considered a result consistent with recombination. Potential recombination events were also assessed by phylogenetic and alignment consistency examinations. Each program's default settings were used, except as specified: Bootscan, number of bootstrap replicates, 500, window size, 100 bp, with step size, 10 bp; SiScan, window size, 100 bp, with step size, ten bp.

3. Results

3.1. Viral Detection

During the period of the study, 103 children were presented with acute wheezing linked to acute bronchiolitis. The parents of 93 (90.3%) of these children gave consent, making their children eligible for the collection of nasopharyngeal samples. A single specimen from each child on the same date was included to establish the rates of viral detection, and 91 samples were appropriately stored for viral detection. The total viral positivity rate was 79/91 (86.8%). The most frequently detected pathogen was RSV (42, 46.2%), followed by HRV (15, 16.5%), and FLU (13, 14.3%). Sixteen children (17.6%) were infected with dual viruses (Table 2). The baseline characteristics, clinical manifestations at enrolment, and clinical course for each of the children with any of the different etiologies were comparable (Tables 3 and 4).

Table 2. The frequency of the respiratory viruses detected in the study population (n = 91).

Aetiology	Total n (%)	Age, n (%)		
		1–6 Months n = 24	>6–12 Months n = 35	>12–24 Months n = 32
Overall viral detection	79 (86.8%)	17	32	30
ADV	3 (3.3%)	1	1	1
BOV	1 (1.1%)	0	0	1
COV	1 (1.1%)	0	0	1
FLU	13 (14.3%)	2	4	7
HRV	15 (16.5%)	3	4	8
MPV	3 (3.3%)	1	2	0
PF	1 (1.1%)	0	0	1
RSV	42 (46.2%)	10	21	11
Overall dual detection	16 (17.6%)	4	3	9
RSV + HRV	7 (7.7%)	1	1	5
RSV + FLU	4 (4.4%)	1	1	2
HRV + FLU	5 (5.5%)	2	1	2
Not found	12 (13.2%)	7	3	2

Abbreviations: "ADV: adenovirus; BOV: bocavirus; COV: coronavirus; FLU: influenza; MPV: metapneumovirus; PF: parainfluenza; HRV: human rhinovirus; RSV: Respiratory Syncytial Virus".

Table 3. Baseline characteristics of the included children with the three common etiologies.

Characteristics	Total n = 79	RSV n = 42	HRV n = 15	FLU n = 13
Male, n (%)	45 (62.9)	23 (59.1)	8 (51.6)	9 (70.0)
Body weight (kg), Mean ± SD	8.30 ± 1.82	8.09 ± 1.82	8.52 ± 1.84	8.82 ± 1.86
Breastfeeding, n (%)	76 (94.1)	42 (92.7)	14 (96.8)	10 (93.3)
Duration of breastfeeding (months)	4	4	3	4
First relative atopy, n (%)	25 (31.6)	18 (20.9)	5 (19.4)	4 (26.7)

Abbreviations: "FLU: influenza; HRV: human rhinovirus; RSV: Respiratory Syncytial Virus".

Table 4. Clinical features at presentation and clinical course of acute bronchiolitis.

Characteristics	Total $n = 79$	RSV $n = 42$	HRV $n = 15$	FLU $n = 13$
History of fever, n (%)	72 (91.1)	38 (90.5)	11 (73.4)	12 (92.3)
Temperature, °C Mean ± SD	38.8 ± 0.9	38.2 ± 0.9	37.9 ± 0.9	38.2 ± 0.8
95% CI	37.8–38.3	37.8–38.4	37.7–38.2	38.2–38.8
Duration of fever, days Mean ± SD	4.5 ± 3.0	4.4 ± 2.8	2.9 ± 2.9	4.5 ± 3.3
95% CI	3.9–4.7	3.8–4.8	1.8–3.4	3.2–5.7
SpO$_2$ < 95%, n (%)	105 (61.8)	68 (61.8)	18 (58.1)	20 (66.7)
SpO$_2$, % Min–Max	69–99	69–99	71–99	87–99
Mean ± SD	93.6 ± 4.7	93.7 ± 4.9	94.1 ± 4.8	94.0 ± 3.2
95% CI	93.1–94.4	92.8–94.6	92.3–95.9	92.8–95.2

Abbreviations: "FLU: influenza; HRV: human rhinovirus; RSV: Respiratory Syncytial Virus; SpO$_2$: oxygen saturation".

3.2. Real-Time qPCR for the Template Samples

Using real-time qPCR, the cycle threshold (C_t) value range for the 15 tested respiratory specimens was 18.06 to 33.07. We used these samples' four highest copy numbers (the four lowest C_t values) for PCR optimization.

3.3. HRV Detection Rate of First- and Second-Round PCR Assays Using Gel Electrophoresis

Lacking consistency was one of the features of the results from Stage A of the research (which was performed using the DST-purified primers) (Figure S1), and it was also the case that certain PCR products were non-specific. As for Stage B, combined with the negative control, 15 respiratory samples were analyzed by employing first- and second-round PCR assays. Figure S2, a gel picture, illustrates a first-round PCR product from a single sample, whereas Figure S3 illustrates the second-round products. Considering Figure S4, the suggestion is that the semi-nested and nested assays employed in this research could valuably aid the genotyping of HRV. For example, the gel-check outcomes of 10 assays for a pair of samples are given, with one characterized by an elevated C_t value (namely, 33.00). Noteworthy, several PCR products associated with specimens displaying a C_t value exceeding 30.00 were observed with respect to more than one assay, thereby emphasizing the effectiveness of this research's assays.

We also compared the performance of the LightCycler® Multiplex DNA master (Roche, UK, cat. no. 07339 577001) and the Platinum® SYBR® Green qPCR SuperMix-UDG (Thermo Fisher, UK, cat. no. 11733038). The Platinum® SYBR® Green qPCR SuperMix-UDG gave a better resolution on the gel for most of the tested PCR products. However, both gave the same positivity rate.

The degree to which assays (with various primers) successfully detected the viral capsid proteins (VPs) encoding genes is overviewed in Table S9. The level of positive results has been calculated by dividing the total number of positive samples by the total number of tested samples. Regarding PCR product positivity, the greatest detection rate among the second-round PCR assays was associated with the nested assay "Y:Z" (87%), which targeted the VP4/VP2 region. In turn, VP1 region assays, including the "A:D" semi-nested assay (40%), the "B:E" nested assay (30%), and the "W:X" nested assay (27%), followed this in terms of the next-highest level of positivity. The greatest detection rate among the first-round PCR assays was associated with "Y", at a level of 53%; this assay targeted the VP4/VP2 region, followed by the "A" assay (40%), which targeted the VP3/VP1 region. Figure 3 illustrates the first and second PCR products for the optimal assays in this research, their lengths, and the VP target regions for the HRV genome. In Figure 4, the guidance workflow is given for sequencing all positive HRV respiratory specimens.

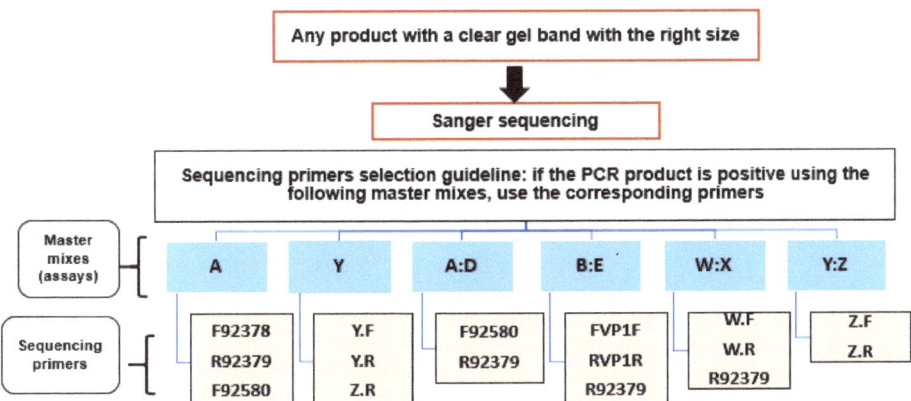

Figure 3. Sequencing primers' selection guideline.

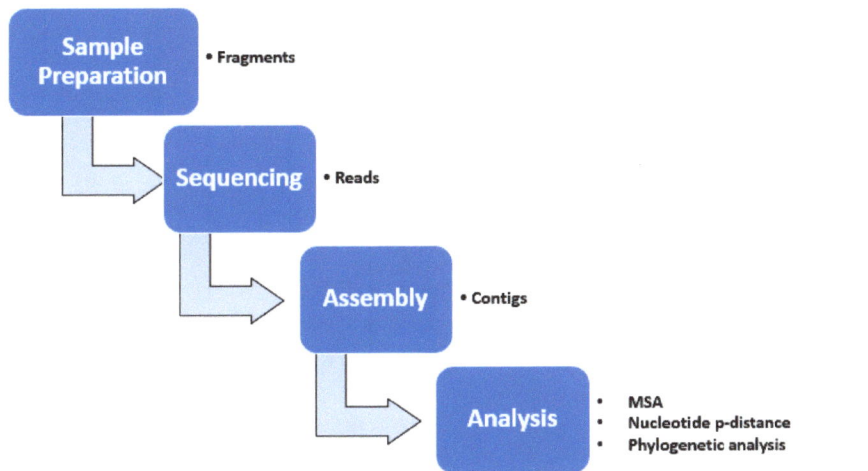

Figure 4. Summary of the analysis steps of HRV genotyping. The boxes represent the main steps, while the points beside the boxes summarize the output. MSA: multiple sequence alignment.

3.4. Sequencing and Sequence Analysis

Using the six assays with a total of 11 primers, sequencing reactions were successful in 95/119 reactions (80%) (Table S10). Lasergene SeqMan Pro version 15 (DNASTAR Inc., Madison, WI, USA) with the Pro Assembler algorithm implemented within the software created contigs in 8/15 samples (Table S11). Trim-ends of low-quality sequences and nucleotides were applied to end up with a mean/median quality (Q) of 24 (Table S12).

3.5. Pairwise Nucleotide p-Distances of HRVs

The distinction between intra-type and inter-type HRV was assisted by the inclusion of reference sequences of assigned genotypes, allowing the distributions of the intra- and inter-pairwise distances to be identified for VP4/VP2 (Figures S5 and S6) and VP3/VP1 (Figures S7 and S8) regions. Divergence values were calculated as distance values × 100%.

Among the strains detected in our study and the reference strains in the VP4/VP2 region, the p-distances (mean ± SD) for HRV-A, HRV-B, and HRV-C were 0.268 ± 0.062, 0.221 ± 0.036, and 0.336 ± 0.111, respectively (Figure S5A–C). Among our study strains and the VP3/VP1 region reference strains, the p-distances (mean ± SD) were 0.278 ± 0.066 for HRV-A and 0.518 ± 0.123 for HRV-C (Figure S6A,B).

The distributions of pairwise nucleotide p-distances were constructed. They showed a maximum within-species divergence of 44%, 31%, and 60%, respectively, for HRV-A, -B, and -C of the VP4/VP2 region (Figure S5), and 43% and 70%, respectively, for HRV-A and -C of the VP3/VP1 region (Figure S7).

When HRV sequences from all three species were compared, the pairwise nucleotide p-distances revealed that, as expected, the lowest values (15%) represented comparisons within the same type. In contrast, the highest (between 30% and 80% divergence) represented comparisons between isolates of different species. The vast number of comparisons ranging from 15% to 45% divergence indicate isolates of the same species but of various types. The minimum between-species divergence values for both regions were between 30% and 40% (Figures S5 and S7).

3.6. HRV Genotype Identification and Phylogenetic Analysis

All HRV sequences were classified into groups based on bootstrap-supported phylogenetic clades that closely matched types assigned by sequence distances (Figure 5). Based on the phylogenetic tree reconstruction of 38 sequences, the 15 clinical isolates were assigned to seven different genotypes and strongly supported with highly significant bootstrap values (70–100%, Tables S13 and 5). The data were bootstrap resampled 500 times to assess the robustness of the branches. Eight HRVs did not significantly match a specific genotype with >15% nucleotide divergence from the nearest reference HRVs. However, they had a high identity and very low E values with reference sequences in the corresponding region.

Table 5. Identification of HRV clinical isolates by BLASTN, BLASTX, phylogenetic tree construction, and p-distance.

Specimen ID	C_t Value	Genotype-BLASTN	E-Value	Genotype-BLASTX	E-Value	Genotype-Phylogeny	Bootstrap	Distance
V14002321	18.06	HRV-A_21	0	HRV-A_21	2.1×10^{-117}	HRV-A_21	100	0.059
V14001831	18.10	HRV-C_32	0	HRV-C	1.8×10^{-93}	HRV-C_32	100	0.047
V14001545	19.08	HRV-B	0	HRV-B	2.2×10^{-94}	HRV-B_79	55	0.150
V14000746	19.12	HRV-A_40	0	HRV-A	2.3×10^{-96}	HRV-A_40	96	0.055
V17004616	33.00	HRV-A	0	HRV-A	4.7×10^{-31}	HRV-A_98	<50	0.173
V17004470	31.10	HRV-A	6.6×10^{-52}	HRV-A	9.7×10^{-19}	HRV-A_13	<50	0.236
V17005728	26.69	HRV-C	0	HRV-C	2.1×10^{-86}	HRV-C_45	73	0.289
V17006129	31.90	HRV-C_7	0	HRV-C	1.4×10^{-137}	HRV-C_7	99	0.098
V17006131	29.91	HRV-C	0	HRV-C	1.5×10^{-96}	HRV-C_45	<50	0.296
V17006286	33.07	HRV-A	4.2×10^{-69}	HRV-A	5.6×10^{-21}	HRV-A_50	50	0.264
V17004189	28.88	HRV-A	2×10^{-25}	HRV-A	5.2×10^{-7}	NA	NA	NA
V17003665	30.09	HRV-C	1.7×10^{-46}	HRV-C	2×10^{-17}	HRV-C_24	69	0.268
V17004870	21.09	HRV-C	3×10^{-20}	NA	NA	HRV-C_32	<50	0.927
V17005031	31.54	HRV-A	1.4×10^{-121}	HRV-A	1.4×10^{-53}	HRV-A_47	52	0.087
V17004381	28.75	HRV C	9×10^{-66}	HRV C	7×10^{-30}	HRV-C_36	100	0.066

Some HRV-type sequences (4 HRV-A and 1 HRV-C) violated the VP1 threshold of 13% proposed in an earlier study [61] (Tables 5 and S13). However, most sequences showed a minimum inter-clade VP divergence (with the nearest neighbor type group) greater than the proposed threshold (Figures S6 and S8).

3.7. Recombination Analysis within the VP4/VP2 and VP3/VP1 Regions

Analysis with the RDP software package highlighted no significant evidence of recombination between the study and reference strains (Table S14). RDP detection programs determine which sequence in the data set contributed the majority of the genome (referred to as the major parent) and which sequence contributed the minor or recombinant region (referred to as the minor parent). None of the recombinant sequences was detected by more than two programs, with average *p*-values of recombination events of $<1.00 \times 10^{-5}$.

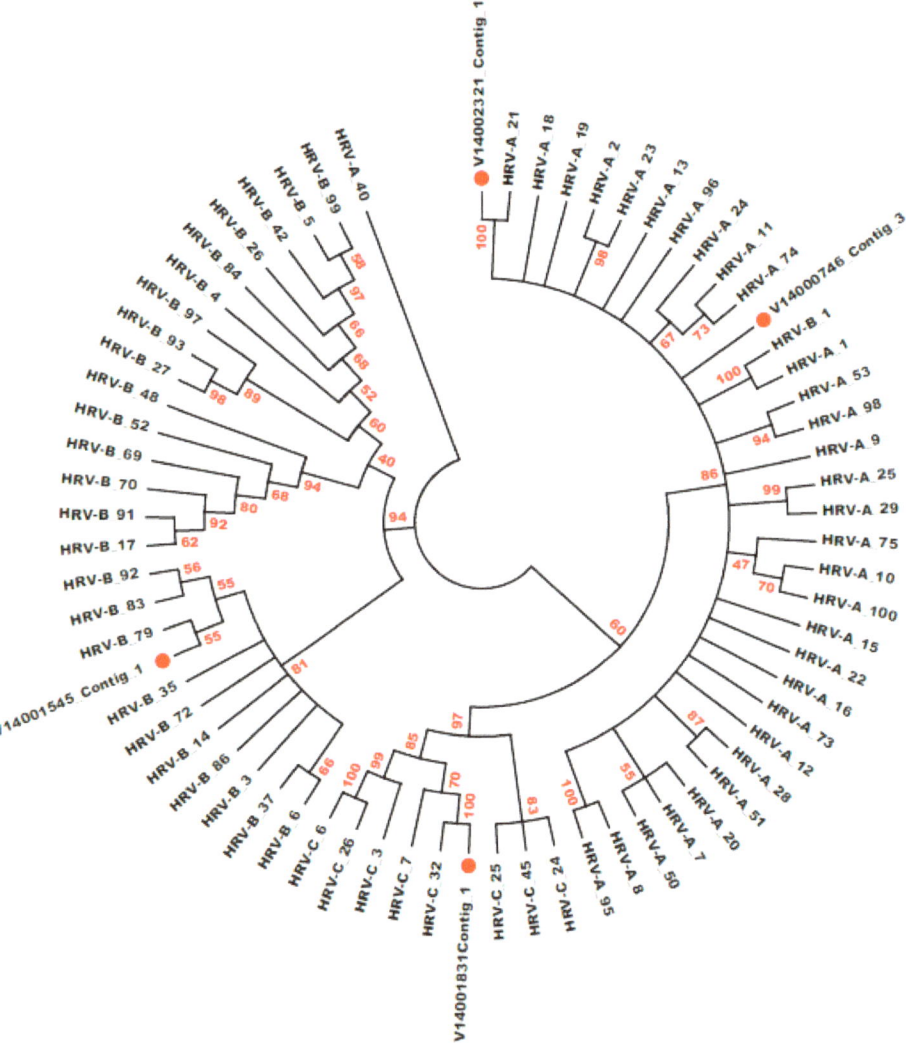

Figure 5. Phylogenetic analysis of HRVs based on the VP4/VP2 region nucleotide sequences (MSA 2). By employing the VP4/VP2 MSA 2 (545 nucleotides), it was possible to complete the neighbor-joining analysis by employing the maximum composite likelihood model. In addition, by employing bootstrapping computed using 500 replicates, it was possible to evaluate the confidence of the sequence clustering. In addition, the branches and those bootstrap values that exceeded 40% are given, and phylogenetic analyses were completed by employing MEGA7. HRV strains in this research are circled in red. The ideal tree (with the sum of the branch lengths = 7.964) is given. Seventy nucleotide sequences were incorporated into the analysis, and positions containing insufficient information, such as gaps, were removed. Therefore, the data set included 417 positions in total.

4. Discussion

According to this study, HRV was the second-most common pathogen (after RSV) causing acute bronchiolitis in Jordanian children. As a result, HRV is an important risk factor for wheezing and acute bronchiolitis. HRV can infect the lower airway directly (it is not limited to the upper airway as previously thought), and multiple epidemiologic studies have shown that HRV is a primary source of lower respiratory infection in children [4–15]. This virus is responsible for many lower respiratory disorders, including pneumonia and asthma exacerbations [49,62,63].

As determined by molecular techniques, the prevalence of HRV in young children three years old with acute lower respiratory infections is between 17 and 35% [4,5,7,9,10,64,65]. This percentage was slightly higher than what we identified in our research. The age range and diagnoses of the research participants may account for the disparity. Acute bronchiolitis is a disease that primarily affects children under the age of two. Jartti et al. found that RSV was more prevalent in infants younger than one year, whereas HRV was more prevalent in older children [4].

Our results demonstrated that the variations in etiology, clinical presentation, and severity were not statistically significant. Children infected with HRV had a higher mean age and less fever than children infected with RSV or another virus. These data are comparable to those from Finland [8] and Thailand [66] but differ from those of France [5], which showed that RSV-infected children had significantly higher coughing and feeding difficulties and required more oxygen delivery than HRV-infected children.

Aeroallergen sensitization and virus-induced wheezing in childhood are recognized to be important risk factors for the development of asthma later in life, and children who have both risk factors are at an exceptionally high risk of acquiring asthma by the time they reach school age [11,14,67–69]. Prior to the discovery of HRV, the most prevalent infection causing wheeze and subsequent asthma was assumed to be RSV [70,71].

Recent studies have used cluster analysis to investigate the interplay between major bacterial species, their functions, and the host response to bronchiolitis in infants. This information, along with clinical, virus, and proteome data, was used to identify biologically distinct endotypes of bronchiolitis with differential risks of asthma development [72–76].

For the purpose of determining the degree to which the HRVs were genetically diverse, respiratory samples were applied in order to characterize the HRV variants in genetic terms. A range of primer combinations (including nested primers) were employed to achieve this, thereby efficiently amplifying the VP4/VP2, VP3/VP1, and VP1 regions of the HRV species and genotypes. Aside from Wisdom et al. [34], which investigated the role played by nested HRV detection assays, the literature about assay technique details is limited, thus motivating the present study.

The researchers understood that finding one assay with an HRV detection rate of 100% would be unlikely. This expectation stems from the recognition that the HRV genome's regions interacted with each other throughout the study and were characterized by a high level of variance. In view of this, the optimal assays would be those that were operable for the greatest number of samples, and in an ideal case, those reflecting elevated C_t values.

The conclusion of the analysis of all available data in this study divided sequences into 7 HRV-A, 1 HRV-B, and 7 HRV-C types based on the VP4/VP2 and VP3/VP1 sequences. The nucleotide divergence between the clinical samples and the corresponding reference strains was lower in the VP4/VP2 region than in the VP3/VP1 region.

When HRV sequences from all three species were compared, the pairwise nucleotide p-distances revealed that, as expected, the lowest values were for comparisons within the same species or genotypes. At the same time, the largest (between 30% and 80% divergence) represented comparisons between isolates of different species. Many comparisons involving 15% to 45% divergence include isolates of the same species but different types. These findings show that HRV-C deviates slightly from the previously stated conclusion and warrants additional examination. A clear inter-species p-distance threshold supports the idea that HRV species can be characterized by nucleotide divergence in the capsid region. The most diverse strains are only represented by a few sequences in each case. As a result, it was difficult to identify whether these were variants that happened to be at the extreme end of the distribution of intra-type divergence values or variants that were midway through the process of diverging into a new HRV type. This may become obvious when more data from epidemiological and evolutionary investigations accrues.

Within EV isolates, recombination has been recognized within the capsid coding region [40]. However, recombination within the capsid coding region of HRV is believed to be relatively uncommon [77,78]. Our study's analysis with the RDP software package highlighted no significant evidence of recombination between the study and reference strains. Due to dealing with short sequences (<2000 nucleotides), we cannot confirm that there is no significant recombination between the investigated regions.

4.1. Development of a Method for the Amplification of the VP Region of HRV

Performing genotyping directly from clinical specimens eliminates the necessity of cell culture passage and significantly decreases the time needed for an accurate diagnosis. This advancement has been successfully demonstrated in studies focusing on EV [79,80]. The assays developed in this research enable the amplification of specific regions of HRV's VP from respiratory specimens, which typically have low viral concentrations. However, due to the extensive genetic variability, creating a single assay capable of simultaneously amplifying all three HRV species was not feasible. Even within a single HRV species, maintaining the necessary balance between primer degeneracy for amplifying all types and avoiding non-specific amplification posed a challenge.

When designing novel methods, PCR optimization is a fundamental stage. The individual reaction component concentrations were modified, including temperature and time parameters, which were brought inside the required range (thereby facilitating the adequate amplification of the desired DNA target sequences). Ultimately, this stemmed from the fact that applying one set of conditions for every PCR amplification is not practically possible.

Several studies have supported using a one-step PCR for EV typing, containing only the first round of amplification [81,82], proposing the idea that a "closed system" is less susceptible to contamination. Nevertheless, one of the aforementioned studies indicated that nearly one-third of the examined isolates were not efficiently amplified in the VP1 region, and the successfully amplified ones exhibited a notable presence of non-specific products [81]. Our findings demonstrate that implementing a nested PCR technique significantly decreases non-specific amplification, making it highly effective for amplifying samples with very low viral concentrations. Furthermore, contamination is notably minimized by strictly adhering to a "one-way" system in PCR laboratories, where different areas are spatially separated for nucleic acid extraction, first-round PCR, and second-round PCR.

Including the nested primers is a viable way to promote the degree to which DNA amplification is specific since it reduces the non-specific DNA products. Consequently, the second-round PCR product is not as long as the first. However, its amplification is more accurate since all amplification errors in the first round have a low probability of being replicated in the second PCR. Nevertheless, a key risk factor is the higher likelihood of non-specific contamination when applying the second-round PCR primers [79,83,84].

4.2. Proposed Criteria for HRV Genotyping

Given the well-conserved nature of 5'NCR, sequencing it for genotyping produces little valuable information. Contrastingly, those genes that encode the VPs are highly variable, and the sequences have a determinative impact on the genotype. Therefore, sequencing parts of these VP regions is expected to be useful for genotyping.

Using only capsid coding regions in type assignment should not detract from the value of continuous examination of other genomic regions, particularly where these regions may contribute to the phenotype and disease associations of HRV. In addition, using the VP1 region to identify novel HRV types should not impede the continued use of VP4/VP2 and

5′NCR screening protocols. Screening in these regions increases the likelihood of discovering previously unknown HRV types. In epidemiological studies and clinical associations, VP4/VP2 sequences can be used to identify the type. Recent and rapid accumulation of sequence data of the VP4/VP2 region on GenBank in contrast to sequences of the VP1 region, which are difficult to amplify without type-specific primers. If sequence data from the VP4/VP2 region are to be utilized in epidemiological or clinical studies, it is necessary to confirm that known HRV types can be accurately identified through analysis of this region. We would suggest the combined use of phylogenetic analysis and pairwise p-distance analysis in the classification of all HRV sequences. In cases where nucleotide divergence is insufficient to assign types definitively, phylogenetic relationships may be considered. The guidelines should be further reviewed as additional data becomes available.

Likely, less sizeable fragments of VP3/VP1 and VP4/VP2 are viable candidates for genotyping in HRV. In the study conducted by Oberste et al. [45,82], the researchers found that a 450-base segment at the 3′ end of VP1 can viably be applied for EV typing, and the outcomes were entirely correlated with the neutralization results. In another study, the researchers demonstrated a 100% correlation between a 303 nucleotide stretch of VP1 and neutralization data, but it should be noted that the research was only relevant for 59 GenBank strains [82]. Recently, pyrosequencing was proposed as a straightforward, rapid, and viable way to type EV [85].

4.3. The Importance and Implications of HRV Genotyping

Identifying HRV types by analyzing available sequence data within the capsid region can improve HRV genotyping, making the classification of all detected HRV sequences much more feasible. A global type of identification system should allow large-scale investigations of epidemiology, transmission, and evolution. Classification and centralized reporting of new HRV types improve the ability of researchers to study the distribution of new types quickly. Whereas previously, a considerable period of time would have been necessary while waiting for type-specific antiserum to be developed and dispatched, sequence data for comparison is almost instantly available worldwide.

HRV genotyping can be used to investigate the frequency and genetic diversity of HRV strains among respiratory samples referred for diagnostic testing and their relationship with different respiratory diseases.

Several of the current research's findings could have vital implications. First and foremost, given that genetic variability has an adverse impact on the derivation of HRV vaccines and antiviral therapy, identifying those characterized by higher virulence might serve as a way to promote therapeutic advancement. In addition, despite how HRV infection has been implicated in the exacerbation of COPD and asthma, the information pertaining to the function of the various HRV species in impacting the exacerbation frequency phenotype is unknown. The clinical implications of HRV infection are much more severe than those associated with the common cold; HRV infection contributes to numerous effects, ranging from the absence of symptoms to COPD, pneumonia, and bronchiolitis. The complex nature of naturally occurring instances of COPD exacerbations is well documented. Yet, the information on the pathogenesis of HRV in the course of and following COPD episodes is limited. However, exacerbations are substantial events in COPD, and the possibility exists that HRV infection is associated with these exacerbations. Therefore, the possibility exists that information about the effect of HRV species on exacerbations could contribute to developing targeted therapeutic interventions, thereby counteracting the severity of the pulmonary diseases' exacerbations.

4.4. Limitations and Future Research

The most important limitations of this study that need to be considered can be summarized as follows: First, the numbers of patients and samples were relatively small. Second, the inconsistencies in results are unfortunately unavoidable and should remain in place for clarity due to the nature of VP region variability, sequencing, or assembly errors.

As for the issue of further research, it would be helpful in subsequent studies to identify whether a particular threshold (one that divides pairwise p-distance comparisons into intra- and inter-type values) pertains to all HRV species. This could be achieved by establishing distributions of pairwise nucleotide p-distances using a more extensive data set. In addition, other researchers should consider replicating the present study to determine the degree to which the assay-related outcomes have yielded reliable conclusions. It would be valuable for some studies to employ larger samples. Finally, further research should examine the frequency and genetic diversity of HRV strains in the context of respiratory samples referred to for diagnostic testing and their connection with various respiratory diseases.

5. Conclusions

HRV is ranked second after RSV as the cause of acute bronchiolitis in children. The results of this study demonstrated the potential utility of the VP4/VP2 region in addition to the VP3/VP1 region for differentiating HRV genotypes. Confirmatory outcomes were yielded, indicating how nested and semi-nested PCR can establish practical ways to facilitate HRV sequencing and genotyping. Additionally, by employing a combination of first- and second-round PCR assays, optimal genome assembly can be achieved by targeting numerous HRV variable genome regions (namely the VP4/VP2, VP3/VP1, and the VP1 regions).

Supplementary Materials: The following supporting information can be downloaded at: https://www.mdpi.com/article/10.3390/jcm12123909/s1, Table S1. Primers used for amplification and sequencing of the HRV region [33,43,44,86–88]. Figure S1. Stage A in PCR optimization. Table S2. Master mixes and primer combinations were used to detect the variable regions of the HRV genome. Table S3. The preparation of the first-round PCR master mixes. Table S4. The preparation of the second-round PCR reactions using the LightCycler® Multiplex DNA master mix. Table S5. The preparation of the second-round PCR reactions using the Platinum® SYBR® Green qPCR SuperMix-UDG. Table S6. Thermal cycling conditions used in PCR reactions. Table S7. Reagents used in sequencing reactions. Table S8. Cycling conditions used in sequencing reactions. Figure S2. PCR product representation of master mix A. Figure S3. The second-round PCR product representation of A:D and C:E assays. Figure S4. Gel electrophoresis of first- and second-round PCR products from 10 different assays. Table S9. The PCR product positivity rate of HRV-VP assays using fifteen respiratory samples. Table S10. The successful representation of the Sanger sequencing primers. Table S11. A summary of gel-check, sequencing success, and sequence assembly results of the clinical HRV tested samples. Table S12. Description of the VP regions' sequence assemblies. Figure S5. Distribution of nucleotide p-distances for HRV-A (A), HRV-B (B), and HRV-C (C) detected in the study compared with sequences from reference strains based on the nucleotide sequences of the VP4/VP2 region. Figure S6. Distribution of pairwise nucleotide p-distances for the VP4/VP2 region of all HRV sequences. Figure S7. Distribution of nucleotide p-distances for HRV-A (A) and HRV-C (B) detected in the study compared with sequences from reference strains based on the nucleotide sequences of the VP3/VP1 region. Figure S8. Distribution of pairwise nucleotide p-distances for the VP3/VP1 region of all HRV sequences. Table S13. Multiple sequence alignment (MSA) data and genotype identification. Table S14. A summary of recombination events detected in the multiple sequence alignments.

Author Contributions: Conceptualization, A.R.A.; methodology, A.R.A. and F.A.; software, A.R.A.; validation, A.R.A. and F.A.; formal analysis, A.R.A.; investigation, A.R.A.; resources, A.R.A. and B.A.; data curation, A.R.A.; writing—original draft preparation, A.R.A.; writing—review and editing: all authors; visualization, A.R.A.; supervision, A.R.A.; project administration, A.R.A.; funding acquisition, A.R.A., A.A. and F.A. All authors have read and agreed to the published version of the manuscript.

Funding: This research received no external funding.

Institutional Review Board Statement: The approval of the study was sought and gained from the Research Ethics Board of the Al-Rayhan Medical Center (2021-IRB-7-1; date of approval: July 2021).

Informed Consent Statement: Informed consent was obtained from all subjects parents involved in the study.

Data Availability Statement: Data is unavailable due to privacy and ethical restrictions.

Acknowledgments: A very special thank you goes out to Derek Fairley (United Kingdom) and all our research assistants.

Conflicts of Interest: The authors declare no conflict of interest.

References

1. Smyth, R.L.; Openshaw, P.J.M. Bronchiolitis. *Lancet* **2006**, *368*, 312–322. [CrossRef] [PubMed]
2. Principi, N.; Esposito, S. Emerging role of *Mycoplasma pneumoniae* and *Chlamydia pneumoniae* in paediatric respiratorytract infections. *Lancet Infect. Dis.* **2001**, *1*, 334–344. [CrossRef]
3. van Woensel, J.; van Aalderen, W.; Kimpen, J.L.L. Viral lower respiratory tract infection in infants and young children. *BMJ* **2003**, *327*, 36–40. [CrossRef]
4. Jartti, T.; Lehtinen, P.; Vuorinen, T.; Österback, R.; van den Hoogen, B.; Osterhaus, A.D.; Ruuskanen, O. Respiratory picornaviruses and respiratory syncytial virus as causative agents of acute expiratory wheezing in children. *Emerg. Infect. Dis.* **2004**, *10*, 1095–1101. [CrossRef] [PubMed]
5. Manoha, C.; Espinosa, S.; Aho, S.-L.; Huet, F.; Pothier, P. Epidemiological and clinical features of hMPV, RSV and RVs infections in young children. *J. Clin. Virol.* **2007**, *38*, 221–226. [CrossRef] [PubMed]
6. Jacques, J.; Bouscambert-Duchamp, M.; Moret, H.; Carquin, J.; Brodard, V.; Lina, B.; Motte, J.; Andréoletti, L. Association of respiratory picornaviruses with acute bronchiolitis in French infants. *J. Clin. Virol.* **2006**, *35*, 463–466. [CrossRef]
7. Papadopoulos, N.G.; Moustaki, M.; Tsolia, M.; Bossios, A.; Astra, E.; Prezerakou, A.; Gourgiotis, D.; Kafetzis, D. Association of Rhinovirus infection with increased disease severity in acute bronchiolitis. *Am. J. Respir. Crit. Med.* **2002**, *165*, 1285–1289. [CrossRef] [PubMed]
8. Korppi, M.; Kotaniemi-Syrjänen, A.; Waris, M.; Vainionpää, R.; Reijonen, T. Rhinovirus-associated wheezing in infancy: Comparison with respiratory syncytial virus bronchiolitis. *Pediatr. Infect. Dis. J.* **2004**, *23*, 995–999. [CrossRef]
9. Calvo, C.; García-García, M.L.; Blanco, C.; Pozo, F.; Flecha, I.C.; Pérez-Breña, P. Role of rhinovirus in hospitalized infants with respiratory tract infections in Spain. *Pediatr. Infect. Dis. J.* **2007**, *26*, 904–908. [CrossRef] [PubMed]
10. Pitrez, P.; Stein, R.T.; Stuermer, L.; Macedo, I.S.; Schmitt, V.M.; Jones, M.H.; Arruda, E. Rhinovirus and acute bronchiolitis in young infants. *J. Pediatr.* **2005**, *81*, 417–420. [CrossRef]
11. Kusel, M.M.; de Klerk, N.H.; Kebadze, T.; Vohma, V.; Holt, P.G.; Johnston, S.L.; Sly, P. Early-life respiratory viral infections, atopic sensitization, and risk of subsequent development of persistent asthma. *J. Allergy Clin. Immunol.* **2007**, *119*, 1105–1110. [CrossRef]
12. Lemanske, R.F., Jr.; Jackson, D.J.; Gangnon, R.E.; Evans, M.D.; Li, Z.; Shult, P.A.; Kirk, C.J.; Reisdorf, E.; Roberg, K.A.; Anderson, E. Rhinovirus illnesses during infancy predict subsequent childhood wheezing. *J. Allergy Clin. Immunol.* **2005**, *116*, 571–577. [CrossRef]
13. Singh, A.M.; Moore, P.E.; Gern, J.E.; Lemanske, R.F., Jr.; Hartert, T.V. Bronchiolitis to asthma: A review and call for studies of gene-virus interactions in asthma causation. *Am. J. Respir. Crit. Care Med.* **2007**, *175*, 108–119. [CrossRef]
14. Jackson, D.J.; Gangnon, R.E.; Evans, M.D.; Roberg, K.A.; Anderson, E.L.; Pappas, T.E.; Printz, M.C.; Lee, W.M.; Shult, P.A.; Reisdorf, E.; et al. Wheezing rhinovirus illnesses in early life predict asthma development in high-risk children. *Am. J. Respir. Crit. Care Med.* **2008**, *178*, 667–672. [CrossRef]
15. Bosis, S.; Esposito, S.; Niesters, H.G.; Zuccotti, G.V.; Marseglia, G.; Lanari, M.; Zuin, G.; Pelucchi, C.; Osterhaus, A.D.; Principi, N. Role of respiratory pathogens in infants hospitalized for a first episode of wheezing and their impact on recurrences. *Clin. Microbiol. Infect.* **2008**, *14*, 677–684. [CrossRef]
16. Kotaniemi-Syrjänen, A.; Vainionpää, R.; Reijonen, T.M.; Waris, M.; Korhonen, K.; Korppi, M. Rhinovirus-induced wheezing in infancy—The first sign of childhood asthma? *J. Allergy Clin. Immunol.* **2003**, *111*, 66–71. [CrossRef]
17. Hamparian, V.; Colonno, R.; Cooney, M.; Dick, E.; Gwaltney Jr, J.; Hughes, J.; Jordan Jr, W.; Kapikian, A.; Mogabgab, W.; Monto, A. A collaborative report: Rhinoviruses–extension of the numbering system from 89 to 100. *Virology* **1987**, *159*, 191–192. [PubMed]
18. Alsayed, A.R.; Abed, A.; Khader, H.A.; Al-Shdifat, L.M.; Hasoun, L.; Al-Rshaidat, M.M.; Alkhatib, M.; Zihlif, M. Molecular Accounting and Profiling of Human Respiratory Microbial Communities: Toward Precision Medicine by Targeting the Respiratory Microbiome for Disease Diagnosis and Treatment. *Int. J. Mol. Sci.* **2023**, *24*, 4086. [CrossRef] [PubMed]
19. Oberste, M.S.; Maher, K.; Kilpatrick, D.R.; Pallansch, M.A. Molecular evolution of the human enteroviruses: Correlation of serotype with VP1 sequence and application to picornavirus classification. *J. Virol.* **1999**, *73*, 1941–1948. [CrossRef]
20. Lee, W.-M.; Kiesner, C.; Pappas, T.; Lee, I.; Grindle, K.; Jartti, T.; Jakiela, B.; Lemanske Jr, R.F.; Shult, P.A.; Gern, J.E. A diverse group of previously unrecognized human rhinoviruses are common causes of respiratory illnesses in infants. *PLoS ONE* **2007**, *2*, e966. [CrossRef] [PubMed]
21. Kiang, D.; Kalra, I.; Yagi, S.; Louie, J.K.; Boushey, H.; Boothby, J.; Schnurr, D.P. Assay for 5′ noncoding region analysis of all human rhinovirus prototype strains. *J. Clin. Microbiol.* **2008**, *46*, 3736–3745. [CrossRef] [PubMed]

22. Lu, X.; Holloway, B.; Dare, R.K.; Kuypers, J.; Yagi, S.; Williams, J.V.; Hall, C.B.; Erdman, D.D. Real-time reverse transcription-PCR assay for comprehensive detection of human rhinoviruses. *J. Clin. Microbiol.* **2008**, *46*, 533–539. [CrossRef]
23. Tapparel, C.; Cordey, S.; Van Belle, S.; Turin, L.; Lee, W.-M.; Regamey, N.; Meylan, P.; Mühlemann, K.; Gobbini, F.; Kaiser, L. New molecular detection tools adapted to emerging rhinoviruses and enteroviruses. *J. Clin. Microbiol.* **2009**, *47*, 1742–1749. [CrossRef] [PubMed]
24. Gama, R.E.; Horsnell, P.R.; Hughes, P.J.; North, C.; Bruce, C.B.; al-Nakib, W.; Stanway, G. Amplification of rhinovirus specific nucleic acids from clinical samples using the polymerase chain reaction. *J. Med. Virol.* **1989**, *28*, 73–77. [CrossRef]
25. Ireland, D.C.; Kent, J.; Nicholson, K.G. Improved detection of rhinoviruses in nasal and throat swabs by seminested RT-PCR. *J. Med. Virol.* **1993**, *40*, 96–101. [CrossRef]
26. Andeweg, A.C.; Bestebroer, T.M.; Huybreghs, M.; Kimman, T.G.; de Jong, J.C. Improved detection of rhinoviruses in clinical samples by using a newly developed nested reverse transcription-PCR assay. *J. Clin. Microbiol.* **1999**, *37*, 524–530. [CrossRef] [PubMed]
27. Faux, C.E.; Arden, K.E.; Lambert, S.B.; Nissen, M.D.; Nolan, T.M.; Chang, A.B.; Sloots, T.P.; Mackay, I.M. Usefulness of published PCR primers in detecting human rhinovirus infection. *Emerg. Infect. Dis.* **2011**, *17*, 296–298. [CrossRef] [PubMed]
28. Bochkov, Y.A.; Gern, J.E. Clinical and molecular features of human rhinovirus C. *Microbes Infect.* **2012**, *14*, 485–494. [CrossRef]
29. Huang, T.; Wang, W.; Bessaud, M.; Ren, P.; Sheng, J.; Yan, H.; Zhang, J.; Lin, X.; Wang, Y.; Delpeyroux, F. Evidence of recombination and genetic diversity in human rhinoviruses in children with acute respiratory infection. *PLoS ONE* **2009**, *4*, e6355. [CrossRef]
30. McIntyre, C.L.; Leitch, E.C.M.; Savolainen-Kopra, C.; Hovi, T.; Simmonds, P. Analysis of genetic diversity and sites of recombination in human rhinovirus species C. *J. Virol.* **2010**, *84*, 10297–10310. [CrossRef]
31. Savolainen, C.; Mulders, M.N.; Hovi, T. Phylogenetic analysis of rhinovirus isolates collected during successive epidemic seasons. *Virus Res.* **2002**, *85*, 41–46. [CrossRef] [PubMed]
32. Ledford, R.M.; Patel, N.R.; Demenczuk, T.M.; Watanyar, A.; Herbertz, T.; Collett, M.S.; Pevear, D.C. VP1 sequencing of all human rhinovirus serotypes: Insights into genus phylogeny and susceptibility to antiviral capsid-binding compounds. *J. Virol.* **2004**, *78*, 3663–3674. [CrossRef]
33. Laine, P.; Savolainen, C.; Blomqvist, S.; Hovi, T. Phylogenetic analysis of human rhinovirus capsid protein VP1 and 2A protease coding sequences confirms shared genus-like relationships with human enteroviruses. *J. Gen. Virol.* **2005**, *86*, 697–706. [CrossRef]
34. Wisdom, A.; Leitch, E.M.; Gaunt, E.; Harvala, H.; Simmonds, P. Screening respiratory samples for detection of human rhinoviruses (HRVs) and enteroviruses: Comprehensive VP4-VP2 typing reveals high incidence and genetic diversity of HRV species C. *J. Clin. Microbiol.* **2009**, *47*, 3958–3967. [CrossRef] [PubMed]
35. Oberste, M.S.; Maher, K.; Pallansch, M.A. Molecular phylogeny and proposed classification of the simian picornaviruses. *J. Virol.* **2002**, *76*, 1244–1251. [CrossRef] [PubMed]
36. Oberste, M.S.; Maher, K.; Nix, W.A.; Michele, S.M.; Uddin, M.; Schnurr, D.; al-Busaidy, S.; Akoua-Koffi, C.; Pallansch, M.A. Molecular identification of 13 new enterovirus types, EV79–88, EV97, and EV100–101, members of the species Human Enterovirus B. *Virus Res.* **2007**, *128*, 34–42. [CrossRef] [PubMed]
37. Oberste, M.S.; Michele, S.M.; Maher, K.; Schnurr, D.; Cisterna, D.; Junttila, N.; Uddin, M.; Chomel, J.-J.; Lau, C.-S.; Ridha, W. Molecular identification and characterization of two proposed new enterovirus serotypes, EV74 and EV75. *J. Gen. Virol.* **2004**, *85*, 3205–3212. [CrossRef]
38. Brown, B.A.; Maher, K.; Flemister, M.R.; Naraghi-Arani, P.; Uddin, M.; Oberste, M.S.; Pallansch, M.A. Resolving ambiguities in genetic typing of human enterovirus species C clinical isolates and identification of enterovirus 96, 99 and 102. *J. Gen. Virol.* **2009**, *90*, 1713–1723. [CrossRef]
39. Smura, T.P.; Junttila, N.; Blomqvist, S.; Norder, H.; Kaijalainen, S.; Paananen, A.; Magnius, L.O.; Hovi, T.; Roivainen, M. Enterovirus 94, a proposed new serotype in human enterovirus species D. *J. Gen. Virol.* **2007**, *88*, 849–858. [CrossRef]
40. Bouslama, L.; Nasri, D.; Chollet, L.; Belguith, K.; Bourlet, T.; Aouni, M.; Pozzetto, B.; Pillet, S. Natural recombination event within the capsid genomic region leading to a chimeric strain of human enterovirus B. *J. Virol.* **2007**, *81*, 8944–8952. [CrossRef]
41. Zhang, Y.; Zhu, S.; Yan, D.; Liu, G.; Bai, R.; Wang, D.; Chen, L.; Zhu, H.; An, H.; Kew, O. Natural type 3/type 2 intertypic vaccine-related poliovirus recombinants with the first crossover sites within the VP1 capsid coding region. *PLoS ONE* **2010**, *5*, e15300. [CrossRef] [PubMed]
42. Arola, A.; Santti, J.; Ruuskanen, O.; Halonen, P.; Hyypiä, T. Identification of enteroviruses in clinical specimens by competitive PCR followed by genetic typing using sequence analysis. *J. Clin. Microbiol.* **1996**, *34*, 313–318. [CrossRef] [PubMed]
43. Oberste, M.S.; Maher, K.; Pallansch, M.A. Molecular phylogeny of all human enterovirus serotypes based on comparison of sequences at the 5' end of the region encoding VP2. *Virus Res.* **1998**, *58*, 35–43. [CrossRef]
44. Oberste, M.S.; Maher, K.; Flemister, M.R.; Marchetti, G.; Kilpatrick, D.R.; Pallansch, M.A. Comparison of classic and molecular approaches for the identification of untypeable enteroviruses. *J. Clin. Microbiol.* **2000**, *38*, 1170–1174. [CrossRef] [PubMed]
45. Oberste, M.S.; Maher, K.; Kilpatrick, D.R.; Flemister, M.R.; Brown, B.A.; Pallansch, M.A. Typing of human enteroviruses by partial sequencing of VP1. *J. Clin. Microbiol.* **1999**, *37*, 1288–1293. [CrossRef]
46. Alsayed, A.R.; Hasoun, L.; Khader, H.A.; Abu-Samak, M.S.; Al-Shdifat, L.M.; Al-Shammari, B.; Maqbali, M.A. Co-infection of COVID-19 patients with atypical bacteria: A study based in Jordan. *Pharm. Pract.* **2023**, *21*, 1–5. [CrossRef]

47. Alsayed, A.R.; Abed, A.; Jarrar, Y.B.; Alshammari, F.; Alshammari, B.; Basheti, I.A.; Zihlif, M. Alteration of the Respiratory Microbiome in Hospitalized Patients with Asthma–COPD Overlap during and after an Exacerbation. *J. Clin. Med.* **2023**, *12*, 2118. [CrossRef]
48. Alsayed, A.; Al-Doori, A.; Al-Dulaimi, A.; Alnaseri, A.; Abuhashish, J.; Aliasin, K.; Alfayoumi, I. Influences of bovine colostrum on nasal swab microbiome and viral upper respiratory tract infections–A case report. *Respir. Med. Case Rep.* **2020**, *31*, 101189. [CrossRef]
49. Al-Dulaimi, A.; Alsayed, A.R.; Maqbali, M.A.; Zihlif, M. Investigating the human rhinovirus co-infection in patients with asthma exacerbations and COVID-19. *Pharm. Pr.* **2022**, *20*, 2665. [CrossRef]
50. Alsayed, A.R.; Talib, W.; Al-Dulaimi, A.; Daoud, S.; Al Maqbali, M. The first detection of Pneumocystis jirovecii in asthmatic patients post-COVID-19 in Jordan. *Bosn. J. Basic Med. Sci.* **2022**, *22*, 784–790. [CrossRef]
51. Tapparel, C.; Junier, T.; Gerlach, D.; Van Belle, S.; Turin, L.; Cordey, S.; Mühlemann, K.; Regamey, N.; Aubert, J.-D.; Soccal, P.M. New respiratory enterovirus and recombinant rhinoviruses among circulating picornaviruses. *Emerg. Infect. Dis.* **2009**, *15*, 719. [CrossRef] [PubMed]
52. Miller, E.K.; Khuri-Bulos, N.; Williams, J.V.; Shehabi, A.A.; Faouri, S.; Al Jundi, I.; Chen, Q.; Heil, L.; Mohamed, Y.; Morin, L.-L. Human rhinovirus C associated with wheezing in hospitalised children in the Middle East. *J. Clin. Virol.* **2009**, *46*, 85–89. [CrossRef] [PubMed]
53. McIntyre, C.L.; Knowles, N.J.; Simmonds, P. Proposals for the classification of human rhinovirus species A, B and C into genotypically assigned types. *J. Gen. Virol.* **2013**, *94*, 1791–1806. [CrossRef] [PubMed]
54. Henquell, C.; Mirand, A.; Deusebis, A.-L.; Regagnon, C.; Archimbaud, C.; Chambon, M.; Bailly, J.-L.; Gourdon, F.; Hermet, E.; Dauphin, J.-B. Prospective genotyping of human rhinoviruses in children and adults during the winter of 2009–2010. *J. Clin. Virol.* **2012**, *53*, 280–284. [CrossRef]
55. Arakawa, M.; Okamoto-Nakagawa, R.; Toda, S.; Tsukagoshi, H.; Kobayashi, M.; Ryo, A.; Mizuta, K.; Hasegawa, S.; Hirano, R.; Wakiguchi, H. Molecular epidemiological study of human rhinovirus species A, B and C from patients with acute respiratory illnesses in Japan. *J. Med. Microbiol.* **2012**, *61*, 410–419. [CrossRef] [PubMed]
56. Saitou, N.; Nei, M. The neighbor-joining method: A new method for reconstructing phylogenetic trees. *Mol. Biol. Evol.* **1987**, *4*, 406–425. [PubMed]
57. Tamura, K.; Nei, M.; Kumar, S. Prospects for inferring very large phylogenies by using the neighbor-joining method. *Proc. Natl. Acad. Sci. USA* **2004**, *101*, 11030–11035. [CrossRef]
58. Felsenstein, J. Confidence limits on phylogenies: An approach using the bootstrap. *Evolution* **1985**, *39*, 783–791. [CrossRef]
59. Kumar, S.; Stecher, G.; Tamura, K. MEGA7: Molecular Evolutionary Genetics Analysis version 7.0 for bigger datasets. *Mol. Biol. Evol.* **2016**, *33*, 1870–1874. [CrossRef]
60. Martin, D.P.; Murrell, B.; Golden, M.; Khoosal, A.; Muhire, B. RDP4: Detection and analysis of recombination patterns in virus genomes. *Virus Evol.* **2015**, *1*, vev003. [CrossRef]
61. Simmonds, P.; McIntyre, C.; Savolainen-Kopra, C.; Tapparel, C.; Mackay, I.M.; Hovi, T. Proposals for the classification of human rhinovirus species C into genotypically assigned types. *J. Gen. Virol.* **2010**, *91*, 2409–2419. [CrossRef] [PubMed]
62. Papadopoulos, N.G.; Bates, P.J.; Bardin, P.G.; Papi, A.; Leir, S.H.; Fraenkel, D.J.; Meyer, J.; Lackie, P.M.; Sanderson, G.; Holgate, S.; et al. Rhinoviruses infect the lower airways. *J. Infect. Dis.* **2000**, *181*, 1875–1884. [CrossRef] [PubMed]
63. Jartti, T.; Jartti, L.; Ruuskanen, O.; Söderlund-Venermo, M. New respiratory viral infections. *Curr. Opin. Pulm. Med.* **2012**, *18*, 271–278. [CrossRef] [PubMed]
64. Bezerra, P.G.; Britto, M.C.; Correia, J.B.; Duarte Mdo, C.; Fonceca, A.M.; Rose, K.; Hopkins, M.J.; Cuevas, L.E.; McNamara, P.S. Viral and atypical bacterial detection in acute respiratory infection in children under five years. *PLoS ONE* **2011**, *6*, e18928. [CrossRef]
65. Cheuk, D.K.; Tang, I.W.; Chan, K.H.; Woo, P.C.; Peiris, M.J.; Chiu, S.S. Rhinovirus infection in hospitalized children in Hong Kong: A prospective study. *Pediatr. Infect. Dis. J.* **2007**, *26*, 995–1000. [CrossRef]
66. Teeratakulpisarn, J.; Pientong, C.; Ekalaksananan, T.; Ruangsiripiyakul, H.; Uppala, R. Rhinovirus infection in children hospitalized with acute bronchiolitis and its impact on subsequent wheezing or asthma: A comparison of etiologies. *Asian Pac. J. Allergy Immunol.* **2014**, *32*, 226–234.
67. Nour, A.; Alsayed, A.R.; Basheti, I. Prevalence of Asthma amongst Schoolchildren in Jordan and Staff Readiness to Help. *Healthcare* **2023**, *11*, 183. [CrossRef]
68. Alsayed, A.R. Illustrating How to Use the Validated Alsayed_v1 Tools to Improve Medical Care: A Particular Reference to the Global Initiative for Asthma 2022 Recommendations. *Patient Prefer. Adherence* **2023**, *17*, 1161–1179. [CrossRef]
69. AL-awaisheh, R.a.I.; Alsayed, A.R.; Basheti, I.A. Assessing the Pharmacist's Role in Counseling Asthmatic Adults Using the Correct Inhaler Technique and Its Effect on Asthma Control, Adherence, and Quality of Life. *Patient Prefer. Adherence* **2023**, *17*, 961–972. [CrossRef]
70. Stein, R.T.; Sherrill, D.; Morgan, W.J.; Holberg, C.J.; Halonen, M.; Taussig, L.M.; Wright, A.L.; Martinez, F.D. Respiratory syncytial virus in early life and risk of wheeze and allergy by age 13 years. *Lancet* **1999**, *354*, 541–545. [CrossRef]
71. Sigurs, N.; Aljassim, F.; Kjellman, B.; Robinson, P.D.; Sigurbergsson, F.; Bjarnason, R.; Gustafsson, P.M. Asthma and allergy patterns over 18 years after severe RSV bronchiolitis in the first year of life. *Thorax* **2010**, *65*, 1045–1052. [CrossRef] [PubMed]

72. Zhu, Z.; Camargo, C.A., Jr.; Raita, Y.; Freishtat, R.J.; Fujiogi, M.; Hahn, A.; Mansbach, J.M.; Spergel, J.M.; Pérez-Losada, M.; Hasegawa, K. Nasopharyngeal airway dual-transcriptome of infants with severe bronchiolitis and risk of childhood asthma: A multicenter prospective study. *J. Allergy Clin. Immunol.* **2022**, *150*, 806–816. [CrossRef] [PubMed]
73. Raita, Y.; Pérez-Losada, M.; Freishtat, R.J.; Hahn, A.; Castro-Nallar, E.; Ramos-Tapia, I.; Stearrett, N.; Bochkov, Y.A.; Gern, J.E.; Mansbach, J.M.; et al. Nasopharyngeal metatranscriptome profiles of infants with bronchiolitis and risk of childhood asthma: A multicentre prospective study. *Eur. Respir. J.* **2021**, *60*, 2102293. [CrossRef]
74. Ooka, T.; Raita, Y.; Fujiogi, M.; Freishtat, R.J.; Gerszten, R.E.; Mansbach, J.M.; Zhu, Z.; Camargo, C.A., Jr.; Hasegawa, K. Proteomics endotyping of infants with severe bronchiolitis and risk of childhood asthma. *Allergy* **2022**, *77*, 3350–3361. [CrossRef] [PubMed]
75. Raita, Y.; Pérez-Losada, M.; Freishtat, R.J.; Harmon, B.; Mansbach, J.M.; Piedra, P.A.; Zhu, Z.; Camargo, C.A.; Hasegawa, K. Integrated omics endotyping of infants with respiratory syncytial virus bronchiolitis and risk of childhood asthma. *Nat. Commun.* **2021**, *12*, 3601. [CrossRef]
76. Zhu, Z.; Camargo, C.A., Jr.; Raita, Y.; Fujiogi, M.; Liang, L.; Rhee, E.P.; Woodruff, P.G.; Hasegawa, K. Metabolome subtyping of severe bronchiolitis in infancy and risk of childhood asthma. *J. Allergy Clin. Immunol.* **2022**, *149*, 102–112. [CrossRef]
77. Palmenberg, A.C.; Spiro, D.; Kuzmickas, R.; Wang, S.; Djikeng, A.; Rathe, J.A.; Fraser-Liggett, C.M.; Liggett, S.B. Sequencing and analyses of all known human rhinovirus genomes reveal structure and evolution. *Science* **2009**, *324*, 55–59. [CrossRef]
78. Lewis-Rogers, N.; Bendall, M.L.; Crandall, K.A. Phylogenetic relationships and molecular adaptation dynamics of human rhinoviruses. *Mol. Biol. Evol.* **2009**, *26*, 969–981. [CrossRef]
79. Nix, W.A.; Oberste, M.S.; Pallansch, M.A. Sensitive, seminested PCR amplification of VP1 sequences for direct identification of all enterovirus serotypes from original clinical specimens. *J. Clin. Microbiol.* **2006**, *44*, 2698–2704. [CrossRef]
80. Leitch, E.M.; Harvala, H.; Robertson, I.; Ubillos, I.; Templeton, K.; Simmonds, P. Direct identification of human enterovirus serotypes in cerebrospinal fluid by amplification and sequencing of the VP1 region. *J. Clin. Virol.* **2009**, *44*, 119–124. [CrossRef]
81. She, R.C.; Hymas, W.C.; Taggart, E.W.; Petti, C.A.; Hillyard, D.R. Performance of enterovirus genotyping targeting the VP1 and VP2 regions on non-typeable isolates and patient specimens. *J. Virol. Methods* **2010**, *165*, 46–50. [CrossRef] [PubMed]
82. Kiang, D.; Newbower, E.C.; Yeh, E.; Wold, L.; Chen, L.; Schnurr, D.P. An algorithm for the typing of enteroviruses and correlation to serotyping by viral neutralization. *J. Clin. Virol.* **2009**, *45*, 334–340. [CrossRef] [PubMed]
83. Haff, L.A. Improved quantitative PCR using nested primers. *Genome Res.* **1994**, *3*, 332–337. [CrossRef] [PubMed]
84. McIntyre, C.L. Epidemiology, Classification and Evolution of Human Rhinoviruses. Ph.D. Thesis, University of Edinburgh, Edinburgh, UK, 2013.
85. Silva, P.A.; Diedrich, S.; de Paula Cardoso, D.d.D.; Schreier, E. Identification of enterovirus serotypes by pyrosequencing using multiple sequencing primers. *J. Virol. Methods* **2008**, *148*, 260–264. [CrossRef] [PubMed]
86. Vlasak, M.; Blomqvist, S.; Hovi, T.; Hewat, E.; Blaas, D. Sequence and structure of human rhinoviruses reveal the basis of receptor discrimination. *J. Virol.* **2003**, *77*, 6923–6930. [CrossRef]
87. Lee, W.-M.; Monroe, S.; Rueckert, R. Role of maturation cleavage in infectivity of picornaviruses: Activation of an infectosome. *J. Virol.* **1993**, *67*, 2110–2122. [CrossRef]
88. Hughes, P.J.; North, C.; Jellis, C.H.; Minor, P.D.; Stanway, G. The nucleotide sequence of human rhinovirus 1B: Molecular relationships within the rhinovirus genus. *J. Gen. Virol.* **1988**, *69*, 49–58. [CrossRef]

Disclaimer/Publisher's Note: The statements, opinions and data contained in all publications are solely those of the individual author(s) and contributor(s) and not of MDPI and/or the editor(s). MDPI and/or the editor(s) disclaim responsibility for any injury to people or property resulting from any ideas, methods, instructions or products referred to in the content.

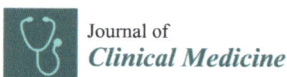

Article

Prevalence of Overweight and Obesity and Their Impact on Spirometry Parameters in Patients with Asthma: A Multicentre, Retrospective Study

Abdullah A. Alqarni [1,*], Abdulelah M. Aldhahir [2], Rayan A. Siraj [3], Jaber S. Alqahtani [4], Hams H. Alshehri [1], Amal M. Alshamrani [1], Ahlam A. Namnqani [1], Lama N. Alsaidalani [1], Mohammed N. Tawhari [2], Omaima I. Badr [5] and Hassan Alwafi [6]

[1] Department of Respiratory Therapy, Faculty of Medical Rehabilitation Sciences, King Abdulaziz University, Jeddah 22230, Saudi Arabia
[2] Respiratory Therapy Department, Faculty of Applied Medical Sciences, Jazan University, Jazan 45142, Saudi Arabia
[3] Department of Respiratory Care, College of Applied Medical Sciences, King Faisal University, Al-Ahsa 31982, Saudi Arabia
[4] Department of Respiratory Care, Prince Sultan Military College of Health Sciences, Dammam 34313, Saudi Arabia
[5] Department of Chest Medicine, Faculty of Medicine, Mansoura University, Mansoura 35516, Egypt
[6] Faculty of Medicine, Umm Al-Qura University, Mecca 21514, Saudi Arabia
* Correspondence: aaalqarni1@kau.edu.sa

Abstract: Introduction: Obesity is a common comorbidity in patients with asthma and has a significant impact on health and prognoses. However, the extent to which overweight and obesity impact asthma, particularly lung function, remains unclear. This study aimed to report on the prevalence of overweight and obesity and assess their impacts on spirometry parameters in asthmatic patients. Methods: In this multicentre, retrospective study, we reviewed the demographic data and spirometry results of all adult patients with confirmed diagnoses of asthma who visited the studied hospitals' pulmonary clinics between January 2016 and October 2022. Results: In total, 684 patients with confirmed diagnoses of asthma were included in the final analysis, of whom 74% were female, with a mean ± SD age of 47 ± 16 years. The prevalence of overweight and obesity among patients with asthma was 31.1% and 46.0%, respectively. There was a significant decline in spirometry results in obese patients with asthma compared with patients with healthy weights. Furthermore, body mass index (BMI) was negatively correlated with forced vital capacity (FVC) (L), forced expiratory volume in one second (FEV_1), forced expiratory flow at 25–75% ($FEF_{25-75\%}$) L/s and peak expiratory flow (PEF) L/s (r = −0.22, $p < 0.001$; r = −0.17, $p < 0.001$; r = −0.15, $p < 0.001$; r = −0.12, $p < 0.01$, respectively). Following adjustments for confounders, a higher BMI was independently associated with lower FVC (B −0.02 [95% CI −0.028, −0.01, $p < 0.001$] and lower FEV_1 (B −0.01 [95% CI −0.01, −0.001, $p < 0.05$]. Conclusions: Overweight and obesity are highly prevalent in asthma patients, and more importantly, they can reduce lung function, characterised mainly by reduced FEV_1 and FVC. These observations highlight the importance of implementing a nonpharmacological approach (i.e., weight loss) as part of the treatment plan for patients with asthma to improve lung function.

Keywords: obesity; overweight; asthma; lung function; BMI; spirometry

1. Introduction

Asthma, a common pulmonary disease, is characterised by airway hyperresponsiveness, inflammation and remodelling, and it is associated with variable airflow limitation and the presence of respiratory symptoms that vary over time and in intensity. Asthma affects around 300 million people worldwide, and it is expected that closer to 400 million people will have this condition by 2025 [1]. Patients with asthma tend to have variable combinations of pulmonary symptoms, including wheeze, cough, shortness of breath and chest tightness. Worsening of these respiratory symptoms (referred to as exacerbation) may lead to frequent visits to emergency departments and impact overall quality of life [2]. Several factors have been suggested to be associated with the exacerbation of asthma symptoms, one of which is obesity.

Obesity is one of the most common asthma comorbidities [2] and is defined as an excessive accumulation of body fat that leads to a generalised increase in body mass or adipose tissue, which increases the risk of health problems [3]. Body mass index (BMI), calculated as weight in kilograms (kg) divided by the square of height in metres (m^2), is the most widely used screening tool to determine overweight and obesity [4]. According to the World Health Organisation (WHO), BMI values of between 25 and 29.9 kg/m^2 are considered to be overweight, while individuals with BMIs of 30 kg/m^2 and higher are classified as obese [5]. Obesity is further classified by the Centres for Disease Control and Prevention (CDC) into three different categories: class I, or mild (30–34.9 kg/m^2), class II, or moderate (35–39.9 kg/m^2), and class III, or morbid (above 40 kg/m^2) [6].

Obesity is prevalent among adults and children with asthma worldwide [2]. Although the prevalence of obesity in patients with physician-diagnosed asthma is unclear, previous studies have shown that the prevalence of obesity in individuals with self-reported asthma ranges from 15% to 52% [7–9]. More importantly, studies suggest that overweight and obesity in conjunction with asthma may lead to deterioration in pulmonary function, which has been shown to be consistent with poor asthma control [10]. In support of this, it has been reported that asthmatic patients who are obese tend to have a four- to six-fold increased risk of hospitalisation compared with non-obese asthmatic patients [11]. Although the exact pathophysiological mechanism remains unknown, it is thought the lung compression caused by accumulation of body fat around the thoracic and abdominal cavities (abdominal obesity) may lead to airway narrowing and increased airway resistance [12]. In addition, it has been suggested that obesity may increase the production of pro-inflammatory mediators that worsen airway inflammation, subsequently causing airway hyperreactivity [13].

Although the impact of obesity on lung function, including spirometry parameters in adults with asthma, has been reported in previous studies, there is still controversy over whether obesity further worsens airway obstruction [7–9]. This controversy is likely due to the fact that some previous studies rely on self-reported asthma diagnoses or self-reported height and weight rather than diagnosis by a physician in clinic or measured height and weight [7–9]. Thus, further studies are warranted to better understand the impact of obesity on a wide range of spirometry parameters: peak expiratory flow (PEF), forced expiratory volume in one second (FEV_1), ratio of FEV_1 to forced vital capacity (FEV_1/FVC), FVC and forced expiratory flow at 25% and 75% of the pulmonary volume ($FEF_{25-75\%}$).

Preliminary reports suggest that both asthma and obesity can lead to worsening of respiratory symptoms and increased risk of hospitalisation. However, the prevalence of obesity and the extent to which overweight and obesity impact lung function, particularly spirometry parameters among patients with asthma in Saudi Arabia, has not been studied. Therefore, this study aimed to report on the prevalence of overweight and obesity and assess their impacts on spirometry parameters in asthmatic patients.

2. Materials and Methods

2.1. Study Design and Settings

This multicentre, retrospective study was conducted to investigate the impact of overweight and obesity on spirometry parameters among patients with asthma. The data collection process was carried out between 1 April 2022 and 31 October 2022 at King Abdulaziz University hospital and two Ministry of Health hospitals in Saudi Arabia.

2.2. Study Population

We retrospectively reviewed the electronic medical records of 1156 outpatients with confirmed asthma diagnoses who had scheduled visits and consultations with specialists and were treated between 1 January 2016 and 31 October 2022. We collected spirometry results and demographic data (e.g., height, weight, BMI, age, gender and smoking status). Demographic data were collected at the time spirometry was performed. Only patients with multidisciplinary-team-confirmed diagnoses of asthma made in accordance with current nationally and internationally accepted criteria were included in the current study [14]. In the final analysis, we only included asthmatic patients with acceptable and reproducible lung function tests at or after age 18, as well as patients without smoking history due to the difficulty in separating asthma from chronic obstructive pulmonary disease in smokers.

2.3. Spirometry Parameters

Only spirometry tests performed in accordance with the current American Thoracic Society/European Respiratory Society guidelines were included in the current study [15]. All spirometry tests were performed in pulmonary clinics by trained pulmonary function technologists. Although the pulmonary function tests were routinely validated by a respiratory consultant, all spirometry tests used in the present study were manually reviewed by two trained senior respiratory therapists (A.A.A. and A.M.A.). The results were not included in the final analysis if the spirometry tests were not acceptable and reproducible. The included spirometry results were obtained using a Sensor Medics Vmax 22 machine (SensorMedics Inc., Anaheim, CA, USA). The following spirometry parameters were recorded and included in the current study: FVC, FEV_1, ratio of FEV_1/FVC, $FEF_{25-75\%}$ and PEF. If the patient had more than one spirometry test performed between 1 January 2016 and 31 October 2022, only the most recent result was included.

2.4. Body Mass Index

Height and weight were routinely measured in the clinics, with patients barefoot and wearing light clothing, using a medical scale (Adam Equipment Inc., Oxford, CT, USA). We only collected BMI values based on the heights and weights measured before spirometry was performed. All asthmatic patients included in the current study were divided into five groups in accordance with WHO and CDC classifications: (1) patients with BMI values of 18.5 to 24.9 kg/m^2 (lean or healthy weight); (2) patients with BMI values of 25 to 29.9 kg/m^2 (overweight); (3) patients with BMI values of 30 to 34.9 kg/m^2 (mild or class I obesity); (4) patients with BMI values of 35 to 39.9 kg/m^2 (moderate or class II obesity); and (5) patients with BMI values of 40 kg/m^2 or above (morbid or class III obesity) [5,6].

2.5. Ethical Considerations

Prior to the start of this study, ethical approval (HA-02-J-008) was obtained from the Unit of Biomedical Ethics Research Committee at the Faculty of Medicine in King Abdulaziz University, Saudi Arabia.

2.6. Statistical Analysis

In this study, Stata (version 16) was used for data management and analysis. Figures were generated using GraphPad Prism (version 9). The results are presented as numbers (%) and arithmetic means $\pm$ SD for categorical and continuous variables, respectively, unless otherwise stated. The normality of the data was graphically assessed. A one-way ANOVA was performed to compare the mean differences between lean, overweight and specifically classed obesity groups. This was followed by an unpaired Student's t test to compare the mean differences between the two independent data sets. The correlation of BMI with spirometry measures (FEV_1, FVC, $FEF_{25-75\%}$ and PEF) was determined using Pearson's correlation coefficient. A multiple linear regression model was also performed to determine the factors associated with spirometry measures. $p < 0.05$ was regarded as statistically significant.

3. Results

3.1. Patient Characteristics

In total, 1156 subjects with confirmed asthma diagnoses were identified from the databases. After excluding patients <18 years old, smokers and those with BMIs <18.5 kg/m^2 or without acceptable spirometry results, a total of 684 asthma patients met our inclusion criteria and were included in the final analysis (Figure 1).

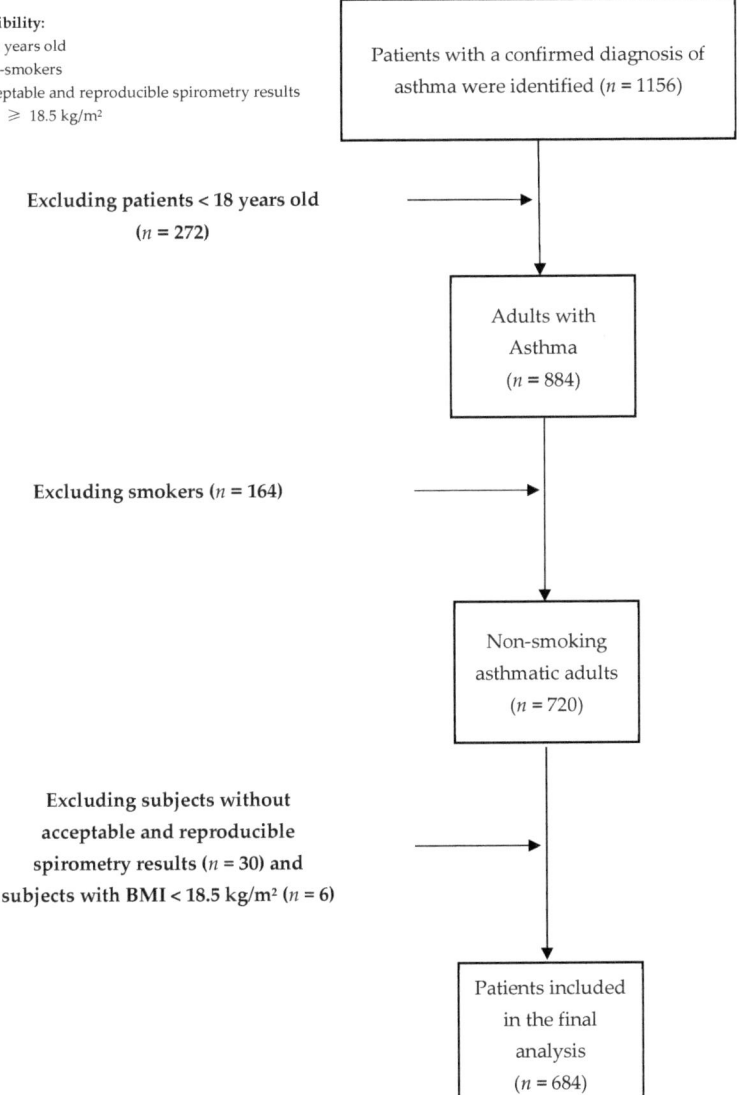

Figure 1. Flow chart of the study.

The mean ± SD age of the study population was 47 ± 16 years, and there were more females (74%) than males. Of the 684 included patients, 23% had BMIs between ≥18.5 and <25 kg/m^2 (lean or healthy weight), 31% had a BMIs between ≥25 and <30 kg/m^2 (overweight) and 46% had BMIs of ≥30 kg/m^2 (all three classes of obesity). The prevalence of obesity alone and obesity including overweight in patients with asthma was 46% and 77%, respectively. The mean ± SD BMI was statistically significantly greater in females than males (30.5 ± 6.9 vs. 28.9 ± 6.1; $p < 0.05$). The proportion of female patients was higher in the overweight (75%) and obesity (87%) groups compared with lean subjects (66%). The baseline characteristics for the study population are shown in Table 1.

Table 1. Patient characteristics ($n = 684$).

Variable	Lean ($n = 157$)	Overweight ($n = 213$)	Class I Obesity ($n = 179$)	Class II Obesity ($n = 82$)	Class III Obesity ($n = 53$)
Age (years)	40 ± 16	47 ± 17	51 ± 15	51 ± 14	53 ± 14
Height (cm)	161 ± 8	163 ± 8	161 ± 10	157 ± 21	156 ± 9
Weight (kg)	59 ± 8	71 ± 8	83 ± 12	90 ± 18	111 ± 16
BMI (kg/m^2)	22 ± 2	27 ± 1	32 ± 1	37 ± 1	46 ± 6
Female, n (%)	104 (66%)	160 (75%)	130 (73%)	69 (84%)	44 (83%)

Data are represented as mean ± SD unless otherwise stated. BMI: body mass index. Obesity is classified based on BMI according to the World Health Organization classification: class I = 30–34.9 kg/m^2, class II = 35–39.9 kg/m^2 and class III = 40 kg/m^2 and greater.

3.2. Associations between BMI and Spirometry Parameters

Pearson correlation analyses were performed to determine whether BMI was associated with spirometry parameters. The results showed that there were statistically significant inverse correlations between BMI and FVC ($r = -0.22$, $p < 0.001$), FEV$_1$ ($r = -0.17$, $p < 0.001$), FEF$_{25-75\%}$ ($r = -0.15$, $p < 0.001$) and PEF ($r = -0.14$, $p < 0.01$) (Figure 2).

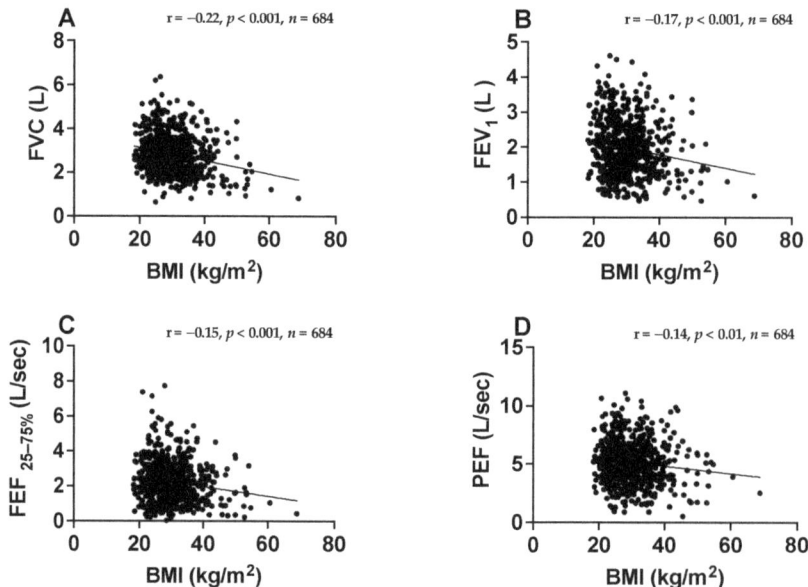

Figure 2. Correlation between body mass index (BMI) and spirometry values among patients with asthma. Correlations between BMI kg/m^2 with forced vital capacity (FVC) L (**A**), forced expiratory volume in one second (FEV$_1$) L (**B**), forced expiratory flow at 25% and 75% of the pulmonary volume (FEF$_{25-75\%}$) L/s (**C**) and peak expiratory flow (PEF) L/s (**D**) were assessed.

3.3. Impact of Overweight and Obesity on Spirometry Parameters

In order to determine whether a progressive decline in spirometry values was observed as BMI increased, we divided asthmatic patients into four different groups based on their

BMI values. A one-way ANOVA showed that the means of the spirometry measures (FVC L, FEV$_1$ L, FEF $_{25-75\%}$ L/s and PEF L/s) differed significantly according to BMI groups ($p < 0.0001$, $p < 0.01$, $p < 0.01$ and $p < 0.05$, respectively) (Figure 3A–D). Unpaired t tests were then performed to assess whether there was a significant difference in each spirometry measure based on the weight category. As shown in Figure 3A, although no difference in the mean FVC was found between normal weight and overweight (3.07 ± 0.06 L and 2.90 ± 0.06 L, respectively), mean FVC was significantly reduced in subjects with class I, class II and class III obesity (2.79 ± 0.06 L, $p < 0.01$, 2.65 ± 0.09 L, $p < 0.001$ and 2.39 ± 0.13 L $p < 0.0001$, respectively) compared with normal weight. In addition, mean FVC was found to be significantly decreased in class II and class III, but not in class I, compared with overweight ($p < 0.05$ and $p < 0.001$, respectively).

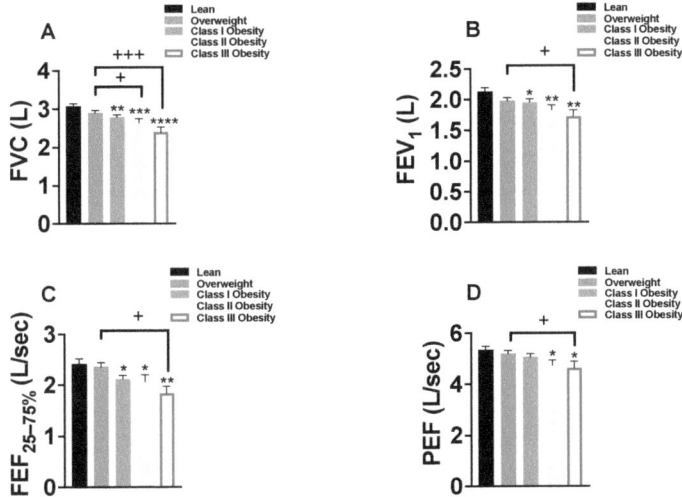

Figure 3. Effect of overweight and obesity on spirometry values in patients with asthma. Patients were divided into four groups based on body mass index (BMI) to assess the impact of overweight and obesity on spirometry values: forced vital capacity (FVC) L (**A**), forced expiratory volume in one second (FEV$_1$) L (**B**), forced expiratory flow at 25% and 75% of the pulmonary volume (FEF $_{25-75\%}$) L/s (**C**) and peak expiratory flow (PEF) L/s (**D**). Patients with BMIs ≥ 18.5 to 24.9 kg/m^2 and BMIs of ≥25 to 29.9 kg/m^2 were classified as lean ($n = 157$) and overweight ($n = 213$), respectively. Obesity was subsequently classified into three different groups: class I (BMI of ≥30 to 34.9 kg/m^2, $n = 179$), class II (BMI of ≥35 to 39.9 kg/m^2, $n = 82$) and class III (BMI of ≥40 kg/m^2 or greater, $n = 53$). Each data point represents mean ± SEM. * $p < 0.05$, ** $p < 0.01$, *** $p < 0.001$, **** $p < 0.0001$ compared with lean; + $p < 0.05$, +++ $p < 0.001$ compared with overweight.

Similar to the FVC findings, mean FEV$_1$ did not significantly differ between asthmatic patients with normal weight and overweight (2.13 ± 0.06 L and 1.98 ± 0.05 L, respectively) (Figure 3B). However, mean FEV$_1$ was found to be significantly lower in all classes of obesity (class I, class II and class III) (1.95 ± 0.05 L, $p < 0.05$, 1.83 ± 0.07 L, $p < 0.01$ and 1.72 ± 0.10 L $p < 0.01$, respectively) compared with normal BMI. When compared with overweight patients, mean FEV$_1$ remained unchanged in those with class I and class II obesity but was significantly reduced in asthmatic patients with class III obesity ($p < 0.05$) (Figure 3B). Furthermore, mean FEF $_{25-75\%}$ was significantly reduced in class I, class II and class III obesity (2.11 ± 0.07 L/s, $p < 0.05$, 2.07 ± 0.13 L/s, $p < 0.05$ and 1.83 ± 0.13 L/s, $p < 0.05$, respectively) but not in overweight patients as compared with normal weight (2.41 ± 0.10 L/s) (Figure 3C). Interestingly, we found that mean PEF did not differ in patients with overweight and class I obesity but was significantly reduced in asthmatic patients with class I and II obesity (4.73 ± 0.19 L/s, $p < 0.05$ and 4.62 ± 0.26 L/s, $p < 0.05$, respectively) compared with normal weight (5.33 ± 0.14 L/s). It was also interesting to find that PEF only decreased in patients with class III obesity when compared with overweight patients ($p < 0.05$) (Figure 3D).

A multiple linear regression model was performed to assess the independent associations of BMI with spirometry measures. BMI was significantly associated with FVC (L) and FEV_1 (L) following adjustments for age and gender (adjusted β: −0.02; 95% CI: −0.028 to −0.01; $p < 0.001$) and (adjusted β: −0.01; 95% CI: −0.01 to −0.001; $p < 0.05$), respectively. In addition, simple regression models showed that BMI was associated with $FEF_{25-75\%}$ (β: −0.03; 95% CI: −0.04 to −0.014; $p < 0.001$) and PEF (β: −0.03; 95% CI: −0.05 to −0.01; $p < 0.01$). However, the associations were nullified upon further adjustments for age and gender (Table 2).

Table 2. Analysis of the associations of BMI with spirometry measures.

Independent Variable	BMI	
	β (95% CI; *p*-Value)	Adjusted β (95% CI; *p*-Value)
FVC L	−0.03 (−0.04 to −0.02; $p < 0.001$)	−0.02 (−0.028 to −0.01; $p < 0.001$) [1]
FEV_1 L	−0.02 (−0.028 to −0.01; $p < 0.05$)	−0.01 (−0.01 to −0.001; $p < 0.05$) [1]
FEF (25–75%) L/s	−0.03 (−0.04 to −0.014; $p < 0.001$)	−0.012 (−0.025 to 0.001; $p = 0.058$) [1]
PEF L/s	−0.03 (−0.05 to −0.01; $p < 0.01$)	−0.014 (−0.03 to 0.01; $p = 0.179$) [1]

[1] Adjusted for age and gender. FVC: forced vital capacity. FEV_1: forced expiratory volume in one second. $FEF_{25-75\%}$: forced expiratory flow at 25% and 75% of the pulmonary volume. PEF: peak expiratory flow. BMI: body mass index.

4. Discussion

To the best of our knowledge, this study is the first to determine overweight and obesity prevalence in asthmatic patients and to assess the impact of overweight and obesity on spirometry measures among asthmatic patients in Saudi Arabia. The main findings of the current study showed that the prevalence of overweight and obesity among patients with asthma was 31% and 46%, respectively. Our findings also demonstrated that there was a significant decline in spirometry results (FEV_1, FVC, PEF and $FEF_{25-75\%}$) in obese patients with asthma compared with normal-weight asthma patients. In addition, we found that BMI was negatively correlated with all spirometry measures and that a higher BMI was independently associated with lower FVC and lower FEV_1. These findings suggest that obesity can reduce lung function, ultimately leading to poor asthma control, and also highlight the importance of using a nonpharmacological approach (e.g., healthy diet and weight loss) as part of the treatment plan for patients with asthma to improve lung function and, ultimately, asthma management and overall quality of life.

Obesity is one of the most common asthma comorbidities and is associated with increased risks of exacerbation and hospitalisation. Our findings that overweight (31%) and obesity (46%) are prevalent in patients with asthma are similar to a previous study reporting that the prevalence of obesity among patients with asthma is 52% in the Netherlands [8] but contrasts with studies demonstrating a low prevalence of obesity (15% and 27%) among asthmatic patients in Taiwan [16] and Norway [9], respectively. This disparity is most likely attributable to the fact that the selection of asthma patients in the previous studies was based on self-reported asthma [9,16], whereas in the current study, only patients with multidisciplinary-team-confirmed diagnoses of asthma carried out in accordance with current nationally and internationally accepted criteria were included. In addition, the fact that the prevalence of obesity has been increasing in recent years among the general population in Saudi Arabia [17] may explain the high obesity prevalence observed in the current study. Despite the differences in prevalence rates, our finding that 77% of asthmatic patients are obese or at risk of obesity (overweight) is alarming and suggests that early identification of obesity and overweight, through a regular screening tool, should be implemented in asthma clinics in order to reduce the risk associated with obesity.

Although the mechanism that links asthma with obesity is not fully understood, it has been reported that obesity may be a consequence of asthma maintenance therapies. For instance, evidence suggests that the use of oral and inhaled corticosteroids is associated with increased body weight [18,19]. On the other hand, several studies describe obesity as a risk factor for asthma [20], indicating that obese patients are at a higher risk of developing the condition, leading to a novel disease phenotype (obesity-associated asthma) that requires careful evaluation and management. Further studies are needed to better understand the characteristics of this phenotype and its main underlying mechanisms.

Obesity has been suggested to be associated with an increased asthma exacerbation rate, but it is unclear whether airflow obstruction is directly responsible for the deterioration of asthma symptoms. Our findings demonstrated a reduction in spirometry parameters (FEV_1, FVC, PEF and $FEF_{25-75\%}$) in asthmatic patients with obesity compared with patients with normal weight, suggesting that obesity may ultimately impair lung function in patients with asthma. This is likely due to the fact that obesity can cause mechanical compression of the diaphragm, as well as the chest cavity [13], which may lead to a reduction in lung function. In addition, it has been reported that excess adipose tissue in obese individuals can further increase inflammatory mediators (e.g., interleukin 6) [21], which have been shown to be associated with impaired lung function [22,23].

Although the impact of overweight and obesity on PEF and $FEF_{25-75\%}$ values has not been reported, our findings are supported by a previous study that reported a reduction in FEV_1 and FVC in self-reported asthma subjects with overweight and obesity as compared with normal weight [9]. This is further strengthened by the findings of this study that a higher BMI is independently associated with lower FVC and FEV_1 even after adjustments for known confounders. A previous study demonstrated that an intensive six-month weight-loss programme was correlated with improvement in FVC and FEV_1 in women with BMIs >30 kg/m^2 [24]. Our findings, together with these observations, suggest that obesity can cause a decline in lung function, which can be reversed by weight loss. Thus, a screening tool to identify asthmatic patients at high risk for obesity should be implemented in order to improve overall quality of life in patients with asthma.

It is also worth noting that we demonstrated that obesity and overweight, in general, are more prevalent among female asthmatic patients (75% and 77%, respectively) than male patients. This finding is supported by a previous study conducted in the US, showing that overweight and obesity are more prevalent in females with asthma (63% and 82%, respectively) than in males [23]. Overweight and obesity have also been reported to be more prevalent in females (54% and 66%, respectively) than males in Norwegian patients with self-reported asthma [9]. Our findings, together with these previous observations, may be explained by the fact that the proportion of asthma, regardless of subjects' body weight and geographical location, is found to be higher in female than male subjects in the current study (74% prevalence), as well as in a previous study (65% prevalence) [25]. In addition, obesity without asthma has been reported to be higher in female than male subjects. A high rate of asthma with obesity in adult women suggests that sex hormones and nutrition quality may play a role in the presence and severity of asthma in obese patients.

4.1. Strengths

This study has a number of strengths. First, most studies have assessed the impact of overweight and obesity on lung function in patients with self-reported asthma. The current study only included patients whose diagnoses of asthma were made and confirmed in accordance with current nationally and internationally accepted criteria. Second, we only included patients with spirometry tests performed in accordance with the current American Thoracic Society/European Respiratory Society guidelines. In addition, two trained respiratory therapists reviewed all spirometry tests and further excluded tests that were not acceptable and reproducible. Third, some previous studies have relied on self-reported height and weight. In the current study, BMI was calculated based on height and weight measured using medical scales in pulmonary clinics under the supervision of a trained nurse or respiratory therapist.

4.2. Limitations

The current study is not without limitations. First, we were unable to study lung volumes and diffusion capacity as these tests are either unavailable or not routinely performed in our pulmonary clinics for patients with asthma. Second, it is known that the use of asthma maintenance therapies (e.g., inhaled corticosteroids) can lead to better asthma control and improvement in asthma symptoms and lung function. In the current study, all patients were on inhaled corticosteroids as a maintenance therapy to control asthma symptoms. However, it remains critical in the current study to determine the doses of inhaled corticosteroids, the levels of patient adherence to therapies and whether those patients were on other asthma control therapies due to the unavailability of these data. Thus, it is important to acknowledge that spirometry parameters can also be affected by patient non-adherence to therapies and/or types of therapy added on to existing inhaled corticosteroid treatment. Third, the prevalence of overweight and obesity was assessed in this study based on BMIs calculated from height and weight measured before spirometry was performed. Although BMI is currently considered to be the gold standard and is used by international organisations (e.g., WHO and CDC) to classify overweight and obesity, it should be noted that it lacks the ability to differentiate between fat and lean mass and does not take into account the differences in fat distribution. This is unlikely to affect the results of this study, as previous studies have shown that abdominal and thoracic fat have a differential effect on lung volumes [26]. There is no evidence to suggest that spirometry parameters are affected by differences in fat distribution. Fourth, our entire study population was diagnosed with asthma in Saudi Arabia. Thus, the findings may not translate to individuals with other chronic pulmonary and non-pulmonary diseases and/or other ethnic groups.

4.3. Practical Implementation

Obesity is an asthma comorbidity that can eventually contribute to worsening respiratory symptoms. We report here that the prevalence of obesity and overweight in asthmatic patients is high, and that obesity can lead to a reduction in lung function in patients with asthma. In addition to pharmacological therapies, our findings highlight the importance of using non-pharmacological add-on therapies (e.g., physical exercise, healthy diet and weight loss) as part of the treatment plan for patients with asthma to improve lung function and, ultimately, asthma symptoms and overall quality of life. Further studies are needed to explore the impact of different lifestyle strategies on the treatment of asthma patients.

5. Conclusions

Overweight and obesity are highly prevalent in asthma patients, and, more importantly, they can reduce lung function, characterised mainly by reduced FEV_1 and FVC. These observations suggest that weight loss may reduce the severity of asthma and that early obesity prevention and healthy lifestyles should be implemented through routine screening in primary care to improve lung function, thereby leading to improvements in asthma management, as well as quality of life.

Author Contributions: The study was designed by A.A.A. and A.M.A. (Abdulelah M. Aldhahir); statistical methodology was performed by J.S.A., H.A. and R.A.S.; data collection was performed by H.A., O.I.B., H.H.A., A.M.A. (Amal M. Alshamrani), A.A.N., L.N.A. and M.N.T.; formal analysis was performed by A.A.A. and R.A.S.; original draft of the manuscript was prepared by A.A.A., A.M.A. (Abdulelah M. Aldhahir) and R.A.S. and reviewed and edited by all authors. All authors have read and agreed to the published version of the manuscript.

Funding: This research work was funded by Institutional Fund Projects under grant no. (IFPIP:993-883-1443). The authors gratefully acknowledge the technical and financial support provided by the Ministry of Education and King Abdulaziz University, DSR, Jeddah, Saudi Arabia.

Institutional Review Board Statement: The study was conducted in accordance with the Declaration of Helsinki and approved by the Unit of Biomedical Ethics Research Committee at the Faculty of Medicine at King Abdulaziz University, Saudi Arabia (HA-02-J-008).

Informed Consent Statement: Not applicable.

Data Availability Statement: All data generated and analysed during this study are available from the corresponding author upon reasonable request.

Acknowledgments: The authors would like to thank Husam Alahmadi for his professional critique of the work presented here and for providing technical assistance in the analyses.

Conflicts of Interest: The authors declare no conflict of interest. The funder had no role in the design of the study; in the collection, analyses, or interpretation of data; in the writing of the manuscript; or in the decision to publish the results.

References

1. Masoli, M.; Fabian, D.; Holt, S.; Beasley, R. Global Initiative for Asthma P. The global burden of asthma: Executive summary of the GINA Dissemination Committee report. *Allergy* **2004**, *59*, 469–478. [CrossRef] [PubMed]
2. Reddel, H.K.; Bacharier, L.B.; Bateman, E.D.; Brightling, C.E.; Brusselle, G.G.; Buhl, R.; Cruz, A.A.; Duijts, L.; Drazen, J.M.; FitzGerald, J.M.; et al. Global Initiative for Asthma Strategy 2021. Executive Summary and Rationale for Key Changes. *Arch. Bronconeumol.* **2022**, *58*, 35–51. [CrossRef]
3. Lim, Y.; Boster, J. *Obesity and Comorbid Conditions*; StatPearls: Treasure Island, FL, USA, 2022.
4. Ghesmaty Sangachin, M.; Cavuoto, L.A.; Wang, Y. Use of various obesity measurement and classification methods in occupational safety and health research: A systematic review of the literature. *BMC Obes.* **2018**, *5*, 28. [CrossRef]
5. World Health Organization. Obesity and Overweight. Available online: https://www.who.int/news-room/fact-sheets/detail/obesity-and-overweight (accessed on 13 January 2023).
6. Defining Adult Overweight & Obesity by Centers for Disease Control and Prevention. Available online: https://www.cdc.gov/obesity/basics/adult-defining.html?CDC_AA_refVal=https%3A%2F%2Fwww.cdc.gov%2Fobesity%2Fadult%2Findex.html#print (accessed on 13 January 2023).
7. Sin, D.D.; Jones, R.L.; Man, S.F. Obesity is a risk factor for dyspnea but not for airflow obstruction. *Arch. Intern. Med.* **2002**, *162*, 1477–1481. [CrossRef]
8. Kasteleyn, M.J.; Bonten, T.N.; de Mutsert, R.; Thijs, W.; Hiemstra, P.S.; le Cessie, S.; Rosendaal, F.R.; Chavannes, N.H.; Taube, C. Pulmonary function, exhaled nitric oxide and symptoms in asthma patients with obesity: A cross-sectional study. *Respir. Res.* **2017**, *18*, 205. [CrossRef]
9. Klepaker, G.; Henneberger, P.K.; Hertel, J.K.; Holla, O.L.; Kongerud, J.; Fell, A.K.M. Influence of asthma and obesity on respiratory symptoms, work ability and lung function: Findings from a cross-sectional Norwegian population study. *BMJ Open Respir. Res.* **2021**, *8*, e000932. [CrossRef]
10. Reddel, H.; Ware, S.; Marks, G.; Salome, C.; Jenkins, C.; Woolcock, A. Differences between asthma exacerbations and poor asthma control. *Lancet* **1999**, *353*, 364–369. [CrossRef] [PubMed]
11. Holguin, F.; Bleecker, E.R.; Busse, W.W.; Calhoun, W.J.; Castro, M.; Erzurum, S.C.; Fitzpatrick, A.M.; Gaston, B.; Israel, E.; Jarjour, N.N.; et al. Obesity and asthma: An association modified by age of asthma onset. *J. Allergy Clin. Immunol.* **2011**, *127*, 1486–1493.e2. [CrossRef] [PubMed]
12. Dixon, A.E.; Peters, U. The effect of obesity on lung function. *Expert Rev. Respir. Med.* **2018**, *12*, 755–767. [CrossRef]
13. Peters, U.; Dixon, A.E.; Forno, E. Obesity and asthma. *J. Allergy Clin. Immunol.* **2018**, *141*, 1169–1179. [CrossRef] [PubMed]
14. Al-Moamary, M.S.; Alhaider, S.A.; Alangari, A.A.; Idrees, M.M.; Zeitouni, M.O.; Al Ghobain, M.O.; Alanazi, A.F.; Al-Harbi, A.S.; Yousef, A.A.; Alorainy, H.S.; et al. The Saudi Initiative for Asthma—2021 Update: Guidelines for the diagnosis and management of asthma in adults and children. *Ann. Thorac. Med.* **2021**, *16*, 4–56. [CrossRef] [PubMed]
15. Graham, B.L.; Steenbruggen, I.; Miller, M.R.; Barjaktarevic, I.Z.; Cooper, B.G.; Hall, G.L.; Hallstrand, T.S.; Kaminsky, D.A.; McCarthy, K.; McCormack, M.C.; et al. Standardization of Spirometry 2019 Update. An Official American Thoracic Society and European Respiratory Society Technical Statement. *Am. J. Respir. Crit. Care Med.* **2019**, *200*, e70–e88. [CrossRef] [PubMed]
16. Huang, Y.J.; Chu, Y.C.; Huang, H.L.; Hwang, J.S.; Chan, T.C. The Effects of Asthma on the Association Between Pulmonary Function and Obesity: A 16-Year Longitudinal Study. *J. Asthma Allergy* **2021**, *14*, 347–359. [CrossRef]
17. Althumiri, N.A.; Basyouni, M.H.; AlMousa, N.; AlJuwaysim, M.F.; Almubark, R.A.; BinDhim, N.F.; Alkhamaali, Z.; Alqahtani, S.A. Obesity in Saudi Arabia in 2020: Prevalence, Distribution, and Its Current Association with Various Health Conditions. *Healthcare* **2021**, *9*, 311. [CrossRef] [PubMed]

18. Price, D.B.; Trudo, F.; Voorham, J.; Xu, X.; Kerkhof, M.; Jie, J.L.Z.; Tran, T.N. Adverse outcomes from initiation of systemic corticosteroids for asthma: Long-term observational study. *J. Asthma Allergy* **2018**, *11*, 193–204. [CrossRef] [PubMed]
19. Peerboom, S.; Graff, S.; Seidel, L.; Paulus, V.; Henket, M.; Sanchez, C.; Guissard, F.; Moermans, C.; Louis, R.; Schleich, F. Predictors of a good response to inhaled corticosteroids in obesity-associated asthma. *Biochem. Pharmacol.* **2020**, *179*, 113994. [CrossRef] [PubMed]
20. Gibeon, D.; Batuwita, K.; Osmond, M.; Heaney, L.G.; Brightling, C.E.; Niven, R.; Mansur, A.; Chaudhuri, R.; Bucknall, C.E.; Rowe, A.; et al. Obesity-associated severe asthma represents a distinct clinical phenotype: Analysis of the British Thoracic Society Difficult Asthma Registry Patient cohort according to BMI. *Chest* **2013**, *143*, 406–414. [CrossRef]
21. Jeong, K.Y.; Lee, J.; Li, C.; Han, T.; Lee, S.B.; Lee, H.; Back, S.K.; Na, H.S. Juvenile obesity aggravates disease severity in a rat model of atopic dermatitis. *Allergy Asthma Immunol. Res.* **2015**, *7*, 69–75. [CrossRef]
22. Neveu, W.A.; Allard, J.L.; Raymond, D.M.; Bourassa, L.M.; Burns, S.M.; Bunn, J.Y.; Irvin, C.G.; Kaminsky, D.A.; Rincon, M. Elevation of IL-6 in the allergic asthmatic airway is independent of inflammation but associates with loss of central airway function. *Respir. Res.* **2010**, *11*, 28. [CrossRef]
23. Dixon, A.E.; Shade, D.M.; Cohen, R.I.; Skloot, G.S.; Holbrook, J.T.; Smith, L.J.; Lima, J.J.; Allayee, H.; Irvin, C.G.; Wise, R.A. American Lung Association-Asthma Clinical Research C. Effect of obesity on clinical presentation and response to treatment in asthma. *J. Asthma* **2006**, *43*, 553–558. [CrossRef]
24. Aaron, S.D.; Fergusson, D.; Dent, R.; Chen, Y.; Vandemheen, K.L.; Dales, R.E. Effect of weight reduction on respiratory function and airway reactivity in obese women. *Chest* **2004**, *125*, 2046–2052. [CrossRef] [PubMed]
25. Disease, G.B.D.; Injury, I.; Prevalence, C. Global, regional, and national incidence, prevalence, and years lived with disability for 328 diseases and injuries for 195 countries, 1990–2016: A systematic analysis for the Global Burden of Disease Study 2016. *Lancet* **2017**, *390*, 1211–1259.
26. Mehari, A.; Afreen, S.; Ngwa, J.; Setse, R.; Thomas, A.N.; Poddar, V.; Davis, W.; Polk, O.D.; Hassan, S.; Thomas, A.V. Obesity and Pulmonary Function in African Americans. *PLoS ONE* **2015**, *10*, e0140610. [CrossRef] [PubMed]

Disclaimer/Publisher's Note: The statements, opinions and data contained in all publications are solely those of the individual author(s) and contributor(s) and not of MDPI and/or the editor(s). MDPI and/or the editor(s) disclaim responsibility for any injury to people or property resulting from any ideas, methods, instructions or products referred to in the content.

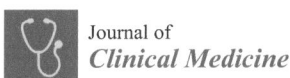

Systematic Review

Effects of Prenatal Paracetamol Exposure on the Development of Asthma and Wheezing in Childhood: A Systematic Review and Meta-Analysis

Agnieszka Barańska [1,*], Wiesław Kanadys [2], Artur Wdowiak [3], Maria Malm [1], Agata Błaszczuk [4], Urszula Religioni [5], Anita Wdowiak-Filip [6] and Małgorzata Polz-Dacewicz [4]

1. Department of Medical Informatics and Statistics with e-Health Laboratory, Medical University of Lublin, 20-954 Lublin, Poland
2. Specialistic Medical Center Czechow, 20-848 Lublin, Poland
3. Chair of Obstetrics and Gynecology, Medical University of Lublin, 20-081 Lublin, Poland
4. Department of Virology with SARS Laboratory, Medical University of Lublin, 20-093 Lublin, Poland
5. School of Public Health, Centre of Postgraduate Medical Education of Warsaw, 01-826 Warsaw, Poland
6. Department of Cosmetology and Aesthetic Medicine, Medical University of Lublin, 20-093 Lublin, Poland
* Correspondence: agnieszkabaranska@umlub.pl

Abstract: The aim of the report was to evaluate whether in utero exposure to paracetamol is associated with risk towards developing respiratory disorders such as asthma and wheeze after birth. MEDLINE (PubMed), EMBASE and Cochrane Library databases were searched for articles published in English to December 2021. The study involved 330,550 women. We then calculated the summary risk estimates and 95% CIs and plotted forest plots using random effect models (DerSimonian–Laird method) and fixed effect models. We also performed a systematic review of the chosen articles and a meta-analysis of studies based on the guidelines outlined in the PRISMA statement. Accordingly, maternal exposure to paracetamol during pregnancy was associated with a significant increased risk of asthma: crude OR = 1.34, 95% CI: 1.22 to 1.48, $p < 0.001$; and significant increased risk of wheeze: crude OR = 1.31, 95% CI: 1.12 to 1.54, $p < 0.002$. Results of our study confirmed that maternal paracetamol use in pregnancy is associated with an enhanced risk of asthma and wheezing in their children. We believe paracetamol should be used with caution by pregnant women, and at the lowest effective dose, and for the shortest duration. Long-term use or the use of high doses should be limited to the indications recommended by a physician and with the mother-to-be under constant supervision.

Keywords: paracetamol; asthma; wheeze; prenatal exposure; pregnancy; acetaminophen

1. Introduction

Paracetamol, also called "acetaminophen" or "N-acetyl-p-aminophenol" (APAP), is a mild-to-moderate antipyretic/analgesic drug widely used across the world, among a wide range of populations (from pregnant, pediatric and adult, to elderly people). At therapeutic doses, paracetamol is metabolized mainly by the formation of conjugates by glucuronidation and sulphation and is then excreted in the urine. Around 10% of all paracetamol is metabolized by cytochrome P450 (CYP) enzymes to form n-acetyl-p-benzoquinoneimine (NAPQI), which is subsequently conjugated with intracellular glutathione, and ultimately excreted as cysteine and mercapturic acid conjugates. Less than 5% is excreted unchanged [1–3].

Pregnancy is a special period in a woman's life, characterized not only by metabolic and physiological changes in her organism, but also by the possibility of susceptibility to pathological conditions. This may have consequences for the fetus, as well as affect the further health of the woman [4]. Use of over-the-counter medications or drugs for acute/short-term illnesses and chronic/long-term disorders, as well as for temporary pain control, is common in pregnancy [5]. One of the more frequently employed drugs as an analgesic and antipyrotic during this period is paracetamol [6].

Cytochrome P450s metabolizes endogenous and exogenous substrates and is involved in metabolizing toxins and procarcinogens [7]. Therefore, paracetamol must be metabolized either to sulfate via sulfation or to N-acetyl-p-benzoquinone imine (NAPQI) via cytochrome P450s in early pregnancy [8,9]. Paracetamol freely crosses the placenta [10]; however, the fetus has a limited ability to metabolize paracetamol through glucoronidation. Detoxification of paracetamol may deplete stores of glutathione, leading to increased oxidative damage to the lung epithelium and, thus, contributing to wheezing or asthma [11–13].

The aim of this review and meta-analysis is to assess the relationship between prenatal paracetamol exposure and wheezing or asthma in children.

2. Methods

We performed a systematic review of articles and a meta-analysis studies based on the guidelines outlined in the PRISMA statement [14].

2.1. Search Strategy

We considered all epidemiological studies that compared the risk of asthma or wheeze in childhood with prenatal paracetamol use. There were no limitations in searching for articles of interest in assessing the dependencies between prenatal paracetamol exposure and asthma or wheeze risk in childhood [15].

A thorough search was conducted in the electronic databases MEDLINE (PubMed), EMBASE and Cochrane to identify relevant research. Studies published up to December 2021 were included. The following search terms were used for all databases in various combinations: "asthma" or "wheeze" AND "paracetamol" or "acetaminophen" AND "prenatal" or "pregnancy". Taking into account the possibility of not finding all the articles of interest to us during the database search, references lists of relevant articles were additionally analyzed. The search results were compared with previously published meta-analyses on this topic. All data were extracted by two investigators (A.B. and W.K.), and disagreements were resolved in discussion with a third investigator (A.W.).

2.2. Eligibility Criteria

Definitions that were adopted in our analysis include: "wheeze"—definition characterized by paroxysmal transient or persistent, symptoms affecting breathing, such as noisy breathing ("wheezing" or "whistling"), shortness of breath, or a troublesome cough affecting sleep or everyday activity; "asthma"—definition established by doctor's diagnosis, clinical symptoms (shortness of breath, chest tightness or pain, cough, wheezing episodes) and/or use of asthma medication (note: certain differences in the definitions contained in some works made it difficult to qualify them to the finale definitions we have adopted).

The following inclusion criteria were established in the selection of studies: (i) trials that involve the comparison of women who used paracetamol during pregnancy with an observational group; (ii) studies evaluating the effect of prenatal paracetamol use on offspring, using wheeze or asthma as a primary outcomes; (iii) structure interview and clinical research; (iv) articles written in English; (v) data included in the articles were sufficient to calculate the odds ratio (OR) and 95% confidence interval (CI) and (vi) if there was an overlap in the cases included, only the latest and most comprehensive data were selected.

The exclusion criteria were as follows: (i) insufficient quantitative data (not possible to extract sufficient data for statistical calculations); (ii) duplicate reports; (iii) articles published in languages other than English and (iv) publications that were reviews, commentaries/letters, editorials, conference abstracts, cross-sectional studies.

Full texts of potential articles were selected for evaluation on the basis of a review of the titles and/or abstracts of all identified studies. After analyzing the selected works, a decision was made to include or exclude them. Papers meeting these conditions were qualified for meta-analysis, data collection on clinical characteristics and for test statistics.

2.3. Data Abstraction

Extracted data included: age of children's diagnosis and number of children with asthma or wheeze; number of women using paracetamol during pregnancy; trimester of pregnancy in which paracetamol use took place, and number of pregnant women in a particular trimester (if recorded).

2.4. Quality Assessment

The Newcastle-Ottawa Scale (NOS) was applied to assess the methodological quality of all the included studies [16]. The NOS included three categorical criteria with a maximum score of 9 points: (1) selection of the study group; (2) comparability of the groups; and (3) identification of the exposure for studies. The quality of each study was rated using the following scoring algorithms: ≥ 7 points were considered as "high", 4 to 6 points were considered as "moderate", and ≤ 3 point was considered as "low".

2.5. Statistical Analysis

The distribution of cases, ORs and 95% CIs were separately identified based on the risk of childhood wheezing/asthma and prenatal exposure to paracetamol (ever or never) and use of paracetamol in each trimester (if available).

We calculated the summary risk estimates and 95% CIs and plotted forest plots using random-effects models (DerSimonian–Laird method) and fixed effect models for the association between prenatal paracetamol exposure and wheeze/asthma in childhood. The value of I^2 statistics was adopted as a criterion—in the case of $I^2 < 50$, we used a fixed effect model, and when $I^2 \geq 50$, a random effect model. The results indicated that the taking of paracetamol may have a high probability of increase in risk if OR was above 1, compared with non-use of paracetamol [17].

Heterogeneity among articles was estimated by engaging the I^2 statistic and p values associated with Q statistics. Herein, I^2 statistic indicates the percentage of total variability explained by heterogeneity, and values of $\leq 25\%$, 25%–75%, and $\geq 75\%$ are arbitrarily considered as indicative of low, moderate, and high heterogeneity, respectively [18].

To explain the possible presence of publication bias, Begg's test (a rank correlation method based on Kendall's tau) and Egger's test (a linear regression method) were applied [19,20]. We also checked for funnel plot symmetry. Here, in the absence of bias, the plots will resemble a symmetrical funnel, as the results of minor studies will scatter at the left side of the plot and the spread will narrow among the major studies on the right side of the plot [21]. Meta-analysis of summary statistics from individual studies was performed through Statistica 13.3 software (StatSoft Poland, Kraków, Poland), using the Medical Package program.

3. Results

As result of the search of electronic databases, 532 citations were identified. Titles and abstracts were checked in the initial selection phase, in which 424 items were excluded due to irrelevance. In the second phase, 108 articles with potentially significant studies were identified and submitted for full-text assessment. There were 96 papers which did not meet all the inclusion criteria, contained duplicate publications, and the required data were missing, amongst others. We identified twelve articles fulfilling the criteria for inclusion, in which the effect of paracetamol exposure during pregnancy on disorders of the respiratory system in children was analyzed [22–33]. The outcome of the search strategy is shown in Figure 1.

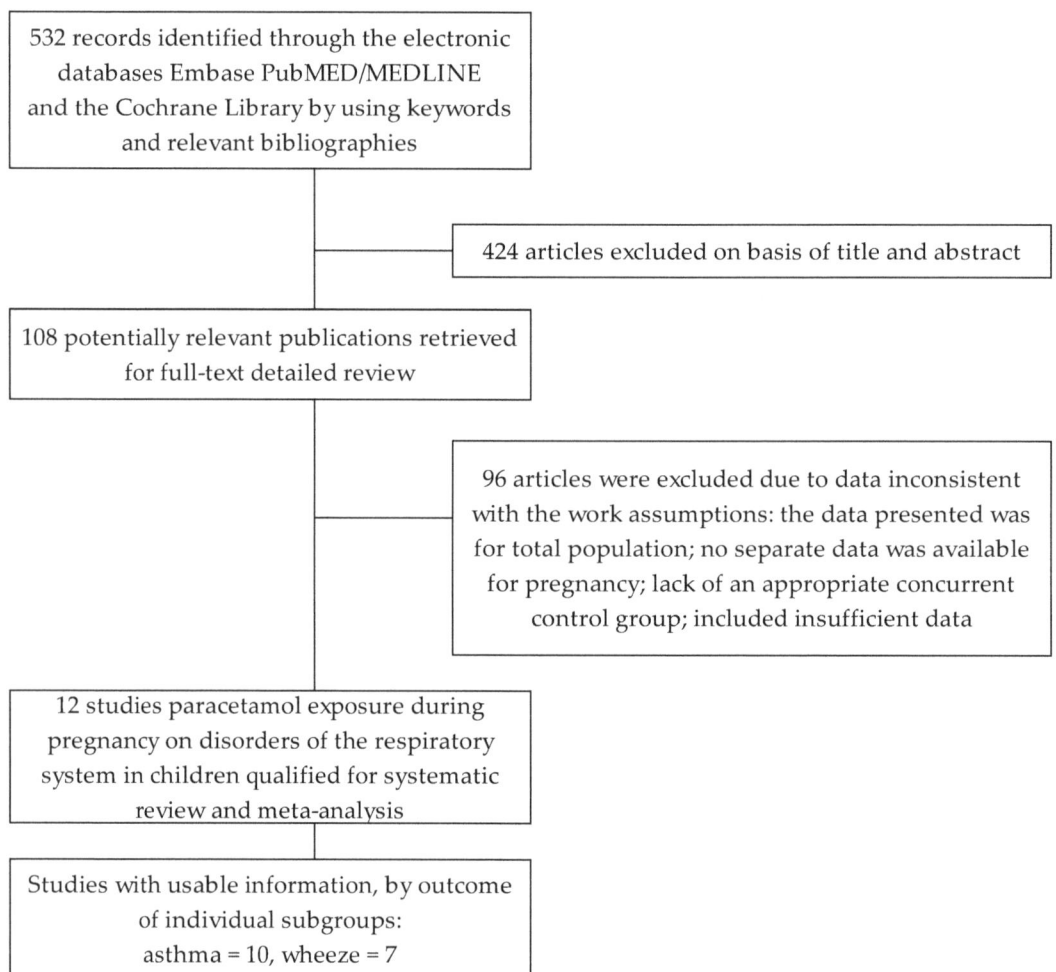

Figure 1. Flow diagram of literature search and research selection procedure.

The studies involved 330,550 women and 44,502 women intake of paracetamol during pregnancy. Table 1 presents a tabular summary of the individual clinical–control studies discussed in this review. All studies included were in accordance with NOS scale and all studies were defined as high-quality. The average value was 8.03.

Table 1. Characteristics of included studies evaluating the association between prenatal paracetamol intake and asthma or wheezing risk in childhood.

	Author, Year Country	Study	Exposure Classification Research Period (Years)	The Children's Respiratory Disorders	Age of Children's Diagnosis	Population: Paracetamol Use	Child With Asthma or Wheezing	Outcome Period (Months)	Nos Scale
				Studies Included in Meta-Analysis					
1.	Liew [22], 2021 USA	Environment and Pregnancy Outcomes Study	Paracetamol use during pregnancy: 1st trimester, 2nd trimester, 3rd trimester, ever. 2003–2007	Asthma: diagnosed by medical professional Wheezing	early childhood	958	Asthma: 118 Wheeze: 304	48	9
2.	Piler [23], 2018 Czech Republic/Brno and Znojmo regions	Cohort study Czech European Longitudinal Study of Pregnancy and Childhood	Paracetamol use during pregnancy. 1991–1992	Paediatrician-diagnosed asthma	3, 5, 7 and 11 years	1105	Asthma: 41	132	9
3.	Magnus [24], 2016 Norway	Norwegian Mother and Child Cohort Study	Paracetamol use during pregnancy. 1999–2014	Childhood asthma	3 years; 7 years	34,703	Asthma: 1751	36	9
4.	Liu [25], 2016 Denmark	Danish National Birth Cohort	Paracetamol use during pregnancy: 1st trimester, 2nd trimester, 3rd trimester, ever. 1996–2010	Asthma: at least two prescriptions for inhalants or cases diagnosed by a hospital doctor.	3 years or later	63,652	Asthma: 7644	36	8
5.	Migliore [26], 2015 Italy	Nascita e INFanzia: Effeti dell Ambiente study	Paracetamol use during pregnancy: 1st trimester, 3rd trimester. 2005–2013	Asthma: diagnosed by doctor Wheezing or whistling: at least one episode	18 months	3358	Asthma: 185 Wheeze 535	18	7
6.	Andersen [27], 2012 Denmark	Danish Medical Birth Registry	Paracetamol use during pregnancy: 1st trimester, both 2nd and 3rd trimesters, ever. 1996–2008	Asthma: hospital diagnosed, anti-asthmatic drug prescription	median—6.8 years	197,060	Asthma: 24,506	~82	8
7.	Goksör [28], 2011 Sweden	Swedish Medical Birth Register	Paracetamol use during pregnancy. 2003	Asthma: Inhaled corticosteroid-treated Wheezing: three or more episodes	6, 12 months and 4, 5 years	4496	Asthma: 258 Wheeze: 235	54	7
8.	Perzanowski [29], 2010 USA	Columbia Center for Children's Environmental Health	Paracetamol used during pregnancy by low-income women. 1998–2006	Asthma: self-reported Wheezing: self-reported	5 years	297	Asthma: 99 Wheeze: 99	60	7
9.	Kang [30], 2009 USA	The Yale Study	Paracetamol used in 1st and 3rd trimesters pregnancy. 1997–2000	Asthma: diagnosed by a doctor or health professional	6 years +/− 3 months	1505	Asthma: 172	72	7
10.	Garcia-Marcos [31], 2009 Spain	Murcia (Spain) Study	Paracetamol use during pregnancy.	Wheezing: self-reported	4.08 +/− 0.8 (3–4 years)	1741	Wheeze: 341	36–60	8
11.	Rebordosa [32], 2008 Denmark	Danish National Birth Cohort study	Paracetamol use during pregnancy: 1st trimester, 2nd trimester, 3rd trimester, ever. 1996–2003	Asthma: symptoms reported, physician-diagnosed Wheezing: self-reported	18 months—wheeze; 7 years—asthma	12,733	Asthma: 12,530 Wheeze: 11,980	84	9
12.	Saheen [33], 2002 UK	Avon Longitudinal Study of Parents and Children	Paracetamol use during pregnancy. 1992–1999	Wheezing: self-reported	30–42 months	8942	Wheeze: 1195	30–42	9

3.1. Sensitivity Analysis

In the study on the relationship between childhood asthma and paracetamol use (ever vs. never) during pregnancy and each trimester of pregnancy, sensitivity analysis showed that in the case of a total study and 3rd trimester, removing any of the studies would not significantly affect the result of the meta-analysis. However, in the case of the 1st trimester, deleting one of the studies: Andersen [27], Liu [25], Migliore [26] or Rebordosa [32] would change the result of the meta-analysis to be statistically insignificant. On the other hand, in the case of the 2nd trimester, the result of the meta-analysis would be statistically insignificant after excluding the study of Liu [25] or Rebordosa [32].

In the study on the relationship between childhood wheeze and paracetamol use (ever vs. never) during pregnancy and each trimester of pregnancy, sensitivity analysis for total study, 2nd trimester and 3rd trimester indicated that the results would not change significantly after excluding any of the studies. In turn, in the 1st trimester, the exclusion of the Liew study [22] would change the result of the meta-analysis to a statistically significant one.

3.2. Association between Paracetamol Exposure during Pregnancy and Asthma in Children

The present meta-analysis was conducted on the basis of data from ten studies [22–30,32] assessing the effect of paracetamol exposure in pregnancy on the risk of occurrence of asthma in children. Paracetamol was taken at any time during the trimesters of pregnancy. The crude OR amounted to 1.34, 95% CI: 1.22 to 1.48, p <0.001, with moderate heterogeneity of I^2 = 64.75% (Figure 2). The Begg and Mazumdar's test for rank correlation did not indicate evidence of publication bias (Kendall's tau = 0.142, z = 0.495, p < 0.622; similarly, Egger's test: b0 = 0.966, 95% CI − 0.748 to 2.681, t = 1.299, p < 0.231).

Results of five studies [22,25–27,32] analyzing the relationship between of intake of paracetamol during first trimester and childhood asthma pointed to increased risk (crude OR = 1.21, 95% CI: 1.01 to 1.45, p < 0.035, I^2 = 79.48%), (Figure 2). The Begg Mazumdar's test and Egger's test did not indicated evidence of publication bias (Kendall's tau b = −1.000, z = −1.567, p < 0.118 and b0 = −1.288, 95% CI: −7.752 to 5.177, t = −0.634, p < 0.572, respectively). The major problem indicated by this analysis is the large heterogeneity of effect of paracetamol.

Further analysis involving three studies [22,25,32] also suggested that use of paracetamol during the second trimester of pregnancy was associated with increased childhood asthma risk (crude OR = 1.10, 95% CI: 1.01 to 1.19, p < 0.030, I^2 = 0.00%), (Figure 2). Evidence of publication bias was not shown in the Begg and Mazumdar's test (Kendall's tau = 0.333, z = 0.522, p < 0.603); or in the Egger's test (b0 = −0.237, 95% CI: −6.686 to 6.212, t = −0.468, p < 0.723).

In turn, meta-analysis based on the results of four studies [22,25,26,32] showed that paracetamol intake by women in the third trimester of pregnancy was associated with an enhanced risk of asthma in the child (crude OR = 1.18, 95% CI: 1.11 to 1.26, p < 0.001, I^2 = 0.00%), (Figure 2). The Begg and Mazumdar's test and Egger's test did not indicate evidence of publication bias (Kendall's tau = −0.667, z = −1.359, p = 0.174 and b0 = 0.966, 95% CI: −0.748 to 2.681, t = 1.299, p < 0.231, respectively).

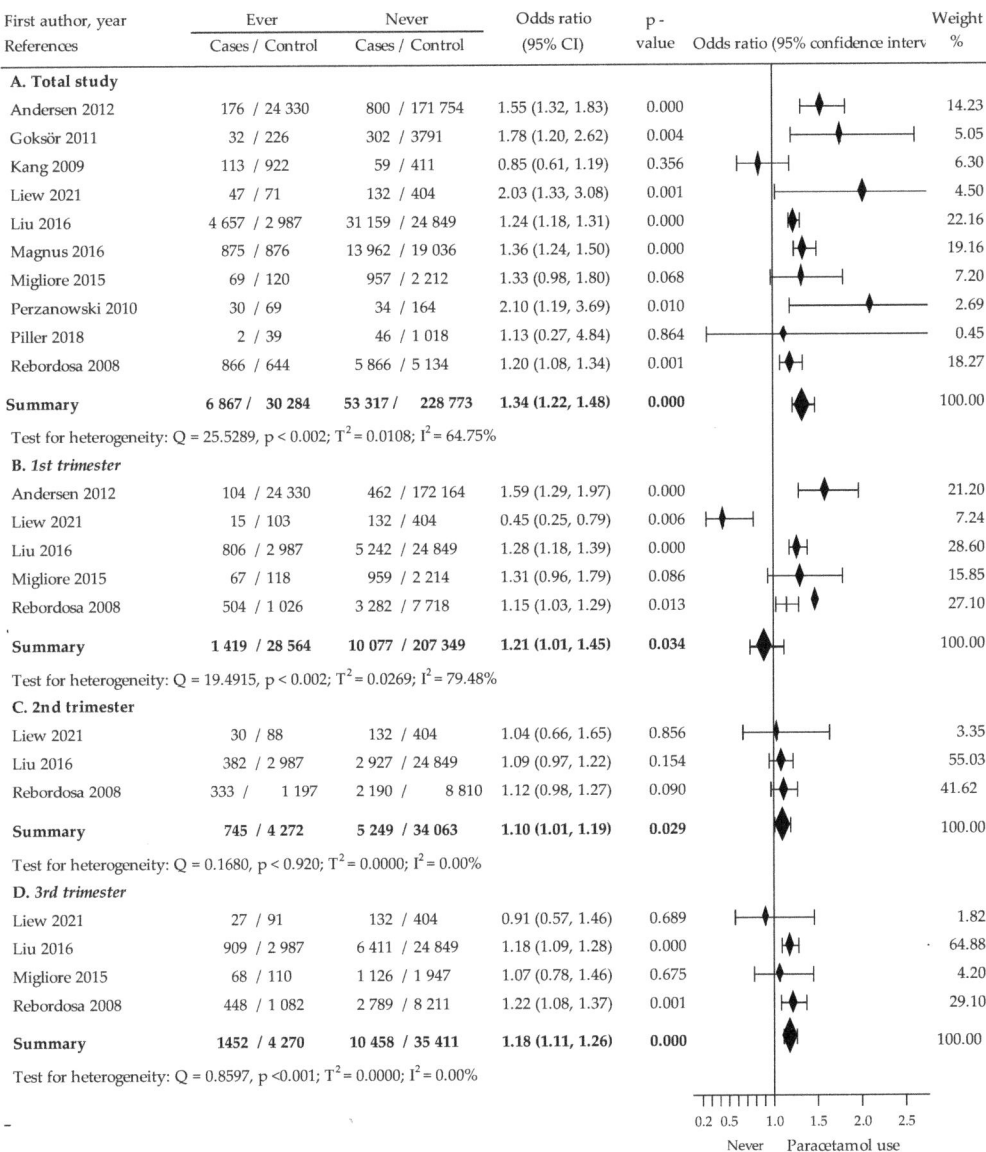

Figure 2. The crude relationship between childhood asthma and paracetamol use (ever vs. never) during pregnancy and each trimester of pregnancy [22–30,32].

3.3. Association between Paracetamol Exposure during Pregnancy and Wheezing in Children

In the eight studies [22,26,28–33] analyzed in order to assess prenatal paracetamol exposure during any time of pregnancy, we noted a significant increased risk of childhood wheeze (crude OR = 1.31, 95% CI: 1.12 to 1.54, $p < 0.002$; with relatively high heterogeneity, $I^2 = 75.29\%$), (Figure 3). The Begg and Mazumdar's test for rank correlation indicated no evidence of publication bias (Kendall's tau b = 0.333, z = 0.939, $p < 0.349$). Egger's test for regression intercept also demonstrated no evidence of publication bias (b0 = 2.161 (95% CI: −1.775 to 6.097), t = 1.344, $p < 0.229$).

The use of paracetamol in the first trimester of pregnancy in three studies [22,26,32] indicated a marginal, insignificant increase in the risk of wheezing in childhood (crude OR = 1.04, 95% CI: 0.78 to 1.37, $p > 0.801$, $I^2 = 80.73\%$), (Figure 3). The results of Begg's test were inaccessible. Egger's test did not indicate evidence of publication bias (b0 = −3.819, 95% CI: −56.874 to 49.237, t = −0.915, $p > 0.529$).

Two studies [22,32] have been identified that meet the inclusion criteria, in assessing the association between paracetamol exposure during the second trimester of pregnancy and childhood wheezing revealed convergent results (OR = 0.95, 95% CI: 0.68 to 1.32, $p > 0.760$ and OR = 0.95, 95% CI: 0.80 to 1.12, $p > 0.517$; respectively), (Figure 3). However, it is difficult to draw reliable result on their basis.

The crude odds ratio (OR) for the risk of wheezing in children of mothers using paracetamol in the third trimester of pregnancy was 1.11, 95% CI: 0.92 to 1.34, $p < 0.266$, $I^2 = 57.80\%$, based on three studies [22,26,32], (Figure 2). Egger's test did not indicate evidence of publication bias (b0 = −0.277, 95% CI: −55.078 to 54.525, t = −0.0641, $p < 0.959$). Results of Begg's test were inaccessible.

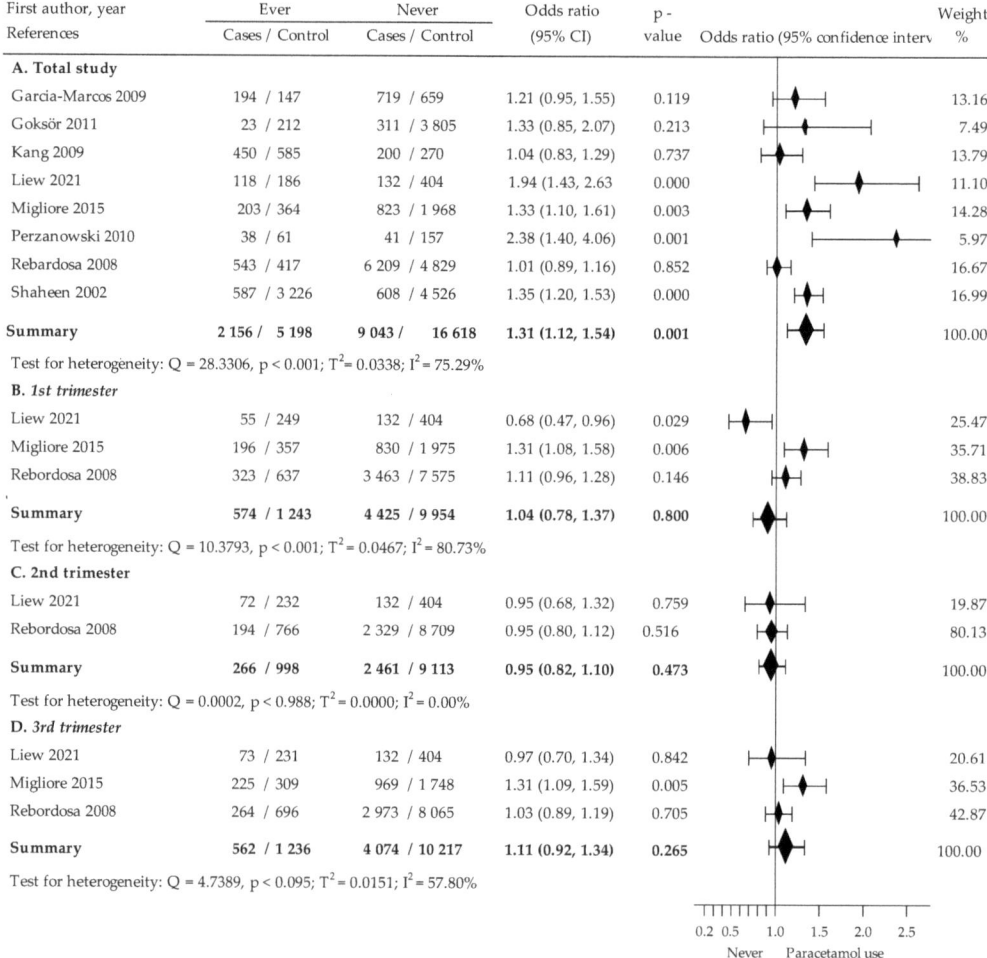

Figure 3. The crude relationship between childhood wheeze and paracetamol use (ever vs. never) during pregnancy and each trimester of pregnancy [22,26,28–33].

4. Discussion

The aim of our systematic review with meta-analysis was to summarize the current evidence on the exposures associated with paracetamol use in utero, focusing on postnatal breathing disorders in children. The study is important for the development of clinical recommendations regarding the consumption of paracetamol during pregnancy. The results of our systematic review and performed meta-analysis indicate a significant increase of the risk of asthma (crude OR = 1.34, 95% CI: 1.22 to 1.48, $p > 0.001$); or wheezing (crude OR = 1.31, 95% CI: 1.12 to 1.54, $p > 0.002$) among children with a history of prenatal exposure to paracetamol.

Singh et al. [34] noted that the odds ratio for the asthma outcome in the offspring of mothers who used paracetamol in the prenatal period in any trimester of pregnancy was 1.28, 95% CI: 1.13 to 1.39. Fan et al. [35] also held the opinion that prenatal paracetamol exposure was significantly associated with the increased risk of child asthma. In their work, OR = 1.19, 95% CI: 1.12 to 1.27. In turn, Eyers et al. [36] showed increased risk of recurrent wheeze in the children of women who were exposed to paracetamol during pregnancy. In their study, OR was 1.21, 95% CI: 1.24 to 1.44. Paracetamol use during pregnancy can affect both the mother and the fetus. Researches of fetal exposure to paracetamol have concerns on: premature birth [37], neurological development [38] low birth weight [39], hyperactivity disorder/hyperkinetic disorder or adverse development issues [40,41], and other birth defects [42,43]

Several limitations should be identified with regard to our study. Firstly, various prenatal ailments and illnesses may themselves have an impact on the risk of postnatal respiratory disorders. In addition, from the studies included into our meta-analysis, it was not possible to obtain confounding factor data that could have an impact on the final results of our analysis. It is difficult to conclude at what age prenatal paracetamol exposure affects children. Secondly, these are observational studies extended over time. During their duration, we cannot avoid the influence of various factors that may affect the final result. Furthermore, the study drug may have been administered to the children post-partum, as mothers who take paracetamol in pregnancy may be more likely to give paracetamol to their children. There are a number of other methodological problems that are also relevant for the interpretation of the results. Firstly, as a meta-analysis of observational studies, it was prone to the bias (e.g., recall and selection bias) inherent in the original studies. Secondly, most of the studies were observational in nature, did not establish a dose–response relationship, and were conceived to be subject to numerous errors and misleading outcomes regarding period of administration. Indeed, in some studies, a progressive increase in risk associated with increasing number of days of prenatal paracetamol exposure, or increased frequency of use, was observed [29,31–33]. Moreover, a limitation may posed by publication high statistical heterogeneity.

5. Conclusions

In summary, the results of our study confirmed that maternal paracetamol use in pregnancy is associated with an increased risk of asthma or wheezing in their children. The current findings are consistent with results of previous meta-analyses showing increase in asthma/wheeze symptoms from paracetamol exposure. We believe paracetamol should be used with caution by pregnant women, and at the lowest effective dose, for the shortest duration. Long-term use or the use of high doses should be limited to the indications recommended by a physician, while the mother-to-be should be under constant supervision.

Author Contributions: Conceptualization, W.K., A.B. (Agnieszka Barańska), A.B. (Agata Błaszczuk); data curation, W.K.; formal analysis, M.P.-D.; funding acquisition, A.W.; investigation, A.B. (Agnieszka Barańska); methodology, W.K., M.M., A.B. (Agnieszka Barańska); project administration, W.K., A.B. (Agnieszka Barańska); resources, W.K., A.B. (Agata Błaszczuk); software, U.R.; supervision, A.W.-F., validation, A.W-F.; visualization, W.K., A.B. (Agnieszka Barańska), A.B. (Agata Błaszczuk), M.M.; writing—original draft, W.K., A.B. (Agnieszka Barańska); writing—review and editing, A.B.

(Agnieszka Barańska), A.W-F. All authors have read and agreed to the published version of the manuscript.

Funding: This research received no external funding.

Institutional Review Board Statement: Not applicable.

Informed Consent Statement: Not applicable.

Data Availability Statement: The data are available upon request from the corresponding author.

Conflicts of Interest: The authors declare no conflict of interest.

References

1. Mazaleuskaya, L.L.; Sangkuhl, K.; Thorn, C.F.; FitzGerald, G.A.; Altman, R.B.; Klein, T.E. PharmGKB summary: Pathways of acetaminophen metabolism at the therapeutic versus toxic doses. *Pharm. Genom.* **2015**, *25*, 416–426. [CrossRef] [PubMed]
2. McCrae, J.C.; Morrison, E.E.; MacIntyre, I.M.; Dear, J.W.; Webb, D.J.B. Long-term adverse effects of paracetamol-a review. *Br. J. Clin. Pharmacol.* **2018**, *84*, 2218–2230. [CrossRef] [PubMed]
3. Nuttall, S.L.; Khan, J.N.; Thorpe, G.H.; Langford, N.; Kendall, M.J. The impact of therapeutic doses of paracetamol on serum total antioxidant capacity. *J. Clin. Pharm. Ther.* **2003**, *28*, 289–294. [CrossRef]
4. Williams, M.A. Pregnancy complications. In *Reproductive and Perinatal Epidemiology*; Louis, G.M.B., Platt, R.W., Eds.; Oxford University Press: London, UK, 2011; pp. 101–128.
5. Lupattelli, A.; Spigset, O.; Twigg, M.J.; Zagorodnikova, K.; Mårdby, A.C.; Moretti, M.E.; Drozd, M.; Panchaud, A.; Hämeen-Anttila, K.; Rieutord, A.; et al. Medication use in pregnancy: A cross-sectional, multinational web-based study. *BMJ Open* **2014**, *4*, e004365. [CrossRef] [PubMed]
6. Ishitsuka, Y.; Kondo, Y.; Kadowaki, D. Toxicological Property of Acetaminophen: The Dark Side of a Safe Antipyretic/Analgesic Drug? *Biol. Pharm. Bull.* **2020**, *43*, 195–206. [CrossRef] [PubMed]
7. Ryu, R.; Hebert, M.F. Impact of pregnancy on maternal pharmacokinetics of medications. In *Clinical Pharmacology during Pregnancy*; Academic Press: Cambridge, MA, USA, 2022; pp. 19–46. [CrossRef]
8. Pacifici, G.M.; Allegaert, K. Clinical Pharmacology of Paracetamol in Neonates: A Review. *Curr. Ther. Res.* **2015**, *77*, 24–30. [CrossRef] [PubMed]
9. Mian, P.; Allegaert, K.; Conings, S.; Annaert, P.; Tibboel, D.; Pfister, M.; van Calsteren, K.; Anker, J.N.V.D.; Dallmann, A. Integration of Placental Transfer in a Fetal–Maternal Physiologically Based Pharmacokinetic Model to Characterize Acetaminophen Exposure and Metabolic Clearance in the Fetus. *Clin. Pharmacokinet.* **2020**, *59*, 911–925. [CrossRef]
10. Nitsche, J.F.; Patil, A.S.; Langman, L.J.; Penn, H.J.; Derleth, D.; Watson, W.J.; Brost, B.C. Transplacental Passage of Acetaminophen in Term Pregnancy. *Am. J. Perinatol.* **2017**, *34*, 541–543. [CrossRef]
11. Chiew, A.L.; Gluud, C.; Brok, J.; Buckley, N.A. Interventions for paracetamol (acetaminophen) overdose. *Cochrane Database Syst. Rev.* **2018**, *23*, CD003328. [CrossRef]
12. Rahman, I.; MacNee, W. Oxidative stress and regulation of glutathione in lung inflammation. *Eur. Respir. J.* **2000**, *16*, 534–554. [CrossRef]
13. Hehua, Z.; Qing, C.; Shanyan, G.; Qijun, W.; Yuhong, Z. The impact of prenatal exposure to air pollution on childhood wheezing and asthma: A systematic review. *Environ. Res.* **2017**, *159*, 519–530. [CrossRef] [PubMed]
14. Moher, D.; Liberati, A.; Tetzlaff, J.; Altman, D.G.; PRISMA Group. Preferred reporting items for systematic reviews and meta-analyses: The PRISMA statement. *PLoS Med.* **2009**, *6*, e1000097. [CrossRef] [PubMed]
15. Higgins, J.P.T.; Thomas, J.; Chandler, J.; Cumpston, M.; Li, T.; Page, M.J.; Welch, V.A. (Eds.) *Cochrane Handbook for Systematic Reviews of Interventions*; John Wiley & Sons: Hoboken, NJ, USA, 2019.
16. Stang, A. Critical evaluation of the Newcastle-Ottawa scale for the assessment of the quality of nonrandomized studies in meta-analyses. *Eur. J. Epidemiol.* **2010**, *25*, 603–605. [CrossRef] [PubMed]
17. DerSimonian, R.; Laird, N. Meta-analysis in clinical trials revisited. *Contemp. Clin. Trials* **2015**, *45*, 139–145. [CrossRef] [PubMed]
18. Higgins, J.P.T.; Thompson, S.G. Quantifying heterogeneity in a meta-analysis. *Stat. Med.* **2002**, *21*, 1539–1558. [CrossRef]
19. Begg, C.B.; Mazumdar, M. Operating characteristics of a rank correlation test for publication bias. *Biometrics* **1994**, *50*, 1088–1101. [CrossRef]
20. Egger, M.; Smith, G.D.; Schneider, M.; Minder, C. Bias in meta-analysis detected by a simple, graphical test. *BMJ* **1997**, *315*, 629–634. [CrossRef]
21. Duval, S.; Tweedie, R. Trim and Fill: A Simple Funnel-Plot-Based Method of Testing and Adjusting for Publication Bias in Meta-Analysis. *Biometrics* **2000**, *56*, 455–463. [CrossRef]
22. Liew, Z.; Yuan, Y.; Meng, Q.; von Ehrenstein, O.S.; Cui, X.; Flores, M.E.S.; Ritz, B. Prenatal Exposure to Acetaminophen and Childhood Asthmatic Symptoms in a Population-Based Cohort in Los Angeles, California. *Int. J. Environ. Res. Public Health* **2021**, *18*, 10107. [CrossRef]
23. Piler, P.; Švancara, J.; Kukla, L.; Pikhart, H. Role of combined prenatal and postnatal paracetamol exposure on asthma development: The Czech ELSPAC study. *J. Epidemiol. Community Health* **2018**, *72*, 349–355. [CrossRef]

24. Magnus, M.C.; Karlstad, Ø.; Håberg, S.E.; Nafstad, P.; Smith, G.D.; Nystad, W. Prenatal and infant parace-tamol exposure and development of asthma: The Norwegian Mother and Child Cohort Study. *Int. J. Epidemiol.* **2016**, *45*, 512–522. [CrossRef] [PubMed]
25. Liu, X.; Liew, Z.; Olsen, J.; Pedersen, L.H.; Bech, B.H.; Agerbo, E.; Yuan, W.; Li, J. Association of prenatal exposure to ac-etaminophen and coffee with childhood asthma. *Pharmacoepidemiol. Drug Saf.* **2016**, *25*, 188–195. [CrossRef] [PubMed]
26. Migliore, E.; Zugna, D.; Galassi, C.; Merletti, F.; Gagliardi, L.; Rasero, L.; Trevisan, M.; Rusconi, F.; Richiardi, L. Prenatal Paracetamol Exposure and Wheezing in Childhood: Causation or Confounding? *PLoS ONE* **2015**, *10*, e0135775. [CrossRef] [PubMed]
27. Andersen, A.B.; Farkas, D.K.; Mehnert, F.; Ehrenstein, V.; Erichsen, R. Use of prescription paracetamol during pregnancy and risk of asthma in children: A population-based Danish cohort study. *Clin. Epidemiol.* **2012**, *4*, 33–40. [CrossRef] [PubMed]
28. Goksör, E.; Thengilsdottir, H.; Alm, B.; Norvenius, G.; Wennergren, G. Prenatal paracetamol exposure and risk of wheeze at preschool age. *Acta Paediatr.* **2011**, *100*, 1567–1571. [CrossRef] [PubMed]
29. Perzanowski, M.S.; Miller, R.L.; Tang, D.; Ali, D.; Garfinkel, R.S.; Chew, G.L.; Goldstein, I.F.; Perera, F.P.; Barr, R.G. Prenatal acetaminophen exposure and risk of wheeze at age 5 years in an urban low-income cohort. *Thorax* **2010**, *65*, 118–123. [CrossRef]
30. Kang, E.M.; Lundsberg, L.S.; Illuzzi, J.L.; Bracken, M.B. Prenatal Exposure to Acetaminophen and Asthma in Children. *Obstet. Gynecol.* **2009**, *114*, 1295–1306. [CrossRef]
31. Garcia-Marcos, L.; Sanchez-Solis, M.; Perez-Fernandez, V.; Pastor-Vivero, M.D.; Mondejar-Lopez, P.; Valverde-Molina, J. Is the effect of prenatal paracetamol exposure on wheezing in preschool children modified by asthma in the mother? *Int. Arch. Allergy Immunol.* **2009**, *149*, 33–37. [CrossRef]
32. Rebordosa, C.; Kogevinas, M.; Sørensen, H.T.; Olsen, J. Pre-natal exposure to paracetamol and risk of wheezing and asthma in children: A birth cohort study. *Int. J. Epidemiol.* **2008**, *37*, 583–590. [CrossRef]
33. Shaheen, S.O.; Newson, R.B.; Sherriff, A.; Henderson, A.J.; Heron, J.E.; Burney, P.G.J.; Golding, J.; ALSPAC Study Team. Paracetamol use in pregnancy and wheezing in early childhood. *Thorax* **2002**, *57*, 958–963. [CrossRef]
34. Singh, M.; Varukolu, S.; Chauhan, A.; Jaiswal, N.; Pradhan, P.; Mathew, J.L.; Singh, M. Paracetamol exposure and asthma: What does the evidence say? An overview of systematic reviews. *Pediatr. Pulmonol.* **2021**, *56*, 3189–3199. [CrossRef] [PubMed]
35. Fan, G.; Wang, B.; Liu, C.; Li, D. Prenatal paracetamol use and asthma in childhood: A systematic review and meta-analysis. *Allergol. Immunopathol.* **2017**, *45*, 528–533. [CrossRef] [PubMed]
36. Eyers, S.; Weatherall, M.; Jefferies, S.; Beasley, R. Paracetamol in pregnancy and the risk of wheezing in offspring: A systematic review and meta-analysis. *Clin. Exp. Allergy* **2011**, *41*, 482–489. [CrossRef] [PubMed]
37. Sujan, A.C.; Quinn, P.D.; Rickert, M.E.; Wiggs, K.K.; Lichtenstein, P.; Larsson, H.; Almqvist, C.; Öberg, A.S.; D'Onofrio, B.M. Maternal prescribed opioid analgesic use during pregnancy and associations with adverse birth outcomes: A population-based study. *PLoS Med.* **2019**, *16*, e1002980. [CrossRef] [PubMed]
38. de Fays, L.; Van Malderen, K.; De Smet, K.; Sawchik, J.; Verlinden, V.; Hamdani, J.; Dogné, J.-M.; Dan, B. Use of paracetamol during pregnancy and child neurological development. *Dev. Med. Child Neurol.* **2015**, *57*, 718–724. [CrossRef] [PubMed]
39. Arneja, J.; Hung, R.J.; Seeto, R.A.; Knight, J.A.; Hewko, S.L.; Bocking, A.; Lye, S.J.; Brooks, J.D. Association between maternal acetaminophen use and adverse birth outcomes in a pregnancy and birth cohort. *Pediatr. Res.* **2020**, *87*, 1263–1269. [CrossRef] [PubMed]
40. Thompson, J.M.D.; Waldie, K.E.; Wall, C.R.; Murphy, R.; Mitchell, E.A.; ABC Study Group. Associations between Acetaminophen Use during Pregnancy and ADHD Symptoms Measured at Ages 7 and 11 Years. *PLoS ONE* **2014**, *9*, e108210. [CrossRef] [PubMed]
41. Liew, Z.; Ritz, B.; Rebordosa, C.; Lee, P.-C.; Olsen, J. Acetaminophen Use during Pregnancy, Behavioral Problems, and Hyperkinetic Disorders. *JAMA Pediatr.* **2014**, *168*, 313–320. [CrossRef]
42. Cooper, M.; Langley, K.; Thapar, A. Antenatal acetaminophen use and attention-deficit/hyperactivity disorder: An interesting observed association but too early to infer causality. *JAMA Pediatr.* **2014**, *168*, 306–307. [CrossRef]
43. Bauer, A.Z.; Swan, S.H.; Kriebel, D.; Liew, Z.; Taylor, H.S.; Bornehag, C.-G.; Andrade, A.M.; Olsen, J.; Jensen, R.H.; Mitchell, R.T.; et al. Paracetamol use during pregnancy—A call for precautionary action. *Nat. Rev. Endocrinol.* **2021**, *17*, 757–766. [CrossRef]

Disclaimer/Publisher's Note: The statements, opinions and data contained in all publications are solely those of the individual author(s) and contributor(s) and not of MDPI and/or the editor(s). MDPI and/or the editor(s) disclaim responsibility for any injury to people or property resulting from any ideas, methods, instructions or products referred to in the content.

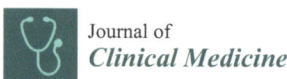
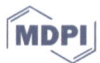

Article

Association between Exposure to Selected Heavy Metals and Blood Eosinophil Counts in Asthmatic Adults: Results from NHANES 2011–2018

Jun Wen [†], Mohan Giri [†], Li Xu and Shuliang Guo *

Department of Respiratory and Critical Care Medicine, The First Affiliated Hospital of Chongqing Medical University, Chongqing Medical University, Chongqing 400016, China
* Correspondence: guoshul666@163.com; Tel.: +86-131-0136-3078
† These authors contributed equally to this work.

Abstract: (1) Background: Heavy metals are widely used and dispersed in the environment and people's daily routines. Many studies have reported an association between heavy metal exposure and asthma. Blood eosinophils play a crucial role in the occurrence, progression, and treatment of asthma. However, there have thus far been few studies that aimed to explore the effects of heavy metal exposure on blood eosinophil counts in adults with asthma. Our study aims to discuss the association between metal exposure and blood eosinophil counts among asthmatic adults. (2) Methods: A total of 2026 asthmatic individuals were involved in our research from NHANES with metal exposure, blood eosinophils, and other covariates among the American population. A regression model, the XGBoost algorithm, and a generalized linear model (GAM) were used to explore the potential correlation. Furthermore, we conducted a stratified analysis to determine high-risk populations. (3) Results: The multivariate regression analysis indicated that concentrations of blood Pb (log per 1 mg/L; coefficient β, 25.39; $p = 0.010$) were positively associated with blood eosinophil counts. However, the associations between blood cadmium, mercury, selenium, manganese, and blood eosinophil counts were not statistically significant. We used stratified analysis to determine the high-risk group regarding Pb exposure. Pb was identified as the most vital variable influencing blood eosinophils through the XGBoost algorithm. We also used GAM to observe the linear relationship between the blood Pb concentrations and blood eosinophil counts. (4) Conclusions: The study demonstrated that blood Pb was positively correlated with blood eosinophil counts among asthmatic adults. We suggested that long-time Pb exposure as a risk factor might be correlated with the immune system disorder of asthmatic adults and affect the development, exacerbation, and treatment of asthma.

Keywords: heavy metal; lead (Pb); eosinophil; asthma; National Health and Nutrition Examination Survey (NHANES)

1. Introduction

Asthma is a heterogeneous disease characterized by chronic airway inflammation and respiratory symptoms [1,2]. It is one of the most common chronic respiratory disorders affecting approximately 358 million people worldwide [3,4], and 250,000 deaths are directly caused by asthma every year. The prevalence of asthma has increased in many countries in recent decades, and the prevalence of asthma in children and adults is estimated to be 8.1% and 7.9% in America, respectively [3,5]. According to a report, the US treatment and mortality costs for asthma have been estimated at USD 81 billion during 2008–2013 [6].

For many years, the presence of eosinophils in asthmatic inflammation has been recognized as an essential factor in the pathophysiology of the disease [7], and eosinophils are key inflammatory cells of "T2 high" asthma [8]. When monitoring patients with asthma, measurement of blood eosinophil counts is often used in clinical practice. As is known to us, the blood eosinophil count is a readily available biomarker, and existing research demonstrates that the blood eosinophil correlates reasonably well with sputum eosinophilia [9–11]. Among patients with asthma, elevated blood eosinophil counts have been associated with increased mortality [12] and are used to adjust treatment with corticosteroids, anti-IL-5, anti-IL-5-receptor-alpha or anti-IL-4 receptor alpha antibodies in asthma, resulting in improved asthma control and reduced exacerbation frequency [13–20]. Additionally, a high blood eosinophil count has been shown to be a risk factor for future asthma exacerbations in adults with persistent asthma [14,21–23]. In conclusion, blood eosinophils play a crucial role in the occurrence, progression, and treatment of asthma.

Heavy metals are widely used and dispersed in the environment, including the air, water, soil, dust, diet, and the manufacturing industry [24]. The general population is usually exposed to low concentrations of metals by ingesting contaminated water and food or inhaling environmental air pollution [25]. According to the Agency for Toxic Substances and Disease Registry, lead (Pb), cadmium (Cd), mercury (Hg), and so on are the top-priority contaminants. Heavy metals exposed to the environment may adhere to fine particles in the air and cause asthma as environmental allergens [26]. Previous studies observed that asthma induced by heavy metals was triggered by the immune system, indicating that heavy metals have great inflammatory potential and immunomodulatory effects on individuals [27,28]. Many studies have reported the association between heavy metals (Pb, Cd, Hg and Mn) and asthma [24,29–33].

In addition, some studies still demonstrated the correlation between common heavy metals (Pb, Hg, Cd, etc.) and blood eosinophil counts [34–41]. For example, previous studies have demonstrated that Pb exposure was implicated in alterations in humoral and cell-mediated immunity and the development of allergic conditions, including the production of serum IgE, eosinophil migration and proliferation, activation of Th2 cytokines, as well as an abnormality of bronchial responsiveness [37,38]. An experimental animal study in Iran indicated levels of total protein, total white blood cell counts, histamine, and eosinophils were elevated after guinea pigs inhaled aerosol Pb, which supported the proinflammatory effect of Pb poisoning [39]. Another experimental animal study demonstrated an elevation of circulating eosinophils after Cd exposure [40]. Additionally, a Korean study found Hg was not associated with blood eosinophil counts in 311 Korean children but was associated with increased blood lymphocyte counts [41]. Chao-Hsin Huang et al. conducted a study in which urine Mn was not associated with blood eosinophil counts among 2447 adults [34]. A small study involving 25 adult asthmatic patients and healthy subjects found that the asthma group had lower serum Se concentrations and higher indicators of oxidative stress [42].

However, there have been few studies that aimed to explore the effects of different kinds of exposure to heavy metals on blood eosinophil counts in adults with asthma so far. To explore the association between heavy metals (Pb, Cd, Hg, Se, and Mn) and blood eosinophil counts, in our study, we used a nationally representative sample of adults who participated in the 2011–2018 NHANES in the USA. We also comprehensively explored whether the association was different in various populations.

2. Materials and Methods

2.1. Data Source

The NHANES, which was conducted by the Centers for Disease Control and Prevention of America, collected information regarding the health and nutritional status of the US population every 2 years. NHANES used a complex, stratified sampling design, which can select representative samples of non-institutionalized civilians. The survey ethics review board of the CDC approved the NHANES procedures and protocols, and all participants provided written informed consent.

2.2. Study Population

Four cycles of NHANES data (2011–2012, 2013–2014, 2015–2016 and 2017–2018) were integrated into our study. These data included demographic data, examination data, laboratory data, and questionnaire data for the second analysis. A total of 39,156 participants were included in the NHANES from 2011 to 2018. We excluded individuals: (1) aged < 18 years old (n = 15331); (2) missing blood eosinophil data (n = 2147); (3) missing blood Pb, Cd, Hg, Se, and Mn data (n = 5573); (4) participants without asthma (n = 13673); (5) missing data about covariates in at least one of following (n = 406): education level, marital status, the ratio of family income to poverty, BMI, smoking status, hypertension history, diabetes history, blood urea nitrogen, blood creatinine and blood cotinine. Eventually, a large nationally representative sample (n = 2026) of American adults with asthma was enrolled in our study. The flow chart of the screening process is shown in Figure 1.

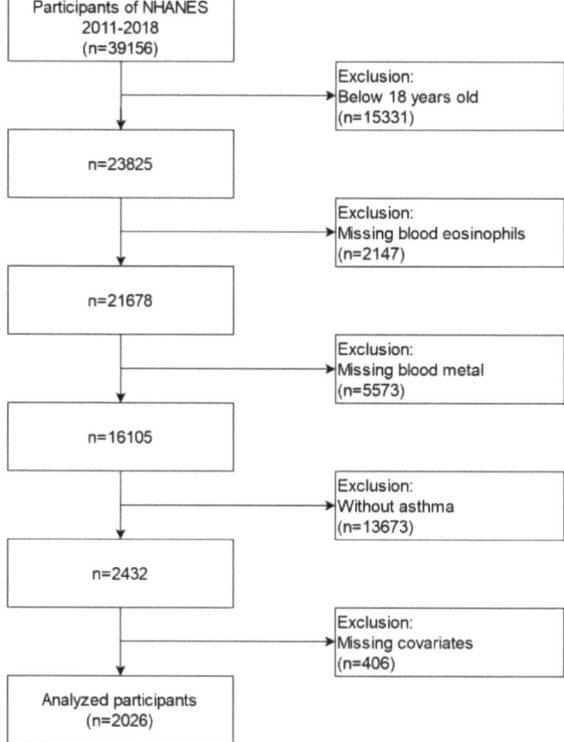

Figure 1. Flowchart for selecting analyzed participants.

2.3. Measurement of Metal Exposures

The measurements of all the exposures of whole-blood lead, cadmium, mercury, selenium, and manganese were tested by inductively coupled plasma-dynamic reaction mass spectrometry (ICP-DRC-MS) on an ELAN 6100 DRC Plus or ELAN DRC II (PerkinElmer Instruments, Headquarters Office, 710 Bridgeport Ave., Shelton, CT 06,484–4794) at the CDC's National Center for Environmental Health. Values of concentrations below the limit of detection (LOD) were imputed values of LOD/sqrt [2]. Detailed information on laboratory quality assurance and monitoring is available on the NHANES website.

2.4. Blood Eosinophil Count Measurement

Blood differential counts were performed in NHANES 2011–2018 using the Beckman Coulter HMX (Beckman Coulter, Fullerton, Calif), a quantitative and automated hematologic analyzer and leukocyte differential cell counter for in vitro diagnostic use in clinical laboratories. A detailed description of the laboratory methods can be found on the NHANES website.

2.5. Covariates and Asthma Assessment

Covariates were chosen a priori based on previous studies. Demographic data included gender, age (years old), race/ethnicity (Mexican American, other Hispanic, non-Hispanic white, non-Hispanic black, others), educational level (less than high school, high school, more than high school), poverty-to-income ratio, and marital status (married, single, living with a partner). Secondly, we also included examination data and personal life history data involving body mass index (kg/m^2), smoking (smoked at least 100 cigarettes in life), diagnosis with hypertension (yes or no), and diagnosis with diabetes (yes, no, or borderline). Finally, variables of laboratory data included blood urea nitrogen (mmol/L), blood creatinine (mol/L), and blood cotinine (ng/mL). The assessment of asthma was based on the information from the questionnaire section of the US National Health Interview Survey. In order to assess asthma, participants were asked, "Has a doctor or other health professional ever told you that you have asthma?" If the participant responded "yes", he or she was regarded as an asthma patient. A more detailed description of variables can be obtained on the NHANES official website (http://www.cdc.gov/nchs/nhanes/, 6 January 2023).

2.6. Statistical Analysis

According to the criteria of the CDC guidelines, we conducted a statistical analysis of blood metal concentration and blood eosinophil count. Blood metal concentration, blood eosinophil count, and other continuous variables were expressed as the mean and 95% CIs. The categorical variables were expressed in frequency or percentage. Firstly, we divided blood eosinophil count as a continuous variable into four quartiles. The weighted chi-square test was used to calculate the *p*-value of the characteristics of the analyzed population's categorical variables. In the case of continuous variables, we used the Kruskal–Wallis rank-sum test to calculate the *p*-value (Table 1). Secondly, all blood metal levels were initially naturally log-transformed for further analysis because their distributions were skewed. We constructed three kinds of weighted multiple linear regression models that adjusted various variables shown in Table 2 to identify the association between the blood metal concentrations and blood eosinophil count (non-adjusted model, minimally adjusted model, and fully adjusted model). Thirdly, we constructed the machine learning XGBoost algorithm model to predict the relative importance of blood metal on the effect of blood eosinophil count (Figure 2). The XGBoost model was used to analyze blood metal contribution (gain) to blood eosinophil count. Next, we found the statistical difference between the blood lead and blood eosinophil count. Therefore, we further conducted a stratified analysis to determine the stratified association between the blood lead and blood eosinophil count through stratified multivariate logistic regression. Finally, based on the penalty spline method, we constructed a smooth curve using a generalized additive model (GAM) model with a fully adjusted model to explore the potential linear relationship between blood lead concentration and blood eosinophil count. A two-piecewise linear regression model was applied if a non-linear correlation was detected to determine the threshold effect of blood lead concentration on blood eosinophil count. When the ratio between blood lead concentration and blood eosinophil count appeared obvious in a smooth curve, the recursive method automatically calculated the inflection point, where the maximum model likelihood was used. To prevent the bias caused by missing data, we curated the NHANES database to improve the accuracy of the analysis by using the MICE package to account for missing data. We found the results of data without missing covariates were basically consistent with those of data with missing covariates and multiple imputation data. All in all, univariate and multiple analysis results were based on the calculated dataset as well as Rubin's rules. All kinds of statistical analyses were performed by R software (Version 4.2.0) using the R package. The software EmpowerStats offered significant help in the analysis process, as well (http://www.empowerstats.com, 6 January 2023, X&Y Solutions, Inc., Boston, MA, USA). In our study, a p-value < 0.05 was considered statistically significant.

Table 1. Clinical characteristics of the study population disaggregated by quartiles of blood eosinophil count.

	Q1	Q2	Q3	Q4	p-Value
Gender (%)					0.039
Male	37.41 (26.44, 49.85)	37.87 (32.63, 43.41)	39.27 (33.83, 44.98)	46.96 (42.24, 51.74)	
Female	62.59 (50.15, 73.56)	62.13 (56.59, 67.37)	60.73 (55.02, 66.17)	53.04 (48.26, 57.76)	
Age, mean (95% CI) (years)	45.46 (41.40, 49.52)	43.48 (41.89, 45.06)	45.41 (43.54, 47.28)	46.64 (44.97, 48.30)	0.038
Race/ethnicity (%)					0.361
Mexican American	4.73 (1.52, 13.79)	4.91 (3.34, 7.16)	6.13 (4.14, 8.99)	7.03 (4.96, 9.88)	
Other Hispanic	6.84 (2.44, 17.76)	6.14 (4.17, 8.96)	7.20 (5.22, 9.86)	6.56 (4.61, 9.24)	
Non-Hispanic White	63.01 (44.80, 78.14)	67.54 (60.54, 73.84)	66.28 (59.36, 72.58)	68.35 (63.38, 72.93)	
Non-Hispanic Black	20.79 (12.00, 33.56)	13.01 (9.69, 17.26)	11.36 (8.75, 14.64)	10.40 (7.98, 13.46)	
Other race	4.63 (1.79, 11.40)	8.40 (5.51, 12.61)	9.02 (6.42, 12.54)	7.66 (5.75, 10.13)	
Education (%)					0.502
Less than high school	16.70 (9.34, 28.08)	10.86 (8.44, 13.86)	14.20 (10.82, 18.42)	13.28 (9.82, 17.72)	
High school	23.31 (12.86, 38.51)	20.27 (16.29, 24.92)	19.30 (14.90, 24.63)	22.88 (18.43, 28.03)	
More than high school	59.98 (44.64, 73.59)	68.88 (63.79, 73.55)	66.49 (60.71, 71.82)	63.84 (57.45, 69.79)	
Marital status (%)					0.501
Married	45.22 (31.88, 59.29)	50.45 (45.43, 55.46)	46.76 (41.46, 52.14)	51.84 (47.29, 56.35)	
Single	50.68 (36.51, 64.74)	41.19 (36.81, 45.73)	46.01 (40.48, 51.64)	40.95 (37.12, 44.89)	
Living with a partner	4.10 (1.21, 13.00)	8.36 (5.87, 11.77)	7.22 (4.98, 10.36)	7.21 (5.06, 10.19)	
Poverty-to-income ratio, mean (95% CI)	2.60 (2.07, 3.13)	2.88 (2.68, 3.08)	2.65 (2.43, 2.88)	2.75 (2.53, 2.96)	0.241
BMI, mean (95% CI) (kg/m^2)	28.05 (25.90, 30.20)	29.41 (28.55, 30.26)	31.03 (29.96, 32.10)	31.70 (30.80, 32.59)	0.001
Smoked at least 100 cigarettes in life (%)					0.224
Yes	50.51 (34.88, 66.05)	43.61 (37.64, 49.77)	45.57 (39.23, 52.06)	51.05 (44.87, 57.20)	
No	49.49 (33.95, 65.12)	56.39 (50.23, 62.36)	54.43 (47.94, 60.77)	48.95 (42.80, 55.13)	
Hypertension (%)					0.003
Yes	36.62 (23.68, 51.82)	29.25 (24.35, 34.68)	37.71 (32.22, 43.53)	41.20 (36.32, 46.25)	
No	63.38 (48.18, 76.32)	70.75 (65.32, 75.65)	62.29 (56.47, 67.78)	58.80 (53.75, 63.68)	
Diabetes (%)					0.394
Yes	13.66 (6.13, 27.72)	8.60 (6.62, 11.09)	12.50 (9.65, 16.04)	13.57 (10.14, 17.92)	
No	82.01 (66.25, 91.36)	88.34 (84.69, 91.22)	85.06 (80.97, 88.39)	84.24 (79.54, 88.03)	
Borderline	4.33 (0.98, 17.18)	3.06 (1.32, 6.94)	2.44 (1.26, 4.67)	2.19 (1.29, 3.70)	
BUN, mean (95% CI) (mmol/L)	4.72 (4.20, 5.24)	4.65 (4.50, 4.80)	4.79 (4.58, 5.00)	4.97 (4.80, 5.15)	0.075
Cr, mean (95% CI) (umol/L)	73.95 (69.17, 78.72)	74.05 (72.23, 75.86)	77.18 (74.93, 79.42)	80.06 (77.99, 82.13)	0.0002
Blood cotinine, mean (95% CI) (ng/mL)	94.98 (52.24, 137.72)	53.90 (38.51, 69.29)	61.44 (49.13, 73.75)	68.29 (51.47, 85.12)	0.200
Blood Pb, mean (95% CI) (ug/dL)	1.20 (0.92, 1.49)	1.00 (0.91, 1.08)	1.03 (0.94, 1.13)	1.17 (1.06, 1.28)	0.007
Blood Cd, mean (95% CI) (ug/dL)	0.56 (0.42, 0.71)	0.46 (0.37, 0.55)	0.49 (0.44, 0.54)	0.59 (0.50, 0.69)	0.106
Blood Hg, mean (95% CI) (ug/dL)	1.53 (1.00, 2.06)	1.40 (1.14, 1.65)	1.24 (1.05, 1.42)	1.13 (0.88, 1.37)	0.126
Blood Se, mean (95% CI) (ug/dL)	197.90 (190.03, 205.77)	194.14 (191.52, 196.75)	192.45 (189.50, 195.40)	194.60 (191.24, 197.97)	0.567
Blood Mn, mean (95% CI) (ug/dL)	9.62 (8.37, 10.88)	10.15 (9.81, 10.49)	10.10 (9.77, 10.42)	9.72 (9.39, 10.06)	0.179

Note: Data are expressed as weighted means (95% Cis) or proportions. Q1–Q4: Grouped by quartile according to the blood eosinophil counts. Our data included blood metal concentrations, blood eosinophil counts, demographic data, examination data, laboratory data, and questionnaire data for the second analysis. BUN: blood urea nitrogen; Cr: blood creatinine; Pb: lead; Cd: cadmium; Hg: mercury; Se: selenium; Mn: manganese.

Table 2. Multivariate weighted linear model analysis reveals the association between the blood metal and blood eosinophil count.

	Non-Adjusted Model	Minimally Adjusted Model	Fully Adjusted Model
	β (95% CI) p value	β (95% CI) p value	β (95% CI) p value
Log blood Pb (ug/dL)	24.76 (8.22, 41.30) 0.005	17.66 (−0.78, 36.09) 0.066	25.39 (6.91, 43.88) 0.010
Log blood Cd (ug/dL)	4.18 (−7.55, 15.91) 0.487	7.18 (−5.56, 19.92) 0.274	17.51 (−0.43, 35.45) 0.063
Log blood Hg (ug/dL)	−1.91 (−11.32, 7.50) 0.693	−4.35 (−14.13, 5.43) 0.387	−3.23 (−13.20, 6.75) 0.530
Log blood Se (ug/dL)	14.48 (−68.49, 97.45) 0.734	−6.99 (−86.32, 72.35) 0.864	−7.60 (−82.84, 67.64) 0.844
Log blood Mn (ug/dL)	−14.27 (−40.80, 12.26) 0.296	−6.18 (−37.67, 25.31) 0.702	−5.87 (−37.43, 25.68) 0.717

Note: Non-adjusted model adjusts for none. Minimally adjusted model adjusts for age, race/ethnicity. Fully adjusted model adjusts for gender, age, race/ethnicity, education level, marital status, poverty to income ratio, BMI, smoked at least 100 cigarettes in life, hypertension, diabetes, blood urea nitrogen, blood creatinine and blood cotinine.

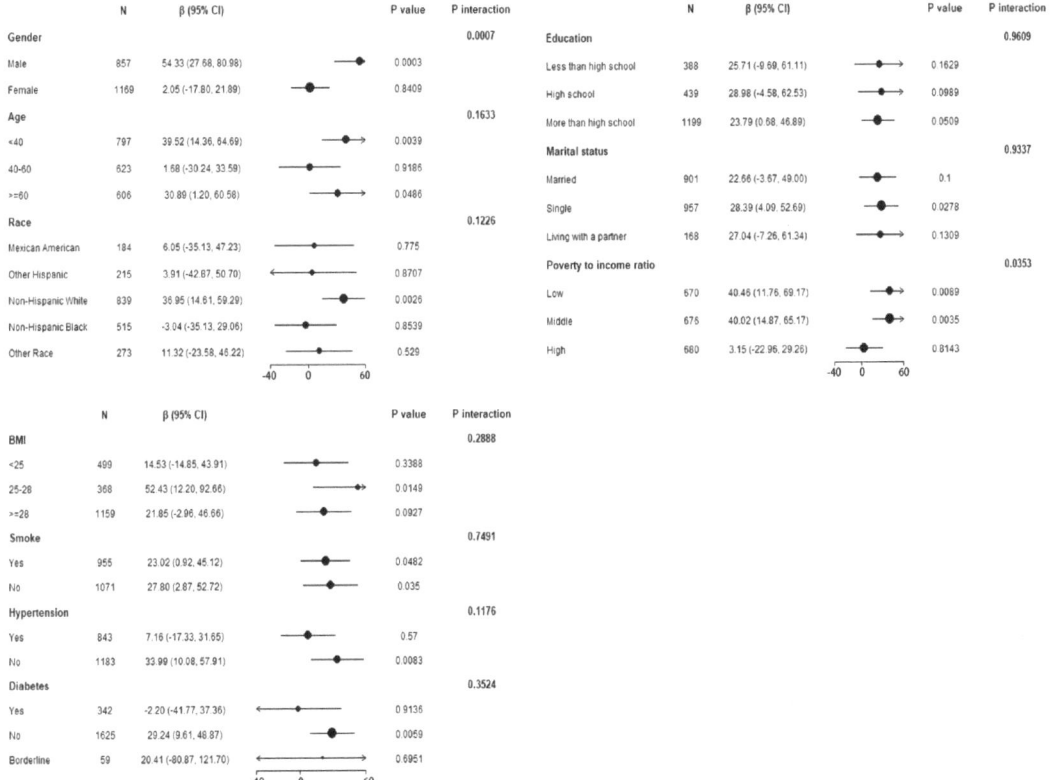

Figure 2. Stratified association of blood Pb on blood eosinophil counts in the prespecified and exploratory subgroups. Above adjusts for gender, age, race/ethnicity, education level, marital status, poverty to income ratio, BMI, smoked at least 100 cigarettes in life, hypertension, diabetes, blood urea nitrogen, blood creatinine and blood cotinine. In each case, the model was not adjusted for the stratification variable itself.

3. Results

3.1. Characteristics of the Participants

The baseline characteristics, which were of a weighted distribution, are shown in Table 1, including the demographic data, examination data, laboratory data, and questionnaire data of selected participants from the NHANES (2011–2018) survey. In our study, the average age of selected participants was 45.46 years old, and non-Hispanic Whites were the main population. Then, we divided different blood eosinophil counts into four quartiles (Q1–Q4). The distribution of race, education, marital status, poverty-to-income ratio, smoking status, diabetes history, blood urea nitrogen and blood cotinine in Q1–Q4 of blood eosinophil count indicated no statistical difference (p-value > 0.05), and gender, age, BMI, hypertension history, blood creatinine showed statistical differences (p-values < 0.05). Compared with the various groups, the distribution difference of blood Pb showed statistical significance, which may indicate a difference in exposure to Pb. However, blood Cd, Hg, Se, and Mn showed no exposure difference between the four quartile groups of blood eosinophil count.

3.2. The Associations between the Blood Metal Concentrations and Blood Eosinophil Counts

After all blood metal concentrations were naturally log-transformed, we applied the weighted multivariate linear regression model to assess the association of blood metal concentrations with blood eosinophil count in three different models (Table 2). According to the results, we found that only blood Pb was positively correlated with blood eosinophil count in the non-adjusted model and fully adjusted model, which was statistically significant. In the non-adjusted model, the blood eosinophil count increased by 24.76 (8.22, 41.30)/uL for each additional unit of blood lead of natural logarithmic conversion (ug/dL) ($p < 0.05$). In the fully adjusted model, which adjusted for gender, age, race/ethnicity, education level, marital status, poverty income ratio, BMI, smoking status, hypertension history, diabetes history, blood urea nitrogen, blood creatinine, and blood cotinine, the blood eosinophil count increased by 25.39 (6.91, 43.88)/uL for each additional unit of blood lead of natural logarithmic conversion (ug/dL) ($p < 0.05$). In the minimally adjusted model, which adjusted for gender, age, race/ethnicity, blood Pb also showed a positive association with blood eosinophil count but without statistical significance ($p > 0.05$). The above results indicated that long-time Pb exposure as an independent risk factor may increase the blood eosinophil counts of adults with asthma.

3.3. Stratified Associations between Blood Pb Concentrations and Blood Eosinophil Counts

To confirm the stability of multivariate linear regression analysis results, we further analyzed stratified associations between the blood Pb concentrations and blood eosinophil counts in a specific subgroup by gender, age, race, education level, marital status, poverty-to-income ratio, BMI, smoking status, hypertension history, and diabetes history (Figure 2). According to stratified analysis results, it was possible that males, age < 40 and ≥60 years old, non-Hispanic Whites, those who declared their marital status to be single, the low and middle group of poverty-to-income ratio, 25 < BMI ≤ 28, those who had smoked <100 cigarettes and ≥100 cigarettes in life, those who were without hypertension, and those who were without diabetes had higher blood eosinophil counts, with increasing blood Pb concentrations displaying a significant trend ($p < 0.05$). Furthermore, we found that the variables of gender, poverty-to-income ratio, and blood Pb may have an interaction effect associated with blood eosinophil counts (p for interaction < 0.05).

3.4. Using Machine Learning from the XGBoost Algorithm Model to Explore the Blood Metals' Relative Importance

To identify which metal exposure affected blood eosinophil counts of adults with asthma most, we constructed the machine learning XGBoost algorithm to determine the relative importance among all selected blood metals. The blood metal variables we selected included blood Pb, Cd, Hg, Se, and Mn. In light of the results of each blood metal's contribution according to the XGBoost model, we observed that blood Pb was the most critical variable in the blood eosinophil counts, followed by blood Se, Mn, Hg, and Cd (Figure 3). The above analysis was conducted using logarithmically transformed blood metal data. Ultimately, blood Pb, as the most relative variable, was further applied to constructing smooth curve models in our study.

3.5. Exploring Dose-Response Relationships of Blood Pb Concentrations with Blood Eosinophil Counts by the Generalized Additive Model (GAM)

The GAM is very sensitive to identifying linear relationships or non-linearity. To verify the reliability and stability of the analysis results, we used the GAM to explore the linear relationship between the blood Pb concentrations and blood eosinophil counts. Based on the fully adjusted model (Figure 4), we constructed a smooth fit curve to reflect the possible association. These analyses were conducted using logarithmically transformed blood Pb data. We observed the linear relationship between blood Pb concentrations with blood eosinophil counts after adjusting gender, age, race/ethnicity, education level, marital status, poverty-to-income ratio, BMI, smoking status, hypertension history, diabetes history, blood urea nitrogen, blood creatinine, and blood cotinine. In addition, we still used the segmented regression model to further verify the linear relationship of blood Pb concentrations with blood eosinophil counts (Table 3). The log-likelihood ratio test showed that p was more than 0.05, indicating that there was no significant difference between model 1 (one-line model) and model 2 (segmented regression model). Thus, it was more suitable to use the one-line model, and the inflection point was not statistically significant. All the above results indicated that the blood Pb concentration was linearly and positively correlated with blood eosinophil counts.

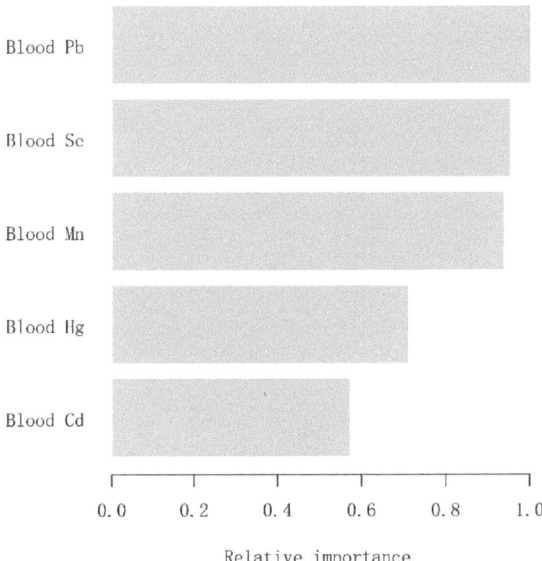

Figure 3. XGBoost model reveals the relative importance of each blood metal on blood eosinophil counts and the corresponding variable importance score. The X-axis is the importance score, the relative number of a variable used to distribute the data; the Y-axis is the blood metal.

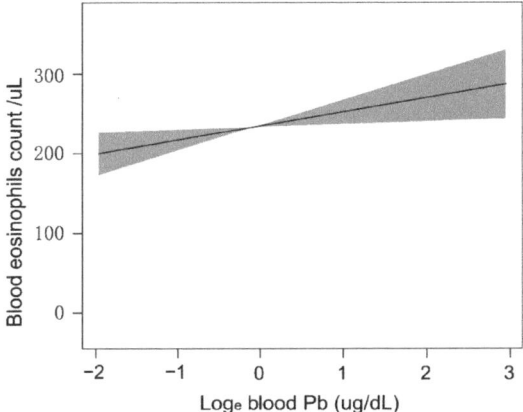

Figure 4. Dose-response relationships of blood Pb concentrations with blood eosinophil counts. The solid line and shadow area represented the corresponding β values and 95% confidence intervals.

Table 3. Threshold effect analysis of between blood Pb and blood eosinophil count using the two-piecewise linear regression model.

	β (95% CI) p-Value
Model I	
Linear effect	25.39 (10.53, 40.26) 0.001
Model II	
Inflection point (K)	−0.87
Log blood Pb < K	56.23 (−5.73, 118.19) 0.075
Log blood Pb > K	21.30 (4.43, 38.18) 0.013
Log likelihood ratio	0.312

Note: Models I and II all adjusted for gender, age, race/ethnicity, education level, marital status, poverty-to-income ratio, BMI, smoking status, hypertension history, diabetes history, blood urea nitrogen, blood creatinine, and blood cotinine.

4. Discussion

Environmental factors were generally considered to be related to the occurrence and progression of asthma. Blood eosinophils play a crucial role in the occurrence, progression, and treatment of asthma [43–47]. However, according to previous studies, the results investigating the correlation between metal elements and the occurrence and progression of asthma were inconsistent [31,48,49]. Meanwhile, the studies on the impact of metal elements on blood eosinophil counts among adults with asthma are few. In this cross-sectional study, we assessed the relationship between blood metal concentrations (Pb, Cd, Hg, Mn and Se) and blood eosinophil counts among 2026 adults with asthma who participated in the NHANES survey from 2011 to 2018 (2011–2012, 2013–2014, 2015–2016, 2017–2018) in the USA. In order to rank the relative importance of exposure to different metals to blood eosinophil counts, we first constructed the machine learning XGBoost model to determine the order of selected metals. We found that blood Pb is the most important metal on blood eosinophil counts, followed by blood Se, Mn, Hg, and Cd. Next, we constructed three weighted linear models (the non-adjusted model, minimally adjusted model, and fully adjusted model) by multivariate regression analysis to determine which metal exposure might be regarded as the independent risk factor. Our study indicated that natural log-transformed blood Pb concentrations were positively associated with blood eosinophil counts in the non-adjusted model and fully adjusted model with statistical significance. In contrast, the association between blood Se, Mn, Hg, Cd, and blood eosinophil counts was not statistically significant in the three models. The above results suggested that long-time Pb exposure as a risk factor might be correlated with the immune system disorder of asthmatic adults and affect the occurrence, development, and exacerbation of asthma.

To our knowledge, Pb is a ubiquitous environmental contaminant with potential immunotoxicity [50]. Though Pb exposures in the environment, as a result of the phase-out of leaded gasoline, have been significantly reduced, Pb is still found in paint, food, and lead-containing consumer products and detected in the general population. Especially among the population of low socioeconomic status, people are increasingly concerned about the possible adverse impacts of exposure to environmental Pb [37]. The immune system is shown to be one of the most sensitive targets for lead toxicity [51]. An epidemiological study in the USA reported that Ellen M. Wells et al. observed a significant association of lead with increased eosinophils among non-Hispanic Whites with asthma after control confounding factors [52]. Additionally, another cross-sectional study involving 2447 participants also observed a positive association between blood Pb concentrations and blood eosinophil counts [34]. However, this cross-sectional study did not conduct stratified analyses in different populations to verify the stability and reliability of this association. In the same way, we found that the association between blood Pb concentrations and blood eosinophil counts demonstrated population differences among American adults with asthma. We identified the high-risk group for Pb exposure through stratified analysis, including males aged less than 40 years old and 60 years old or older, non-Hispanic Whites, those who reported their marital status as single, the low and middle group of the poverty-to-income ratio, those who had a BMI between 25 and 28, non-Hispanic blacks, those who were without hypertension, and those who were without diabetes. Furthermore, we observed a linear relationship between natural log-transformed blood Pb concentrations and blood eosinophil counts, which indicated that the disorder of the immune system might be associated with the accumulation of Pb exposures.

In our study, the selected metal exposure included Cd, Hg, Mn, and Se in addition to lead. However, few studies investigated the associations between Cd, Hg, Mn, and Se exposures and blood eosinophil count. Cd exposure can occur through contaminated water, contaminated food, smoking, and occupational settings [53,54]. In an epidemiological study, Chao-Hsin Huang et al. reported that a high concentration of Cd was associated with a high eosinophil count [34]. Hg is a ubiquitous heavy metal, which is a growing public concern owing to its wide distribution and serious adverse health impacts. Some studies have reported modulatory effects of Hg on the immune system [55,56]. In an experimental animal study, Adam M. Schaefer et al. observed an inverse relationship of blood Hg concentrations with blood eosinophils among free-ranging bottlenose dolphins [57]. Similarly, another American study demonstrated developmental exposure to environmental Hg had no correlation with blood eosinophil counts in childhood. Mn and Se are necessary nutrients, but the intake of these elements' concentrations beyond the homeostatic capacity of the body may cause adverse effects [58]. A previous study including 2447 adults found urine Mn was not associated with blood eosinophil counts [34]. Another small case-control study found that the asthma group had lower serum Se concentrations and higher indicators of oxidative stress [42]. In our study, in three models, we observed that the associations between blood Cd, Hg, Mn, Se, and blood eosinophil counts were not statistically significant among asthmatic adults in the USA.

Compared with previous studies, our study has several advantages. First, our study provides a nationally representative, relatively large sample of asthmatic adults, which includes information on quite a few potential confounders. Second, considering that confounders may affect the results, we identify the high-risk group on the Pb exposures and verify the stability of the results through stratified analysis. Next, we use the machine learning XGBoost algorithm to determine which type of metal exposure affects blood eosinophil counts most. Then, we observed the linear relationship between blood Pb concentrations and blood eosinophil counts by constructing a smooth curve.

Nonetheless, some limitations in interpreting our results need to be taken into account. Though our study is nationally broad, most of the data are based on the American population. Data on populations of countries with less developed economies are still lacking, and heavy metal exposure may be different due to differences in national development. Secondly, this study is a cross-sectional survey, so we cannot distinguish a causal relationship. Thirdly, we cannot determine the drug use of participants. Finally, some other potential confounders, such as information on IgE-dependent sensitization, allergic diseases, parasitic diseases, and so on, may not be taken into consideration. In conclusion, we suggest constructing more predictive models between metal exposures and body biomarkers, including blood eosinophils, in the future clinical setting to guide clinical prevention and therapy.

5. Conclusions

In our study, we observed that blood Pb was positively and independently correlated with blood eosinophil counts among American adults with asthma. We suggested that long-time Pb exposure as a risk factor might be correlated with the immune system disorder of asthmatic adults and affect the occurrence, development, and exacerbation of asthma. Though our study did not elucidate the exact mechanism of action of Pb on the development and exacerbation of asthma, our findings would help to better identify the association of Pb and asthma from an epidemiological perspective. Finally, we wished to attract more attention to the association between metal exposure and asthma.

Author Contributions: Conceptualization and design, M.G., J.W., S.G. and L.X.; Acquisition and analysis of the data, M.G. and J.W.; Interpretation of the data, J.W. and M.G.; Writing—original draft, J.W. and M.G.; Writing—review and editing and critical analysis of the results, J.W., M.G., S.G. and L.X. All authors have read and agreed to the published version of the manuscript.

Funding: Famous talents and teachers in Chongqing (Guo Shuliang).

Institutional Review Board Statement: Not applicable.

Informed Consent Statement: Not applicable.

Data Availability Statement: All data can be obtained on the NHANES official website (http://www.cdc.gov/nchs/nhanes/, 6 January 2023).

Acknowledgments: The NHANES protocol was approved by the NCHS Research Ethics Review Board. The authors also wish to extend their great thanks to Joan, who supported them the most.

Conflicts of Interest: The authors declare that they have no known competing financial interests or personal relationships that could have appeared to influence the work reported in this paper.

References

1. Wenzel, S. Severe asthma: From characteristics to phenotypes to endotypes. *Clin. Exp. Allergy* **2012**, *42*, 650–658. [CrossRef] [PubMed]
2. Chung, K.F.; Wenzel, S.E.; Brozek, J.L.; Bush, A.; Castro, M.; Sterk, P.J.; Adcock, I.M.; Bateman, E.D.; Bel, E.H.; Bleecker, E.R.; et al. International ERS/ATS guidelines on definition, evaluation and treatment of severe asthma. *Eur. Respir. J.* **2014**, *43*, 343–373. [CrossRef] [PubMed]
3. GBD 2015 Chronic Respiratory Disease Collaborators. Global, regional, and national deaths, prevalence, disability-adjusted life years, and years lived with disability for chronic obstructive pulmonary disease and asthma, 1990–2015: A systematic analysis for the Global Burden of Disease Study 2015. *Lancet Res. Med.* **2017**, *5*, 691–706. [CrossRef] [PubMed]
4. Wang, H.; Naghabi, M.; Allen, C.; Barber, R.M.; Bhutta, Z.A.; Carter, A.; Caset, D.C.; Charlson, F.J.; Chen, A.Z.; Coates, A.J.; et al. Global, regional, and national life expectancy, all-cause mortality, and cause-specific mortality for 249 causes of death, 1980–2015: A systematic analysis for the Global Burden of Disease Study 2015. *Lancet* **2016**, *388*, 1459–1544.
5. Pate, C.A.; Zahran, H.S.; Qin, X.; Johnson, C.; Hummelman, E.; Malilay, J. Asthma Surveillance—United States, 2006–2018. Morbidity and mortality weekly report. *Surveill. Summ.* **2021**, *70*, 1–32. [CrossRef] [PubMed]
6. Nurmagambetov, T.; Kuwahara, R.; Garbe, P. The Economic Burden of Asthma in the United States, 2008–2013. *Ann. Am. Thorac. Soc.* **2018**, *15*, 348–356. [CrossRef] [PubMed]
7. Denlinger, L.C.; Phillips, B.R.; Ramratnam, S.; Ross, K.; Bhakta, N.R.; Cardet, J.C.; Castro, M.; Peters, S.P.; Phipatanakul, W.; Aujla, S.; et al. Inflammatory and Comorbid Features of Patients with Severe Asthma and Frequent Exacerbations. *Am. J. Respir. Crit. Care Med.* **2017**, *195*, 302–313. [CrossRef]
8. Carr, T.F.; Zeki, A.A.; Kraft, M. Eosinophilic and Noneosinophilic Asthma. *Am. J. Respir. Crit. Care Med.* **2018**, *197*, 22–37. [CrossRef]
9. Fowler, S.J.; Tavernier, G.; Niven, R. High blood eosinophil counts predict sputum eosinophilia in patients with severe asthma. *J. Allergy Clin. Immunol.* **2015**, *135*, 822–824.e2.
10. Wagener, A.H.; de Nijs, S.B.; Lutter, R.; Sousa, A.R.; Weersink, E.J.; Bel, E.H.; Sterk, P.J. External validation of blood eosinophils, FE(NO) and serum periostin as surrogates for sputum eosinophils in asthma. *Thorax* **2015**, *70*, 115–120. [CrossRef]
11. Hastie, A.T.; Moore, W.C.; Li, H.; Rector, B.M.; Ortega, V.E.; Pascual, R.M.; Peters, S.P.; Meyers, D.A.; Bleecker, E.R. Biomarker surrogates do not accurately predict sputum eosinophil and neutrophil percentages in asthmatic subjects. *J. Allergy Clin. Immunol.* **2013**, *132*, 72–80.e12. [CrossRef] [PubMed]
12. Ulrik, C.S.; Frederiksen, J. Mortality and markers of risk of asthma death among 1,075 outpatients with asthma. *Chest* **1995**, *108*, 10–15. [CrossRef] [PubMed]
13. Kupczyk, M.; Haque, S.; Middelveld, R.J.; Dahlén, B.; Dahlén, S.E. Phenotypic predictors of response to oral glucocorticosteroids in severe asthma. *Respir. Med.* **2013**, *107*, 1521–1530. [CrossRef] [PubMed]
14. Malinovschi, A.; Fonseca, J.A.; Jacinto, T.; Alving, K.; Janson, C. Exhaled nitric oxide levels and blood eosinophil counts independently associate with wheeze and asthma events in National Health and Nutrition Examination Survey subjects. *J. Allergy Clin. Immunol.* **2013**, *132*, 821–827.e5. [CrossRef]
15. Wark, P.A.; McDonald, V.M.; Gibson, P.G. Adjusting prednisone using blood eosinophils reduces exacerbations and improves asthma control in difficult patients with asthma. *Respirology* **2015**, *20*, 1282–1284. [CrossRef]
16. Corren, J.; Weinstein, S.; Janka, L.; Zangrilli, J.; Garin, M. Phase 3 Study of Reslizumab in Patients With Poorly Controlled Asthma: Effects Across a Broad Range of Eosinophil Counts. *Chest* **2016**, *150*, 799–810. [CrossRef]
17. Goldman, M.; Hirsch, I.; Zangrilli, J.G.; Newbold, P.; Xu, X. The association between blood eosinophil count and benralizumab efficacy for patients with severe, uncontrolled asthma: Subanalyses of the Phase III SIROCCO and CALIMA studies. *Curr. Med Res. Opin.* **2017**, *33*, 1605–1613. [CrossRef]

18. Rabe, K.F.; Nair, P.; Brusselle, G.; Maspero, J.F.; Castro, M.; Sher, L.; Zhu, H.; Hamilton, J.D.; Swanson, B.N.; Khan, A.; et al. Efficacy and Safety of Dupilumab in Glucocorticoid-Dependent Severe Asthma. *N. Engl. J. Med.* **2018**, *378*, 2475–2485. [CrossRef]
19. FitzGerald, J.M.; Bleecker, E.R.; Nair, P.; Korn, S.; Ohta, K.; Lommatzsch, M.; Ferguson, G.T.; Busse, W.W.; Barker, P.; Sproule, S.; et al. An anti-interleukin-5 receptor α monoclonal antibody, as add-on treatment for patients with severe, uncontrolled, eosinophilic asthma (CALIMA): A randomised, double-blind, placebo-controlled phase 3 trial. *Lancet* **2016**, *388*, 2128–2141. [CrossRef]
20. Bleecker, E.R.; FitzGerald, J.M.; Chanez, P.; Papi, A.; Weinstein, S.F.; Barker, P.; Sproule, S.; Gilmartin, G.; Aurivillius, M.; Werkström, V.; et al. Efficacy and safety of benralizumab for patients with severe asthma uncontrolled with high-dosage inhaled corticosteroids and long-acting β(2)-agonists (SIROCCO): A randomised, multicentre, placebo-controlled phase 3 trial. *Lancet* **2016**, *388*, 2115–2127. [CrossRef]
21. Vedel-Krogh, S.; Nielsen, S.F.; Lange, P.; Vestbo, J.; Nordestgaard, B.G. Association of Blood Eosinophil and Blood Neutrophil Counts with Asthma Exacerbations in the Copenhagen General Population Study. *Clin. Chem.* **2017**, *63*, 823–832. [CrossRef] [PubMed]
22. Price, D.B.; Rigazio, A.; Campbell, J.D.; Bleecker, E.R.; Corrigan, C.J.; Thomas, M.; Wenzel, S.E.; Wilson, A.M.; Small, M.B.; Gopalan, G.; et al. Blood eosinophil count and prospective annual asthma disease burden: A UK cohort study. *Lancet Respir. Med.* **2015**, *3*, 849–858. [CrossRef] [PubMed]
23. Zeiger, R.S.; Schatz, M.; Dalal, A.A.; Chen, W.; Sadikova, E.; Suruki, R.Y.; Kawatkar, A.A.; Qian, L. Blood Eosinophil Count and Outcomes in Severe Uncontrolled Asthma: A Prospective Study. *J. Allergy Clin. Immunol. Pr.* **2017**, *5*, 144–153.e8. [CrossRef] [PubMed]
24. Wu, K.-G.; Chang, C.-Y.; Yen, C.-Y.; Lai, C.-C. Associations between environmental heavy metal exposure and childhood asthma: A population-based study. *J. Microbiol. Immunol. Infect.* **2019**, *52*, 352–362. [CrossRef] [PubMed]
25. Menke, A.; Guallar, E.; Cowie, C.C. Metals in Urine and Diabetes in U.S. Adults. *Diabetes* **2016**, *65*, 164–171. [CrossRef]
26. Zeng, X.; Xu, X.; Zheng, B.; Reponen, T.; Chen, A.; Huo, X. Heavy metals in PM2.5 and in blood, and children's respiratory symptoms and asthma from an e-waste recycling area. *Environ. Pollut.* **2016**, *210*, 346–353. [CrossRef]
27. Wang, I.J.; Karmaus, W.J.J.; Yang, C.C. Lead exposure, IgE, and the risk of asthma in children. *J. Exp. Sci. Environ. Epidemiol.* **2017**, *27*, 478–483. [CrossRef]
28. Lehmann, I. Environmental pollutants as adjuvant factors of immune system derived diseases. *Bundesgesundheitsblatt, Gesundheitsforschung, Gesundheitsschutz* **2017**, *60*, 592–596. [CrossRef]
29. Feiler, M.O.; Pavia, C.J.; Frey, S.M.; Parsons, P.J.; Thevenet-Morrison, K.; Canfield, R.L.; Jusko, T.A. Early life blood lead levels and asthma diagnosis at age 4–6 years. *Environ. Health Prev. Med.* **2021**, *26*, 108. [CrossRef]
30. Park, S.; Lee, E.-H.; Kho, Y. The association of asthma, total IgE, and blood lead and cadmium levels. *J. Allergy Clin. Immunol.* **2016**, *138*, 1701–1703.e6. [CrossRef]
31. Huang, X.; Xie, J.; Cui, X.; Zhou, Y.; Wu, X.; Lu, W.; Shen, Y.; Yuan, J.; Chen, W. Association between Concentrations of Metals in Urine and Adult Asthma: A Case-Control Study in Wuhan, China. *PloS ONE* **2016**, *11*, e0155818.
32. Rosa, M.J.; Benedetti, C.; Peli, M.; Donna, F.; Nazzaro, M.; Fedrighi, C.; Zoni, S.; Marcon, A.; Zimmerman, N.; Wright, R.; et al. Association between personal exposure to ambient metals and respiratory disease in Italian adolescents: A cross-sectional study. *BMC Pulm. Med.* **2016**, *16*, 6. [CrossRef] [PubMed]
33. Urushidate, S.; Matsuzaka, M.; Okubo, N.; Iwasaki, H.; Hasebe, T.; Tsuya, R.; Iwane, K.; Inoue, R.; Yamai, K.; Danjo, K.; et al. Association between concentration of trace elements in serum and bronchial asthma among Japanese general population. *J. Trace Elements Med. Biol.* **2010**, *24*, 236–242.
34. Huang, C.-H.; Hsieh, C.-Y.; Wang, C.-W.; Tu, H.-P.; Chen, S.-C.; Hung, C.-H.; Kuo, C.-H. Associations and Interactions between Heavy Metals with White Blood Cell and Eosinophil Count. *Int. J. Med Sci.* **2022**, *19*, 331–337. [CrossRef]
35. Oulhote, Y.; Shamim, Z.; Kielsen, K.; Weihe, P.; Grandjean, P.; Ryder, L.P.; Heilmann, C. Children's white blood cell counts in relation to developmental exposures to methylmercury and persistent organic pollutants. *Reprod. Toxicol.* **2017**, *68*, 207–214.
36. Cornwell, C.R.; Egan, K.B.; Zahran, H.S.; Mirabelli, M.C.; Hsu, J.; Chew, G.L. Associations of blood lead levels with asthma and blood eosinophils in US children. *Pediatr. Allergy Immunol.* **2020**, *31*, 695–699.
37. Min, K.-B.; Min, J.-Y. Environmental lead exposure and increased risk for total and allergen-specific IgE in US adults. *J. Allergy Clin. Immunol.* **2015**, *135*, 275–277. [CrossRef]
38. Bellanger, A.-P.; Bosch-Cano, F.; Millon, L.; Ruffaldi, P.; Franchi, M.; Bernard, N. Reactions of airway epithelial cells to birch pollen grains previously exposed to in situ atmospheric Pb concentrations: A preliminary assay of allergenicity. *Biol. Trace Element Res.* **2012**, *150*, 391–395. [CrossRef]
39. Farkhondeh, T.; Boskabady, M.H.; Kohi, M.K.; Sadeghi-Hashjin, G.; Moin, M. Lead exposure affects inflammatory mediators, total and differential white blood cells in sensitized guinea pigs during and after sensitization. *Drug Chem. Toxicol.* **2014**, *37*, 329–335. [CrossRef]
40. Guardiola, F.A.; Cuesta, A.; Meseguer, J.; Martínez, S.; Martínez-Sánchez, M.J.; Pérez-Sirvent, C.; Esteban, M.A. Accumulation, histopathology and immunotoxicological effects of waterborne cadmium on gilthead seabream (Sparus aurata). *Fish Shellfish. Immunol.* **2013**, *35*, 792–800.
41. Kim, J.H.; Lee, K.-H.; Hong, S.-C.; Lee, H.-S.; Lee, J.; Kang, J.W. Association between serum mercury concentration and leukocyte differential count in children. *Pediatr. Hematol. Oncol.* **2015**, *32*, 109–114. [CrossRef] [PubMed]

42. Guo, C.H.; Liu, P.J.; Hsia, S.; Chuang, C.J.; Chen, P.C. Role of certain trace minerals in oxidative stress, in-flam-mation, CD4/CD8 lymphocyte ratios and lung function in asthmatic patients. *Ann. Clin. Biochem.* **2011**, *48 Pt 4*, 344–351. [PubMed]
43. Zeiger, R.S.; Schatz, M.; Li, Q.; Chen, W.; Khatry, D.B.; Gossage, D.; Tran, T.N. The association of blood eo-sinophil counts to future asthma exacerbations in children with persistent asthma. *J. Allergy Clin. Immunol. In Pract.* **2015**, *3*, 283–287.e4. [CrossRef]
44. Foster, P.S.; Hogan, S.P.; Yang, M.; Mattes, J.; Young, I.G.; Matthaei, K.I.; Kumar, R.K.; Mahalingam, S.; Webb, D.C. Interleukin-5 and eosinophils as therapeutic targets for asthma. *Trends Mol. Med.* **2002**, *8*, 162–167. [PubMed]
45. Casciano, J.; Krishnan, J.A.; Small, M.B.; Buck, P.O.; Gopalan, G.; Li, C.; Kemp, R.; Dotiwala, Z. Burden of asthma with elevated blood eosinophil levels. *BMC Pulm. Med.* **2016**, *16*, 100. [CrossRef]
46. Anderson, H.M.; Lemanske, R.F., Jr.; Arron, J.R.; Holweg, C.T.J.; Rajamanickam, V.; Gangnon, R.E.; Gern, J.E.; Jackson, D.J. Relationships among aeroallergen sensitization, peripheral blood eosinophils, and periostin in pediatric asthma development. *J. Allergy Clin. Immunol.* **2017**, *139*, 790–796. [PubMed]
47. Nakagome, K.; Nagata, M. Involvement and Possible Role of Eosinophils in Asthma Exacerbation. *Front. Immunol.* **2018**, *9*, 2220.
48. Thomson, C.D.; Wickens, K.; Miller, J.; Ingham, T.; Lampshire, P.; Epton, M.J.; Town, G.I.; Pattemore, P.; Crane, J. Selenium status and allergic disease in a cohort of New Zealand children. *Clin. Exp. Allergy J. Br. Soc. Allergy Clin. Immunol.* **2012**, *42*, 560–567.
49. Li, X.; Fan, Y.; Zhang, Y.; Huang, X.; Huang, Z.; Yu, M.; Xu, Q.; Han, X.; Lu, C.; Wang, X. Association be-tween selected urinary heavy metals and asthma in adults: A retrospective cross-sectional study of the US National Health and Nutrition Examination Survey. *Environ. Sci. Pollut. Res. Int.* **2021**, *28*, 5833–5844. [CrossRef]
50. Mishra, K.P. Lead exposure and its impact on immune system: A review. *Toxicol. Vitr.* **2009**, *23*, 969–972.
51. Min, J.-Y.; Min, K.-B.; Kim, R.; Cho, S.-I.; Paek, M. Blood lead levels and increased bronchial responsiveness. *Biol. Trace Element Res.* **2008**, *123*, 41–46. [CrossRef] [PubMed]
52. Wells, E.M.; Bonfield, T.L.; Dearborn, D.G.; Jackson, L.W. The relationship of blood lead with immunoglobulin E, eosinophils, and asthma among children: NHANES 2005–2006. *Int. J. Hyg. Environ. Health* **2014**, *217*, 196–204. [CrossRef] [PubMed]
53. Cao, Z.R.; Cui, S.M.; Lu, X.X.; Chen, X.M.; Yang, X.; Cui, J.P.; Zhang, G.H. Effects of occupational cadmium exposure on workers' cardiovascular system. *Zhonghua Lao Dong Wei Sheng Zhi Ye Bing Za Zhi Zhonghua Laodong Weisheng Zhiyebing Zazhi/Chin. J. Ind. Hyg. Occup. Dis.* **2018**, *36*, 474–477.
54. Huo, J.; Huang, Z.; Li, R.; Song, Y.; Lan, Z.; Ma, S.; Wu, Y.; Chen, J.; Zhang, L. Dietary cadmium exposure assessment in rural areas of Southwest China. *PLoS ONE* **2018**, *13*, e0201454. [CrossRef] [PubMed]
55. Nyland, J.F.; Fillion, M.; Barbosa, F., Jr.; Shirley, D.L.; Chine, C.; Lemire, M.; Mergler, D.; Silbergeld, E.K. Bi-omarkers of methylmercury exposure immunotoxicity among fish consumers in Amazonian Brazil. *Environ. Health Perspect.* **2011**, *119*, 1733–1738. [CrossRef]
56. Kim, K.-N.; Bae, S.; Park, H.Y.; Kwon, H.-J.; Hong, Y.C. Low-level Mercury Exposure and Risk of Asthma in School-age Children. *Epidemiology* **2015**, *26*, 733–739. [CrossRef]
57. Schaefer, A.M.; Stavros, H.-C.W.; Bossart, G.D.; Fair, P.A.; Goldstein, J.D.; Reif, J.S. Associations between mercury and hepatic, renal, endocrine, and hematological parameters in Atlantic bottlenose dolphins (Tursiops truncatus) along the eastern coast of Florida and South Carolina. *Arch. Environ. Contam. Toxicol.* **2011**, *61*, 688–695. [CrossRef]
58. Rayman, M.P. Selenium and human health. *Lancet* **2012**, *379*, 1256–1268. [CrossRef]

Disclaimer/Publisher's Note: The statements, opinions and data contained in all publications are solely those of the individual author(s) and contributor(s) and not of MDPI and/or the editor(s). MDPI and/or the editor(s) disclaim responsibility for any injury to people or property resulting from any ideas, methods, instructions or products referred to in the content.

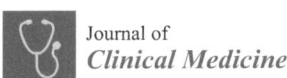

Article

Reduced Skeletal Muscle Mass Is Associated with an Increased Risk of Asthma Control and Exacerbation

Shuwen Zhang [1,2,3,†], Xin Zhang [1,2,3,†], Ke Deng [2,3], Changyong Wang [2,3], Lisa G. Wood [4], Huajing Wan [2,3], Lei Liu [1,2,3], Ji Wang [2,3], Li Zhang [1,2,3], Ying Liu [1,2,3], Gaiping Cheng [5], Peter G. Gibson [6], Brian G. Oliver [7,8], Fengming Luo [2,3], Vanessa M. McDonald [6], Weimin Li [2,9,*] and Gang Wang [2,3,*]

- [1] Pneumology Group, Department of Integrated Traditional Chinese and Western Medicine, West China Hospital, Sichuan University, Chengdu 610041, China
- [2] Department of Respiratory and Critical Care Medicine, Clinical Research Center for Respiratory Disease, West China Hospital, Sichuan University, Chengdu 610041, China
- [3] Laboratory of Pulmonary Immunology and Inflammation, Frontiers Science Center for Disease-Related Molecular Network, Sichuan University, Chengdu 610041, China
- [4] Priority Research Center for Healthy Lungs, Hunter Medical Research Institute, The University of Newcastle, New Lambton, NSW 2308, Australia
- [5] Department of Clinical Nutrition, West China Hospital, Sichuan University, Chengdu 610041, China
- [6] Centre of Excellence in Severe Asthma and Priority Research Centre for Healthy Lungs, Hunter Medical Research Institute, The University of Newcastle, Newcastle, NSW 2300, Australia
- [7] School of Life Sciences, University of Technology Sydney, Ultimo, NSW 2007, Australia
- [8] Woolcock Institute of Medical Research, The University of Sydney, Sydney, NSW 2000, Australia
- [9] Respiratory Microbiome Laboratory, Frontiers Science Center for Disease-Related Molecular Network, Sichuan University, Chengdu 610041, China
- * Correspondence: weimi003@scu.edu.cn (W.L.); wcums-respiration@hotmail.com (G.W.)
- † These authors contributed equally to this work.

Abstract: Background: Skeletal muscle mass (SMM) has been suggested to be associated with multiple health-related outcomes. However, the potential influence of SMM on asthma has not been largely explored. Objective: To study the association between SMM and clinical features of asthma, including asthma control and exacerbation, and to construct a model based on SMM to predict the risk of asthma exacerbation (AEx). Methods: In this prospective cohort study, we consecutively recruited patients with asthma ($n = 334$), classified as the SMM ^{Normal} group ($n = 223$), SMM ^{Low} group ($n = 88$), and SMM ^{High} group ($n = 23$). We investigated the association between SMM and clinical asthma characteristics and explored the association between SMM and asthma control and AEx within a 12-month follow-up period. Based on SMM, an exacerbation prediction model was developed, and the overall performance was externally validated in an independent cohort ($n = 157$). Results: Compared with the SMM ^{Normal} group, SMM ^{Low} group exhibited more airway obstruction and worse asthma control, while SMM ^{High} group had a reduced eosinophil percentage in induced sputum. Furthermore, SMM ^{Low} group was at a significantly increased risk of moderate-to-severe exacerbation compared with the SMM ^{Normal} group (relative risk $_{adjusted}$ 2.02 [95% confidence interval (CI), 1.35–2.68]; $p = 0.002$). In addition, a model involving SMM was developed which predicted AEx (area under the curve: 0.750, 95% CI: 0.691–0.810). Conclusions: Low SMM was an independent risk factor for future AEx. Furthermore, a model involving SMM for predicting the risk of AEx in patients with asthma indicated that assessment of SMM has potential clinical implications for asthma management.

Keywords: asthma; skeletal muscle mass; exacerbation; clinical prediction model

1. Introduction

Asthma is a common chronic respiratory disease affecting 1–18% of the population in different countries [1] Uncontrolled asthma may lead to reduced physical activity in daily life [2]. Lack of physical activity and other risk factors such as aging, nutritional status, and chronic inflammation could contribute to progressive loss of skeletal muscle mass (SMM) [3]. Reduced SMM is related to functional comorbidities, including mobility disorders, risk of falls and fractures, and loss of physical independence in activities of daily living for patients with asthma, which would increase the demand on the healthcare system [3]. Bioelectrical impedance analysis (BIA), as an inexpensive and non-invasive technique, provides measurements of SMM with little complexity [4].

SMM has been shown to affect health outcomes differentially. A decrease in muscle mass has been linked to greater insulin resistance and protection against the development of type 2 diabetes [5]. In contrast, lower amounts of SMM are associated with numerous health problems. A recently published study suggested that a lower muscle mass leads to an increased risk of cardiovascular events [6]. Moreover, the substantial loss of muscle mass relative to fat mass, termed "sarcopenia", has been found to have a negative effect on the quality of life and survival of patients [7–9]. This relationship has been observed not only in the elderly population and in cancer patients, in whom muscle loss is prevalent, but also in the general population [3,10].

There is increasing evidence that the loss of SMM is associated with lung health [11,12]. This may be relevant to asthma and chronic obstructive pulmonary disease (COPD), both of which are chronic inflammatory airway diseases [13]. Reduced SMM has been associated with impaired lung function and poor health status in patients with COPD [14–16]. We and others have shown that various extra-pulmonary traits, including obesity, are associated with asthma control [17–19]. However, to date, no studies have specifically examined SMM as a potential extra-pulmonary treatable trait in asthma outcome in future.

In this prospective cohort study, we explored whether reduced SMM was associated with worse asthma control and exacerbation (AEx). Subsequently, a prediction model involving SMM for identifying the risk of AEx was developed. The relative importance of SMM for all screened predictors in the model for predicting AEx was also assessed.

2. Materials and Methods

2.1. Study Design and Patients

The ASAN (https://www.severeasthma.org.au, accessed on 3 December 2022) is a multicenter clinical research network (Australia, Singapore, China, and New Zealand) in a real-world setting. This prospective cohort study consecutively recruited adult patients (aged $\geq$ 18 years) diagnosed with stable asthma at the West China Hospital, Sichuan University. Asthma was diagnosed based on the Global Initiative for Asthma [1]. Stable asthma was defined as no respiratory tract infections, asthma exacerbations, or systemic corticosteroid (SCS) use in the previous 4 weeks. Patients who were unable to complete the questionnaires, perform spirometry, perform the sputum induction, or were pregnant or breastfeeding were excluded from the study.

We recruited 334 patients (recruitment period: March 2014 to October 2018). According to the age, sex, height, and weight of the individual, the range of normal values for SMM in Asian populations was calculated using a validated equation by multifrequency BIA and classified as SMM^{Normal} group [20,21]. SMM values lower than the 10th percentile of the reference values were classified as SMM^{Low} group and values of SMM equal to or higher than the 90th percentile of the reference values were classified as SMM^{High} group [20,21]. These patients were followed for 12 months to assess the occurrence of AEx. We used these participants as the training cohort to explore the association between SMM and asthma and construct a prediction model.

We independently recruited 157 patients as the validation cohort (recruitment period: November 2018 to October 2020) to validate the prediction model established in the training cohort (Figure 1). As in the training cohort, these patients were also followed up for 12 months to assess the occurrence of AEx. All patients (training and validation cohorts) were included in this study satisfying the above inclusion/exclusion criteria.

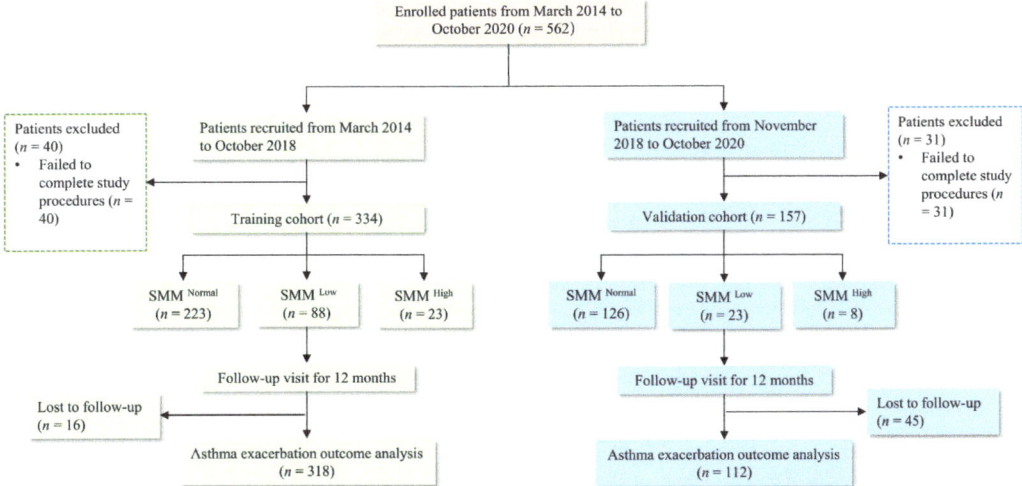

Figure 1. Flowchart for patient inclusion in the training and validation cohorts. SMM, skeletal muscle mass.

All patients provided written informed consent before participating in the study. The study was approved by the Institutional Review Board of West China Hospital, Sichuan University (Chengdu, China) (2014-30) and registered in the Chinese Clinical Trial Registry (ChiCTR-OOC-16009529; http://www.chictr.org.cn, accessed on 3 December 2022).

2.2. Data Collection and Clinical Assessments

Participants were followed up for 1 year with visits at baseline, 1 month, 3 months, 6 months, 9 months and 12 months.

Baseline data of the participants were collected, which included demographics, medications at/prior to study entry, asthma history, atopy, BMI, asthma control questionnaire-6 (ACQ-6), psychological status assessed using the Hospital Anxiety and Depression Scale (HADS) [22]. And all included subjects underwent spirometry, sputum induction, fractional exhaled nitric oxide (FeNO), blood sampling and body composition (BC).

2.3. Anthropometric and BC Assessments

SMM was measured as a parameter in BC assessments at baseline. BC was evaluated using BIA (InBody S10 analyzer; Biospace Co., Ltd., Seoul, Republic of Korea) according to the user manual [20]. Body resistance (R) was used to estimate the total body SMM according to the method previously described by Janssen et al. as follows [21]:

$$\text{SMM (kg)} = [(\text{Ht}^2/R \times 0.401) + (\text{sex} \times 3.825) + (\text{age} \times -0.071)] + 5.102$$

where Ht is height in centimeters and R is BIA resistance in ohms; for sex, men = 1 and women = 0, and age is in years.

Anthropometric and BC assessments were performed by trained nutritionists. The patients had overnight fasting, emptied their bladder by urinating, removed their clothes, and stood during the measurements, during which the ambient temperature remained at 25 degrees centigrade. Height and weight were measured to the nearest 0.1 cm and 0.1 kg when wearing light clothing and no shoes [23]. BMI was calculated (BMI = weight [kg]/height squared [m^2]). Waist circumference and hip circumference were measured at the navel and maximum posterior protuberance of the buttocks, respectively.

BC variables, including visceral fat area (VFA) (cm^2), fat mass (FM) (kg), percentage body fat (PBF), and SMM (kg), were estimated.

2.4. Spirometry and FeNO

Spirometry was performed at baseline according to the American Thoracic Society/European Respiratory Society (ATS/ERS) standards using a spirometer (Med Graphics CPES/D USB, St. Paul, MN, USA) [24]. Pre-bronchodilator FEV_1 and pre-bronchodilator forced vital capacity (FVC) were also measured. The largest pre-bronchodilator FEV_1 and FVC values from the three forced expiratory curves were used for analysis [24]. We measured FeNO before spirometry testing using a NIOX analyzer (Aerocrine, Solna, Sweden) in accordance with the ATS/ERS recommendations [25].

2.5. Sputum and Blood Processing

Sputum induction, processing, and blood analyses were performed at baseline as described in our previous studies [26,27]. The total and differential blood cell counts and serum immunoglobulin E (IgE) levels were measured. Details are provided in the Supplementary Materials.

2.6. Atopy

Atopy was confirmed at baseline by at least one positive skin prick test (SPT) of common allergens, defined as a wheal diameter ≥ 3 mm after 15 min. The details are provided in the Supplementary Materials [28].

2.7. Asthma Control

Asthma control was assessed using the ACQ-6 at baseline [29]. The ACQ score is the mean of the six items and ranges from zero (totally controlled) to six (severely uncontrolled). A mean score of ≥ 0.75 is indicative of partially controlled or uncontrolled asthma. In our study, the patients were dichotomized into 2 groups on the basis of ACQ scores. We labeled those with scores of less than 0.75 as the well-controlled asthma and those with scores of more than 0.75 as the incompletely controlled asthma.

2.8. Asthma Exacerbation

We have collected the exacerbation history of all patients at baseline and follow-up for 1 year at 3 months, 6 months, 9 months and 12 months to assess exacerbations (face-to-face visits or telephone calls if unable to attend). An asthma exacerbation was defined based on ATS/ERS statement [30].

The definition of a severe asthma exacerbation for clinical trials should include at least one of the following: (a) use of SCS (tablets, suspension, or injection), or an increase from a stable maintenance dose, for at least 3 days. For consistency, courses of corticosteroids separated by 1 week or more were treated as separate severe exacerbations and (b) a hospitalization or emergency room (ER) visit because of asthma, requiring SCS [30].

The definition of a moderate asthma exacerbation included one or more of the following: deterioration in symptoms, deterioration in lung function, and increased rescue bronchodilator use. These features lasted for 2 days or more, but not be severe enough to warrant SCS use and/or hospitalization. ER visits for asthma (e.g., for routine sick care) that do not require SCS were classified as moderate exacerbations [30].

2.9. Statistical Analyses

For categorical data, descriptive variables were presented as n (%). Continuous data were presented as means with standard deviations or medians with interquartile ranges, depending on the distribution assessed by the Kolmogorov–Smirnov test. Differences in continuous data between the training and validation cohorts were assessed using the Mann–Whitney U test. The differences between the three groups were evaluated using one-way analysis of variance or Kruskal–Wallis H test for continuous variables, and the Chi-square test or Fisher's exact test for categorical variables, as appropriate.

In addition, post-hoc Bonferroni comparisons were performed, with the cutoff for significance set at α/n ($\alpha = 0.05$, where n is the number of comparisons). Logistic regression was used to assess the associations between SMM and asthma control at baseline (odds ratio [OR], 95% confidence interval [95% CI]), SMM and AEx during follow-up (relative risk [RR], 95% CI). Considering that COPD, obstructive sleep apnea, bronchiectasis, diabetes, obesity, and gastroesophageal reflux disease (GERD) may be confounding factors in the relationship between SMM and AEx [31–33], multivariable logistic regression by backward elimination in a stepwise fashion and sensitivity analysis was used to explore the effect of confounders on the results of the analysis. The above analyses were conducted using SPSS version 26.0 (IBM Corp., Armonk, NY, USA). In all statistical analyses, a p value of less than 0.05 was considered statistically significant.

2.10. Clinical Prediction Model for Predicting AEx

2.10.1. Selection of Variables and Clinical Prediction Model Establishment

We used a logistic model to select the variables to construct a prediction model [34]. We then calculated the area under the receiver operator characteristic (ROC) curve (AUC) to determine how many candidate factors should be chosen [35]. The details are provided in the Supplementary Materials [36].

Multivariable logistic regression was incorporated in the training cohort, combining significant predictors from the least absolute shrinkage and selection operator (LASSO) method into one final model [37]. This model displayed RR and 95% CI. Each predictor's contribution in the full model was measured as the partial chi-square statistic minus the predictor degrees of freedom [38].

2.10.2. Nomogram Establishment of Predicting AEx

Relationships among predictors in the model were visualized using a nomogram [39], which maps the predicted probabilities into points on a scale from 0 to 100 in a user-friendly graphical interface [40]. In this study, we established a nomogram for predicting AEx, named "AEx nomogram". The details are provided in the Supplementary Materials.

2.10.3. Performance of the Model and Clinical Applicability of the Nomogram

The concordance index (C-index), Hosmer–Lemeshow (HL) goodness-of-fit test, and calibration curve were performed in the training and validation cohorts to estimate the prediction performance of the nomogram [41,42]. The internal and external validity of the model was determined. Internal validation was performed using 1000 bootstrap samplings to produce bias-corrected estimates of the model's performance [43]. External validation was performed on a validation cohort. We then set the two models to further explore whether SMM improves the performance of the prediction model. Model 1 was adjusted for all the predictors from a prediction model minus SMM, while Model 2 was adjusted for all the predictors from a prediction model. The net reclassification improvement (NRI) (>0) can be viewed as an improvement in discrimination by adding SMM to the training and validation cohorts. Likewise, integrated discrimination improvement (IDI) (>0) was considered an improvement in discrimination by adding SMM in the two cohorts.

Finally, decision curve analysis (DCA) was conducted to determine the clinical usefulness of the AEx nomogram by quantifying the net benefits at different threshold probabilities in the training cohort [44,45]. To determine the applicability of SMM in the nomogram, we built three models: (A) a model containing only one variable-SMM, (B) an AEx nomogram with subtraction of SMM, and (C) an AEx nomogram. A clinical impact curve (CIC) was developed based on the DCA of a model (C) to visually display the estimated number of patients at a high risk of AEx for each risk threshold [46]. The details are provided in the Supplementary Materials.

Model performance, validation, and applicability were performed using R software (version 4.0.2; R Foundation for Statistical Computing, Vienna, Austria). The "glmnet" package was used for binary LASSO method, "rms" for nomogram and calibration curve plotting, "pROC" for AUC calculation, "PredictABEL" for NRI and IDI calculation, and "DecisionCurve" for decision curve analysis.

3. Results

3.1. Participant Characteristics

A total of 219 participants (65.6%) were female, with a median age of 44.0 (Q1, Q3: 35.0, 55.0) years and a median BMI of 23.02 (20.99, 25.02) kg/m^2. The prevalence of family history of asthma and atopy was 38.5% and 35.9%, respectively. The median scores of HADS-D and HADS-A in these patients were 1.0 (0, 3.0) and 1.0 (0, 4.0), respectively; 6.6% (n = 22) participants had anxiety symptoms, and 7.5% (n = 25) had depression symptoms. There were 149 patients (44.6%) with incompletely controlled asthma and 96 patients (28.7%) had experienced at least one severe exacerbation in the last 12 months. Rhinitis (53.6%) and eczema (20.4%) were the most common comorbidities.

Of the 334 participants, 223 (66.8%) were classified into the SMM ^{Normal} group, 88 (26.3%) were classified into the SMM ^{Low} group, and 23 (6.9%) were classified into the SMM ^{High} group. Compared with the SMM ^{Low} group, SMM ^{High} group had less airway obstruction (1.64 [1.28, 2.49] vs. 2.32 [2.02, 2.65] L, p = 0.013 for pre-bronchodilator FEV$_1$ in liters and 66.0 [47.0, 82.5] vs. 92.0 [78.0, 104.0] %, p < 0.001 for FEV$_1$% predicted) (Table 1).

Table 1. Demographic and clinical characteristics of the included patients grouped by SMM.

Variables	SMM ^{Normal}	SMM ^{Low}	SMM ^{High}	χ^2/H	p Value
n	223	88	23		
Anthropometric/asthma data					
Age, years, median (Q1, Q3)	44.5 (36.8, 62.0)	57.0 (40.0, 69.0)	47.5 (38.3, 53.0)	0.010	0.995
Female/male, n (%)	148 (66.4)/75 (33.6)	58 (65.9)/30 (34.1)	13 (56.5)/10 (43.5)	0.901	0.637
BMI					
kg/m^2, median (Q1, Q3)	24.09 (22.77, 26.37)	20.66 (19.46, 22.77) *	27.85 (27.29, 30.11) *, **	111.165	<0.001
Normal/overweight/obese, n (%)	130 (58.3)/75 (33.6)/17 (7.6)	66 (75.0)/5 (5.7)/0 (0) *	3 (13.0)/8 (34.8)/12 (52.2) *, **	NA	<0.001 §
WHR, median (Q1, Q3)	0.88 (0.84, 0.92)	0.83 (0.79, 0.90) *	0.93 (0.90, 0.95) *, **	29.483	<0.001
Smoking history (n), current/ex/never smoker	18/29/176	6/17/65	4/2/17	5.058	0.281
Pack years & median (Q1, Q3)	13.00 (2.50, 26.00)	21.50 (6.63, 32.00)	18.25 (3.50, 32.00)	1.276	0.528
Asthma duration (y), median (Q1, Q3)	5.0 (2.0, 20)	5.0 (2.0, 19.5)	9.0 (2, 25.0)	0.771	0.680
Early-onset asthma #, n (%)	38 (17.0)	14 (15.9)	6 (26.1)	NA	0.024 §
Atopy status, n (%)	79 (38.3)	35 (44.9)	6 (30.0)	1.812	0.404
Previous upper respiratory infection-induced asthma exacerbations, n (%)	155 (69.8)	67 (76.1)	15 (65.2)	1.652	0.438
Asthma family history, n (%)	73 (32.7)	37 (42.0)	14 (60.9) *	NA	0.031 §
Spirometry					
Pre-bronchodilator FEV$_1$, L, median (Q1, Q3)	2.06 (1.64, 2.85)	1.64 (1.28, 2.49)	2.32 (2.02, 2.65) **	8.632	0.013
Pre-bronchodilator FEV$_1$% predicted, median (Q1, Q3)	76.0 (62.0, 90.0)	66.0 (47.0, 82.5) *	92.0 (78.0, 104.0) **	15.684	<0.001
Pre-bronchodilator FEV$_1$/FVC, %, median (Q1, Q3)	66.01 (57.54, 76.79)	66.41 (55.23, 75.43)	74.43 (59.28, 82.21)	2.316	0.314
Asthma control					
ACQ-6 scores, median (Q1, Q3)	0.5 (0, 1.3)	0.8 (0.3, 1.3)	0.2 (0, 0.6) **	8.384	0.015
Incompletely controlled asthma, n (%) ‡	95 (42.6)	49 (55.7)	5 (21.7) **	9.599	0.008
Health status					
HADS-A					
Median (Q1, Q3)	1.0 (0, 4.0)	1.0 (0, 4.0)	1.0 (0, 2.0)	3.332	0.189
≥8, n (%) ¶	15 (6.7)	6 (6.8)	1 (4.3)	NA	1.000 §
HADS-D					0.504

Table 1. Cont.

Variables	SMM Normal	SMM Low	SMM High	χ^2/H	p Value
Median (Q1, Q3)	1.0 (0, 3.0)	1.0 (0, 3.0)	0 (0, 2.0)	1.370	0.504
≥8, n (%) ¶	16 (7.2)	8 (9.1)	1 (4.3)	NA	0.780 §
Asthma-related medications					
ICS (BDP equivalent) dose (μg/d), median (Q1, Q3)	400.0 (400.0, 1000.0)	500.0 (400.0, 1000.0)	400.0 (200.0, 625.0)	4.064	0.131
ICS/LABA, n (%)	135 (60.5)	44 (50.0)	13 (56.5)	2.877	0.237
OCS use					
n (%)	8 (3.6)	1 (1.1)	2 (8.7)	NA	0.157 §
Days with OCS use for exacerbation, median (Q1, Q3)	7.00 (6.50, 7.00)	7.00	6.00 (2.00, 10.00)	0.084	0.959
Daily doses of OCS equivalent to prednisone †, mg, median (Q1, Q3)	20.00 (20.00, 32.50)	20.00	55.00 (30.00, 80.00)	3.598	0.165
Cumulative doses of OCS equivalent to prednisone †, mg, median (Q1, Q3)	157.50 (140.00, 280.00)	140.00	430.00 (60.00, 800.00)	0.242	0.886
Leukotriene modifier, n (%)	74 (33.2)	24 (27.3)	9 (39.1)	1.584	0.453
Theophylline, n (%)	35 (15.7)	19 (21.6)	3 (13.0)	NA	0.428 §
Exacerbation in the past year, n (%)					
Severe exacerbation	57 (25.6)	29 (33.0)	10 (43.5)	4.303	0.116
Hospitalization	59 (26.5)	22 (25.0)	3 (13.0)	1.994	0.369
Emergency room visit	31 (13.9)	14 (15.9)	2 (8.7)	NA	0.728 §
Unscheduled visit	68 (30.5)	28 (31.8)	5 (21.7)	0.899	0.638
Comorbidity, n (%)					
Rhinitis	129 (57.8)	42 (47.7)	8 (34.8)	6.113	0.047
Bronchiectasis	11 (4.9)	4 (4.5)	0 (0.0)	NA	0.825 §
Sleep apnea	3 (1.3)	0 (0.0)	0 (0.0)	NA	0.646 §
GERD	14 (6.3)	4 (4.5)	1 (4.3)	NA	0.922 §
Eczema	45 (20.2)	17 (19.3)	6 (26.1)	NA	0.750 §
COPD	11 (4.9)	11 (12.5)	0 (0.0)	NA	0.037 §
Diabetes	7 (3.1)	1 (1.1)	1 (4.3)	NA	0.346 §

Abbreviations: SMM, skeletal muscle mass; BMI, body mass index; WHR, waist-to-hip ratio; FEV_1, forced expiratory volume in 1 s; FVC, forced vital capacity; ACQ, asthma control questionnaire; HADS-A, Hospital Anxiety and Depression Scale-Anxiety; HADS-D, Hospital Anxiety and Depression Scale-Depression; ICS, inhaled corticosteroid; BDP, beclomethasone dipropionate; LABA, long-acting beta-agonist; OCS, oral corticosteroid; GERD, gastroesophageal reflux disease; COPD, chronic obstructive pulmonary disease; NA, not applicable; Q1, first quartile; Q3, third quartile. & Never smokers were excluded from the analysis of pack-years. Pack years: the number of cigarettes smoked per day × years of smoking. ‡ Incompletely controlled asthma: ACQ mean scores ≥ 0.75. ¶ Depression or anxiety disorders was defined as a score ≥ 8 on the respective HADS-D or HADS-A domains. # Early-onset asthma (onset before 12 years of age). † The calculations based on the patients of using OCS in the past year. * $p < 0.05$ vs. SMM Normal, ** $p < 0.05$ vs. SMM Low. The significance level is 0.05. Significance values have been adjusted by the Bonferroni correction for multiple tests. § Fisher's exact probability.

In addition, we explored the differences in inflammatory variables among the three groups. Participants with the SMM High group had fewer sputum eosinophils (0 [0, 0.25] vs. 0.25 [0, 3.50] %, $p = 0.016$) than those with the SMM Normal group. The peripheral blood cell counts showed no significant differences among the three groups (all $p > 0.05$). The IgE ($p = 0.217$) and FeNO ($p = 0.464$) levels did not differ significantly among the three groups (Table S1).

3.2. Anthropometric and BC Assessments

Compared with the SMM Normal group, SMM High group had a significantly higher waist-to-hip ratio (WHR) and BMI. The SMM Low group had a significantly lower WHR and BMI, while the SMM ^{Low} group had a significantly lower FM, PBF, and VFA than patients in the SMM ^{Normal} group (Table S2).

3.3. Asthma Control

There were significant differences in asthma control among the three groups. SMM ^{High} group had better asthma control than SMM ^{Low} group (ACQ-6 median scores, 0.2 [0, 0.6] vs. 0.8 [0.3, 1.3], $p = 0.005$). Logistic regression modeling showed that SMM ^{Low} group was at a significantly increased risk of incompletely controlled asthma (OR $_{adj}$ 1.67 [95% CI: 1.01–2.75], $p = 0.045$) (Table 2).

Table 2. Association of SMM with incompletely controlled asthma (ACQ ≥ 0.75) using multivariable logistic regression with adjustment for confounders.

Group	β	SE for β	OR adj	95% CI for OR adj		p Value
				Lower	Upper	
SMM ^{Normal}			Reference			
SMM ^{High}	−0.983	0.523	0.374	0.134	1.044	0.060
SMM ^{Low}	0.512	0.255	1.668	1.012	2.749	0.045

Abbreviations: SMM, skeletal muscle mass; ACQ, asthma control questionnaire; OR, odds ratio. Adjusted for age, sex, BMI, ICS/LABA, cumulative doses of OCS equivalent to prednisone, smoking status, severe asthma exacerbation in the past year, forced expiratory volume in 1 s% predicted.

3.4. Asthma Exacerbation

Compared with the SMM ^{Normal} group, SMM ^{Low} group had a greater proportion of participants experiencing severe AEx (13.6% vs. 24.4%, $p = 0.006$) and moderate-to-severe AEx (25.8% vs. 40.2%, $p = 0.022$) (Table 3).

Table 3. Asthma exacerbation within the 12-month follow-up period grouped by SMM in the training cohort.

Variables	SMM ^{Normal} Group	SMM ^{Low} Group	SMM ^{High} Group	Total	χ^2/H	p Value
n	213	82	23	318		
Moderate-to-severe exacerbation						
n (%)	55 (25.8)	33 (40.2) *	4 (17.4)	92	7.595	0.022
Mean ± SD	0.61 ± 1.40	0.94 ± 1.53 *	0.52 ± 1.24	0.65 ± 1.40	7.149	0.028
Severe exacerbation						
n (%)	29 (13.6)	20 (24.4)	0 (0) **	49	NA	0.006 §
Mean ± SD	0.27 ± 0.84	0.43 ± 0.96	0 ± 0 **	0.28 ± 0.83	9.399	0.009

Abbreviations: SMM, skeletal muscle mass; SD, standard deviation; NA, not applicable. * $p < 0.05$ vs. SMM ^{Normal}, ** $p < 0.05$ vs. SMM ^{Low}. The significance level is 0.05. Significance values have been adjusted by the Bonferroni correction for multiple tests. § Fisher's exact probability.

We further established logistic regression models to analyze the risk of AEx in the three groups. As a result, the SMM ^{Low} group had an increased risk of moderate-to-severe AEx adjusting for age, sex, BMI, smoking status, inhaled corticosteroids (ICS)/long-acting beta-agonist (LABA), cumulative doses of OCS equivalent to prednisone, pre-bronchodilator FEV$_1$% predicted and moderate-to-severe asthma exacerbation last year (SMM ^{Normal} group as the reference; RR $_{adj}$ 2.02 [95% CI: 1.35–2.68]; $p = 0.002$) (Figure 2).

Likewise, the SMM ^{Low} group was still significantly associated with moderate-to-severe AEx compared with the SMM ^{Normal} group adjusting confounders including age, sex, BMI, smoking status, ICS/LABA, cumulative doses of OCS equivalent to prednisone, pre-bronchodilator FEV$_1$% predicted and severe asthma exacerbation last year, COPD, sleep apnea, bronchiectasis, diabetes, obesity, and GERD using multivariate logistic regression analysis with stepwise backward elimination (RR $_{adj}$ 1.72 [95% CI: 1.19–2.29]; $p = 0.006$) (Table S3).

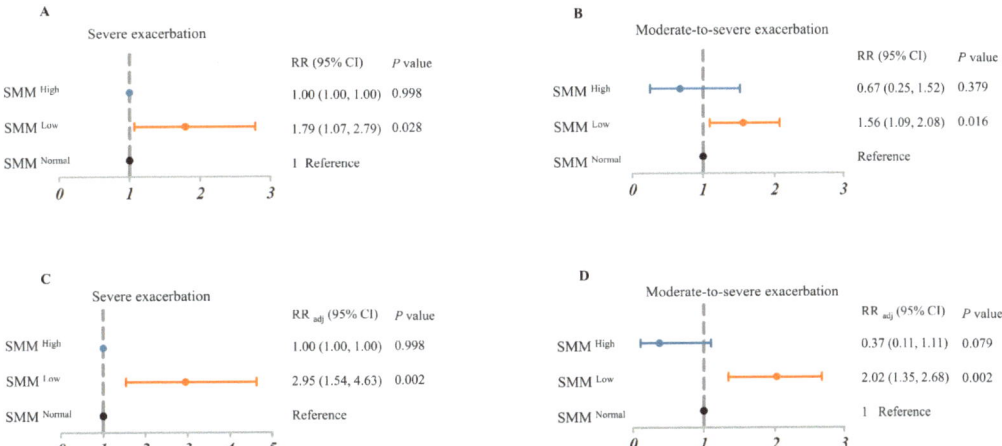

Figure 2. Associations of the SMM (skeletal muscle mass) with (**A**) severe exacerbation; univariate logistic regression analysis, (**B**) moderate-to-severe exacerbation, univariate logistic regression analysis. (**C**) severe exacerbation; multiple logistic regression analysis. Adjusted for age, sex, BMI, smoking status, ICS/LABA, cumulative doses of OCS equivalent to prednisone, severe exacerbation in the past year, pre-bronchodilator forced expiratory volume in 1 s% predicted (**D**) moderate-to-severe exacerbation, multiple logistic regression analysis, with normal SMM as the reference. Adjusted for age, sex, BMI, smoking status, ICS/LABA, cumulative doses of OCS equivalent to prednisone, severe exacerbation in the past year, pre-bronchodilator forced expiratory volume in 1 s% predicted. CI, confidence interval; RR, relative risk; RR $_{adj}$, adjusted relative risk. Blue, SMM ^{High}; Orange, SMM ^{Low}; Black, SMM ^{Normal}.

Additionally, after excluding the patients with COPD, sleep apnea, bronchiectasis, diabetes, obesity, and GERD, our sensitivity analysis indicated that this did not change the association between reduced SMM and AEx in the asthmatics (RR $_{adj}$ 1.77 [95% CI: 1.06–2.53]; $p = 0.032$) (Table S4).

3.5. Clinical Prediction Model

3.5.1. Selection of Variables and Establishment of a Clinical Prediction Model

In the training cohort, there were 17 variables with missing data (missing rates: 0.2% to 40.1%) (Table S5). The associations between 28 potential risk factors are shown in Table S6. Seven variables with nonzero coefficients in the LASSO method remained and were then included in the final multivariate logistic regression model (Figure S1), including low SMM (categorical variable) (RR 2.21 [95% CI: 1.12–3.66]; $p = 0.019$), VFA (categorical variable) (RR 1.78 [95% CI: 1.03–3.08]; $p = 0.039$), sputum eosinophils (continuous variable, %) (RR 1.01 [95% CI: 0.99–1.03]; $p = 0.078$), exacerbation in the past year (categorical variable) (RR 2.21 [95% CI: 1.28–3.81]; $p < 0.001$), rhinitis (categorical variable) (RR 1.42 [95% CI: 0.83–2.44]; $p = 0.114$), previous upper respiratory infection-induced asthma attack (categorical variable) (RR 2.47 [95% CI: 1.20–5.09]; $p = 0.001$), and HADS-D scores (continuous variable, score) (RR 1.06 [95% CI: 0.97–1.15]; $p = 0.116$) (Figure 3).

3.5.2. Nomogram of Predicting AEx

A nomogram containing the seven variables in the logistic regression model was constructed (Figure 4). The importance of each variable in the full model is illustrated (Figure S2). The SMM level had the third-largest predictive value among the seven variables.

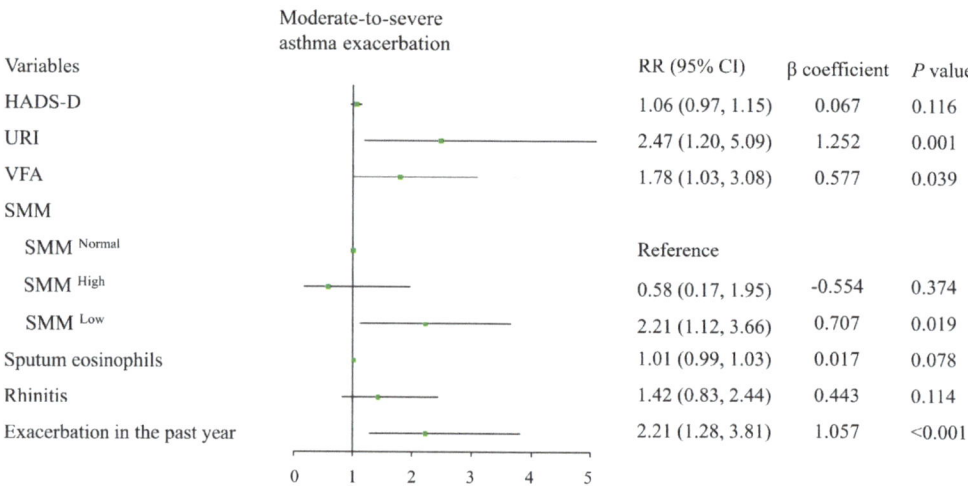

Figure 3. Risk factors in the prediction model for future moderate-to-severe exacerbation of asthma in the following years. Green dot, point estimate; Black line, 95% confidence interval.

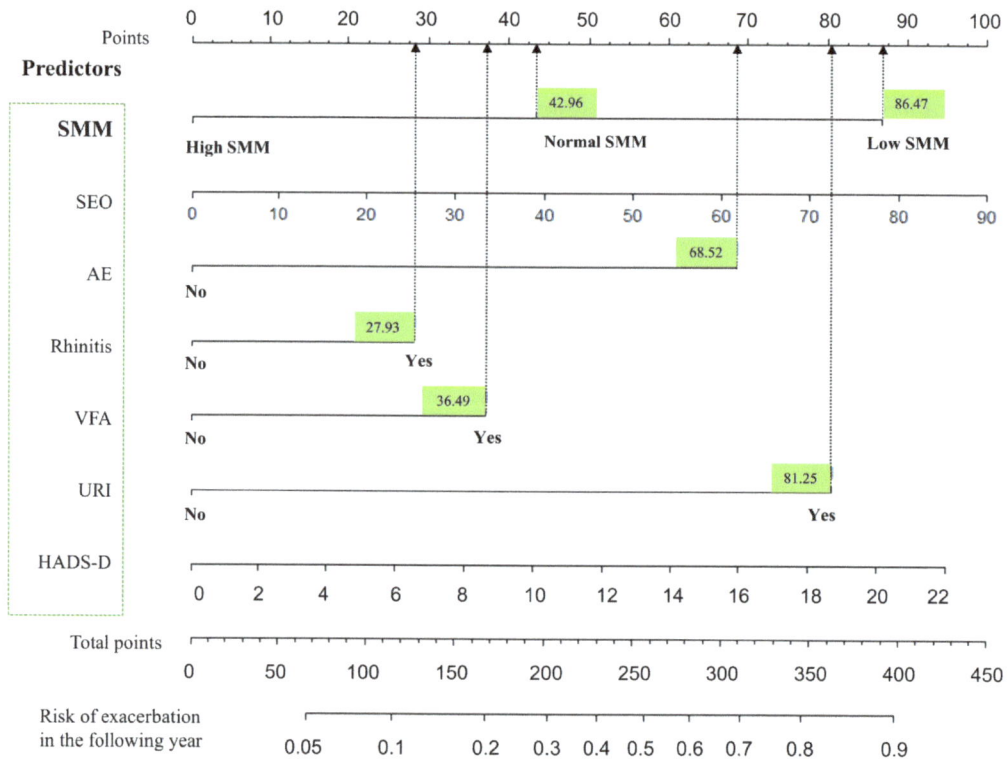

Figure 4. Asthma future exacerbation nomogram. The asthma future exacerbation nomogram was developed on the basis of established multivariable regression models in the whole cohort population. Using the nomogram, the probability of future asthma exacerbation in the following year can be estimated as follows. First, the judgment on predictor variables (e.g., yes or no, SMM [Low] or SMM [High]) can be obtained from patients. Second, if a predictor is judged as "Yes", the value of the

predictor can be designated by drawing an upward straight line from "Yes" up to the "Points" line. Third, add up the points of all the predictors assessed as "Yes" to get the total points. Finally, the probability of future asthma exacerbation in the following year can be obtained by drawing a straight line from the "Total Points line" down to the "Risk of exacerbation in the following year" line. SMM, skeletal muscle mass; VFA, visceral fat area; D, HADS-D; SEO, sputum eosinophils; URI, previous upper respiratory infection induced asthma attack.

3.5.3. Performance of the Prediction Model and Clinical Applicability of the Nomogram

There were no significant differences in sociodemographic characteristics between the training and validation cohorts (Tables S7 and S8). The C-indices of the nomogram in the training and validation cohorts were 0.750 (95% CI: 0.691–0.810) and 0.793 (0.704–0.882), respectively (Figure 5), indicating moderate accuracy. The p values of the HL tests (training cohort: $p = 0.531$; validation cohort: $p = 0.465$) indicated a lack of significance, suggesting no evidence of poor goodness-of-fit for the prediction model in the two cohorts. Likewise, the calibration curves, showed that the observed and predicted future risk of moderate-to-severe AEx in the final multivariate model were in good agreement in the training and validation cohorts (Figure S3). The NRI and IDI values indicated that SMM offered a significant statistical improvement in the performance of the prediction model in both the training and validation cohorts. The NRI was 0.285 (95% CI: 0.061–0.508; $p = 0.013$) in the training cohort (Table S9), whereas in the validation cohort, the NRI was 0.481 (0.100–0.861, $p = 0.013$). Similar results were obtained using IDI.

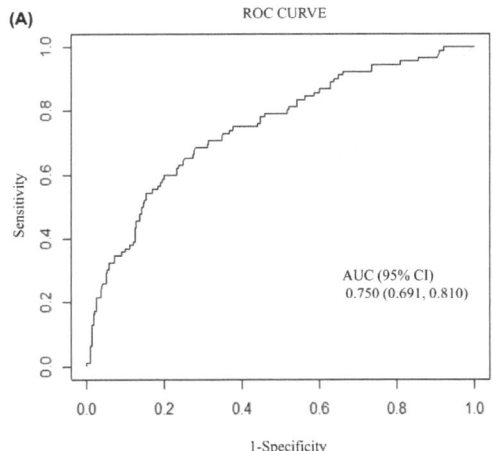
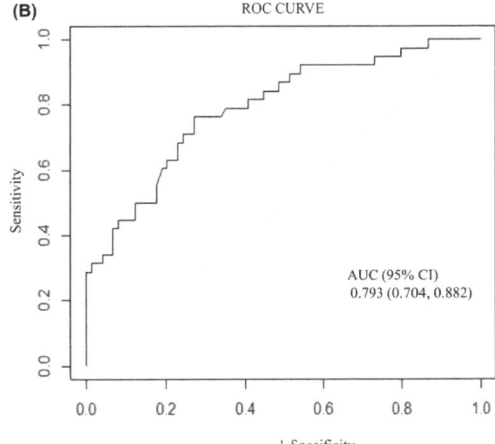

Figure 5. Receiver operating characteristic (ROC) curve for the prediction model for AEx in the training (**A**) and validation (**B**) cohorts. The x-axis, labeled specificity, represents the true-negative rate. The y-axis, labeled sensitivity, represents the true-positive rate. The area under the curve (AUC) and the 95% confidence interval (CI) are shown in the graph. AEx, asthma exacerbation.

Finally, the decision curve showed that using the AEx nomogram model (C) to predict AEx added more benefits than either model (A) or model (B) with different threshold probabilities (Figure S4A). In addition, with a threshold of 0.1 to 0.65, model (C) had the maximum benefits range, as shown in the DCA curve, indicating that SMM played a critical role in the clinical applicability of the prediction model.

The CIC visually shows the proportion of those with true AEx. The CIC also showed that real patients who were at high risk of AEx are included by estimating the number of patients with the risk threshold of 0.1 to 0.65 with the acceptable cost: benefit ratio (Figure S4B).

4. Discussion

To the best of our knowledge, this is the first study to investigate the association between SMM and asthma outcome in future. Even though previous studies have explored the relationship between muscle and asthma [47,48], they aimed to evaluate the peripheral muscle strength or the mechanism of reduced SMM in the patients with asthma, and did not observe the association between SMM and asthma-related outcomes in future.

Our study indicated that patients in the SMM ^{Low} group had a lower BMI and more airway obstruction. Moreover, low SMM as an independent risk factor was associated with poor asthma control and an increased risk of AEx. In contrast, SMM ^{High} group patients had less airway obstruction and sputum eosinophils, in association with better asthma control. Additionally, the prediction model involving SMM for predicting AEx established in our study had moderate discrimination, calibration, and clinical utility and demonstrated that SMM played a critical role in the prediction model. Our study indicated that SMM played an important role in asthma control and exacerbation, and reduced SMM could be a potential extra-pulmonary treatable trait to target in clinical asthma management.

In this study, the SMM ^{Low} group had more airway obstruction, demonstrated by reduced pre-bronchodilator FEV_1% predicted, compared to the SMM ^{High} group. However, there was no difference in pre-bronchodilator FEV_1/FVC, which is consistent with previously published studies [49]. This could be explained by the fact that FEV_1 represents the expiration flow rate; therefore, FEV_1 could be reduced in participants with low SMM because they may have a weakened ability to inflate and deflate their lungs. However, the ratio of FEV_1/FVC may remain constant regardless of the muscle mass.

Previous study indicated that medication use, ICS in particular, significantly reduced sputum eosinophils [50]. Although no significant difference was found in medication use in the three groups, our study still found that the SMM ^{High} group had a lower sputum eosinophils percentage. Two issues that can be explained as follows: SMM myocytes express and secrete numerous cytokines such as IL-6. Steensberg et al. demonstrated that physiological concentrations of IL-6 induce an anti-inflammatory response in humans [51]. Therefore, although we did not measure inflammatory cytokines, according to previous relevant studies, we speculated that the SMM ^{High} group would have increased levels of anti-inflammatory cytokines in circulation, which could inhibit the recruitment of inflammatory cells in the airway [52]. Conversely, the SMM ^{Low} group patients with higher eosinophilic inflammation needed more ICS, indicating that there may be more severe asthma. Hence, further studies are needed to elucidate the mechanisms by which SMM reduces inflammation in asthma.

Low SMM can be considered a potential extra-pulmonary treatable trait because it is clinically relevant, identifiable, measurable, and treatable [53]. It has been shown that most myokines that are regulated by exercise counteract the detrimental effects of adipokines and have beneficial effects on glucose and lipid metabolism and inflammation [54]. In contrast, physical inactivity and muscle disuse lead to the loss of muscle mass and, consequently, to the activation of a network of inflammatory pathways, which promotes the development of a cluster of chronic diseases. Therefore, SMM could potentially provide an important target for clinicians to guide the non-pharmacological treatment of patients with asthma. For example, increasing physical activity can be used to increase SMM, thereby improving asthma control and reducing exacerbations. This is in agreement with a study by McDonald et al. [18], which identified sarcopenia as a potentially treatable trait of asthma.

As is well known, chronic intake of OCS and ICS induced clinically significant muscle hypotrophy for daily treatment [55]. Furthermore, systemic and oral beta-agonists could increase SMM while there has been no evidence to prove the association between inhaled beta-agonists and SMM [56]. Therefore, ICS/LABA and cumulative doses of OCS equivalent to prednisone, as two important confounders, were adjusted to relevant logistic models. We still found the SMM ^{Low} group was still significantly associated with moderate-to-severe AEx. Accordingly, medication use had no effect on the results. This study has several limitations that need to be addressed. Firstly, BC was measured using

BIA only. Dual-energy X-ray absorptiometry is considered a more reliable method for BC assessment. Nevertheless, previous reports have confirmed that multifrequency BIA systems can provide accurate muscle mass and fat mass values that are comparable to those measured using dual-energy X-ray absorptiometry in various populations [57,58]. Secondly, this was a population-based cohort study in China that was specific to the Chinese population. Therefore, the clinical prediction model requires further external validation in multiple centers and different races. Thirdly, although we did not deny that low SMM also could be a consequence of incompletely controlled asthma leading to less physical activity, which formed a vicious circle [2], our prospective cohort study design enabled us to determine the causation that SMM was an exposure factor and AEx were taken as outcomes. Finally, the imbalance of the sample size of a statistical test among the three groups leads to influence the power of a statistical test [59]. Therefore, we calculated the power of the multiple logistic regression for the risk of AEx between the SMM^{Low} and SMM^{Normal} groups. However, the power of the multiple logistic regression was 0.8992. Commonly, the value of power is required to be greater than 0.8 [60]. Thus, the imbalance of sample size was not found to have an influence on the power of the risk of AEx between the SMM^{Low} and SMM^{Normal} groups in our study.

5. Conclusions

We demonstrated that low SMM, as a potential extra-pulmonary treatable trait, is an independent risk factor for asthma control and exacerbation. Furthermore, our model involving SMM for predicting the risk of exacerbation in patients with asthma suggests that SMM may be a suitable therapeutic target for clinical asthma management.

Supplementary Materials: The following supporting information can be downloaded at: https://www.mdpi.com/article/10.3390/jcm11237241/s1, Table S1: Inflammatory characteristics of the included participants in the training cohort grouped by SMM; Table S2: Body composition of the included participants with asthma grouped by SMM; Table S3: Association between SMM and moderate-to-severe asthma exacerbation within the 12-month follow-up period after adjusting for confounders; Table S4: Association between SMM and moderate-to-severe asthma exacerbation within the 12-month follow-up period in sensitive analyses # (n = 252); Table S5: The missing rates of the data set of the variables in our study; Table S6: Correlation between traits, with positive correlations denoted in red and negative correlations in blue (darker = stronger correlation). The symbol (*) placed next to the numbers indicate that the correlation was statistically significant ($p < 0.05$); Table S7: Demographic and clinical characteristics of the included participants in the training and validation cohorts; Table S8: Body composition of the included participants in the training and validation cohorts; Table S9: Assessing improvement of model performance after adding SMM; Figure S1: Predictor selection using the least absolute shrinkage and selection operator (LASSO) binary logistic regression model; Figure S2: The relative importance of variables included in the large model for the prediction of future moderate-to-severe exacerbation of asthma in the following year; Figure S3: Calibration curves for the training (A) and validation (B) cohorts and Figure S4: (A) Decision curves analysis for two risk models for AEx produced with Decision Curve software (B) Clinical impact curve for the SMM-based risk model. Of 1000 patients.

Author Contributions: G.W., W.L., S.Z. and X.Z., conceived the study, performed the data interpretation and manuscript revision, and took accountability for all aspects of the work. S.Z. and X.Z. planned the work, carried out the data analysis and interpretation. S.Z. and X.Z. drafted the manuscript. K.D., C.W., L.L., J.W., L.Z. and Y.L. offered the help of statistical analysis. H.W. performed the laboratory work. G.C. performed BCA. L.G.W., P.G.G., B.G.O., F.L., V.M.M., W.L. and G.W. interpreted the results and contributed to the manuscript revision. All authors have read and agreed to the published version of the manuscript.

Funding: This study was supported by the National Natural Science Foundation of China (81900026, 81920108002, and 81870027), Science and Technology Foundation of Sichuan Province (2022NSFSC1278), Post-Doctor Research Project, West China Hospital, Sichuan University (2019HXBH066), the National Key Development Plan for Precision Medicine Research (2017YFC091004), 1.3.5 project for disciplines of excellence-Clinical Research Incubation Project, West China Hospital, Sichuan

University (2018HXFH016), Science and Technology Bureau of Chengdu City, China (2021-GH03-00007-HZ), Science and Technology Agency of Sichuan Province, China (2022YFS0263).

Institutional Review Board Statement: This study was approved by the Institutional Review Board (IRB) at West China Hospital, Sichuan University (Chengdu, China) (No. 2014–30) and registered at Chinese Clinical Trial Registry (ChiCTR-OOC-16009529; https://www.chictr.org.cn; accessed on 14 June 2022). All participants provided written informed consent.

Informed Consent Statement: Informed consent was obtained from all patients involved in the study.

Data Availability Statement: The data used and analyzed during this research are available from the corresponding author upon reasonable request.

Acknowledgments: The authors are grateful to Michelle Gleeson (Hunter Medical Research Institute, University of Newcastle, Australia), Zhi Lin (West China Hospital, Sichuan University, China) for their blood and sputum processing, and to all patients who volunteered for this study. They also appreciate the advice regarding statistical analysis from Deying Kang (West China Hospital, Sichuan University, China).

Conflicts of Interest: The authors declare no conflict of interest.

Abbreviations

AEx	Asthma exacerbation
ACQ	Asthma Control Questionnaire
ACT	Asthma Control Test
ATS	American Thoracic Society
AUC	Receiver operator characteristic (ROC) curve
BC	Body composition
BMI	Body mass index
BIA	Multifrequency bioimpedance analysis
BDP	Beclomethasone dipropionate
COPD	Chronic obstructive pulmonary disease
CIC	Clinical impact curve
C-index	Concordance index
DCA	Decision curve analysis
ER	Emergency room
ERS	European Respiratory Society
FM	Fat mass
FeNO	Fractional exhaled nitric oxide
FEV_1	Forced expiratory volume in 1 s
FVC	Forced vital capacity
GERD	Gastroesophageal reflux disease
HADS	Hospital Anxiety and Depression Scale
HL	Hosmer–Lemeshow
IgE	Immunoglobulin E
ICS	Inhaled corticosteroid
IDI	Integrated discrimination improvement
LABA	Long-acting β2-agonist
LASSO	Least absolute shrinkage and selection operator
NRI	Net reclassification improvement
OCS	Oral corticosteroid
PBF	Percentage body fat
ROC	Receiver operator characteristic
SMM	Skeletal muscle mass
SPT	Skin prick test
SCS	Systemic corticosteroids
VFA	Visceral fat area

References

1. Global Initiative for Asthma. Global Strategy for Asthma Management and Prevention. 2014. Available online: https://www.ginasthma.org (accessed on 20 August 2020).
2. Abdo, M.; Waschki, B.; Kirsten, A.M.; Trinkmann, F.; Biller, H.; Herzmann, C.; von Mutius, E.; Kopp, M.; Hansen, G.; Rabe, K.F.; et al. Persistent Uncontrolled Asthma: Long-Term Impact on Physical Activity and Body Composition. *J. Asthma Allergy* **2021**, *14*, 229–240. [CrossRef] [PubMed]
3. Tieland, M.; Trouwborst, I.; Clark, B.C. Skeletal muscle performance and ageing. *J. Cachexia Sarcopenia Muscle* **2018**, *9*, 3–19. [CrossRef] [PubMed]
4. Thibault, R.; Pichard, C. The evaluation of body composition: A useful tool for clinical practice. *Ann. Nutr. Metab.* **2012**, *60*, 6–16. [CrossRef] [PubMed]
5. Son, J.W.; Lee, S.S.; Kim, S.R.; Yoo, S.J.; Cha, B.Y.; Son, H.Y.; Cho, N.H. Low muscle mass and risk of type 2 diabetes in middle-aged and older adults: Findings from the KoGES. *Diabetologia* **2017**, *60*, 865–872. [CrossRef] [PubMed]
6. Fiuza-Luces, C.; Santos-Lozano, A.; Joyner, M.; Carrera-Bastos, P.; Picazo, O.; Zugaza, J.L.; Izquierdo, M.; Ruilope, L.M.; Lucia, A. Exercise benefits in cardiovascular disease: Beyond attenuation of traditional risk factors. *Nat. Rev. Cardiol.* **2018**, *15*, 731–743. [CrossRef]
7. Lin, T.Y.; Peng, C.H.; Hung, S.C.; Tarng, D.C. Body composition is associated with clinical outcomes in patients with non-dialysis-dependent chronic kidney disease. *Kidney Int.* **2018**, *93*, 733–740. [CrossRef]
8. Chandra, A.; Neeland, I.J.; Berry, J.D.; Ayers, C.R.; Rohatgi, A.; Das, S.R.; Khera, A.; McGuire, D.K.; de Lemos, J.A.; Turer, A.T. The relationship of body mass and fat distribution with incident hypertension: Observations from the Dallas Heart Study. *J. Am. Coll. Cardiol.* **2014**, *64*, 997–1002. [CrossRef]
9. Ziolkowski, S.L.; Long, J.; Baker, J.F.; Chertow, G.M.; Leonard, M.B. Relative sarcopenia and mortality and the modifying effects of chronic kidney disease and adiposity. *J. Cachexia Sarcopenia Muscle* **2019**, *10*, 338–346. [CrossRef]
10. Gallagher, D.; Ruts, E.; Visser, M.; Heshka, S.; Baumgartner, R.N.; Wang, J.; Pierson, R.N.; Pi-Sunyer, F.X.; Heymsfield, S.B. Weight stability masks sarcopenia in elderly men and women. *Am. J. Physiol. Endocrinol. Metab.* **2000**, *279*, E366–E375. [CrossRef]
11. Bye, A.; Sjøblom, B.; Wentzel-Larsen, T.; Grønberg, B.H.; Baracos, V.E.; Hjermstad, M.J.; Aass, N.; Bremnes, R.M.; Fløtten, Ø.; Jordhøy, M. Muscle mass and association to quality of life in non-small cell lung cancer patients. *J. Cachexia Sarcopenia Muscle* **2017**, *8*, 759–767. [CrossRef]
12. Moon, S.W.; Choi, J.S.; Lee, S.H.; Jung, K.S.; Jung, J.Y.; Kang, Y.A.; Park, M.S.; Kim, Y.S.; Chang, J.; Kim, S.Y. Thoracic skeletal muscle quantification: Low muscle mass is related with worse prognosis in idiopathic pulmonary fibrosis patients. *Respir. Res.* **2019**, *20*, 35. [CrossRef] [PubMed]
13. GBD 2015 Chronic Respiratory Disease Collaborators. Global, regional, and national deaths, prevalence, disability-adjusted life years, and years lived with disability for chronic obstructive pulmonary disease and asthma, 1990-2015: A systematic analysis for the Global Burden of Disease Study 2015. *Lancet Respir. Med.* **2017**, *5*, 691–706. [CrossRef] [PubMed]
14. Jones, S.E.; Maddocks, M.; Kon, S.S.; Canavan, J.L.; Nolan, C.M.; Clark, A.L.; Polkey, M.I.; Man, W.D. Sarcopenia in COPD: Prevalence, clinical correlates and response to pulmonary rehabilitation. *Thorax* **2015**, *70*, 213–218. [CrossRef] [PubMed]
15. Costa, T.M.; Costa, F.M.; Moreira, C.A.; Rabelo, L.M.; Boguszewski, C.L.; Borba, V.Z. Sarcopenia in COPD: Relationship with COPD severity and prognosis. *J. Bras. De Pneumol.* **2015**, *41*, 415–421. [CrossRef]
16. Vestbo, J.; Prescott, E.; Almdal, T.; Dahl, M.; Nordestgaard, B.G.; Andersen, T.; Sørensen, T.I.; Lange, P. Body mass, fat-free body mass, and prognosis in patients with chronic obstructive pulmonary disease from a random population sample: Findings from the Copenhagen City Heart Study. *Am. J. Respir. Crit. Care Med.* **2006**, *173*, 79–83. [CrossRef]
17. Deng, K.; Zhang, X.; Liu, Y.; Cheng, G.P.; Zhang, H.P.; Wang, L.; Wang, L.; Li, W.M.; Wang, G.; Wood, L. Visceral obesity is associated with clinical and inflammatory features of asthma: A prospective cohort study. *Allergy Asthma Proc.* **2020**, *41*, 348–356. [CrossRef]
18. McDonald, V.M.; Clark, V.L.; Cordova-Rivera, L.; Wark, P.A.B.; Baines, K.J.; Gibson, P.G. Targeting treatable traits in severe asthma: A randomised controlled trial. *Eur. Respir. J.* **2019**, *55*, 1901509. [CrossRef]
19. Peters, U.; Dixon, A.E.; Forno, E. Obesity and asthma. *J. Allergy Clin. Immunol.* **2018**, *141*, 1169–1179. [CrossRef]
20. InBody770. Premium Solution for Your Health. Available online: https://www.inbodyusa.com/pages/inbodys10 (accessed on 1 March 2020).
21. Janssen, I.; Heymsfield, S.B.; Baumgartner, R.N.; Ross, R. Estimation of skeletal muscle mass by bioelectrical impedance analysis. *J. Appl. Physiol.* **2000**, *89*, 465–471. [CrossRef]
22. Bjelland, I.; Dahl, A.A.; Haug, T.T.; Neckelmann, D. The validity of the Hospital Anxiety and Depression Scale. An updated literature review. *J. Psychosom. Res.* **2002**, *52*, 69–77. [CrossRef]
23. Harris, T.B. Invited commentary: Body composition in studies of aging: New opportunities to better understand health risks associated with weight. *Am. J. Epidemiol.* **2002**, *156*, 122–124. [CrossRef]
24. Miller, M.R.; Hankinson, J.; Brusasco, V.; Burgos, F.; Casaburi, R.; Coates, A.; Crapo, R.; Enright, P.; van der Grinten, C.P.; Gustafsson, P.; et al. Standardisation of spirometry. *Eur. Respir. J.* **2005**, *26*, 319–338. [CrossRef] [PubMed]
25. Dweik, R.A.; Boggs, P.B.; Erzurum, S.C.; Irvin, C.G.; Leigh, M.W.; Lundberg, J.O.; Olin, A.C.; Plummer, A.L.; Taylor, D.R. An official ATS clinical practice guideline: Interpretation of exhaled nitric oxide levels (FENO) for clinical applications. *Am. J. Respir. Crit. Care Med.* **2011**, *184*, 602–615. [CrossRef] [PubMed]

26. Liu, L.; Zhang, X.; Liu, Y.; Zhang, L.; Zheng, J.; Wang, J.; Hansbro, P.M.; Wang, L.; Wang, G.; Hsu, A.C. Chitinase-like protein YKL-40 correlates with inflammatory phenotypes, anti-asthma responsiveness and future exacerbations. *Respir. Res.* **2019**, *20*, 95. [CrossRef] [PubMed]
27. Wang, G.; Baines, K.J.; Fu, J.J.; Wood, L.G.; Simpson, J.L.; McDonald, V.M.; Cowan, D.C.; Taylor, D.R.; Cowan, J.O.; Gibson, P.G. Sputum mast cell subtypes relate to eosinophilia and corticosteroid response in asthma. *Eur. Respir. J.* **2016**, *47*, 1123–1133. [CrossRef] [PubMed]
28. Zheng, J.; Zhang, X.; Zhang, L.; Zhang, H.P.; Wang, L.; Wang, G. Interactive effects between obesity and atopy on inflammation: A pilot study for asthma phenotypic overlap. *Ann. Allergy Asthma Immunol.* **2016**, *117*, 716–717. [CrossRef]
29. Juniper, E.F.; O'Byrne, P.M.; Guyatt, G.H.; Ferrie, P.J.; King, D.R. Development and validation of a questionnaire to measure asthma control. *Eur. Respir. J.* **1999**, *14*, 902–907. [CrossRef]
30. Reddel, H.K.; Taylor, D.R.; Bateman, E.D.; Boulet, L.P.; Boushey, H.A.; Busse, W.W.; Casale, T.B.; Chanez, P.; Enright, P.L.; Gibson, P.G.; et al. An official American Thoracic Society/European Respiratory Society statement: Asthma control and exacerbations: Standardizing endpoints for clinical asthma trials and clinical practice. *Am. J. Respir. Crit. Care Med.* **2009**, *180*, 59–99. [CrossRef]
31. Gea, J.; Sancho-Muñoz, A.; Chalela, R. Nutritional status and muscle dysfunction in chronic respiratory diseases: Stable phase versus acute exacerbations. *J. Thorac. Dis.* **2018**, *10*, S1332–S1354. [CrossRef]
32. Kim, Y.M.; Kim, J.H.; Baik, S.J.; Jung, D.H.; Park, J.J.; Youn, Y.H.; Park, H. Association between skeletal muscle attenuation and gastroesophageal reflux disease: A health check-up cohort study. *Sci. Rep.* **2019**, *9*, 20102. [CrossRef]
33. Volpato, S.; Bianchi, L.; Lauretani, F.; Lauretani, F.; Bandinelli, S.; Guralnik, J.M.; Zuliani, G.; Ferrucci, L. Role of muscle mass and muscle quality in the association between diabetes and gait speed. *Diabetes Care* **2012**, *35*, 1672–1679. [CrossRef]
34. Iasonos, A.; Schrag, D.; Raj, G.V.; Panageas, K.S. How to build and interpret a nomogram for cancer prognosis. *J. Clin. Oncol. Off. J. Am. Soc. Clin. Oncol.* **2008**, *26*, 1364–1370. [CrossRef] [PubMed]
35. Tang, X.R.; Li, Y.Q.; Liang, S.B.; Jiang, W.; Liu, F.; Ge, W.X.; Tang, L.L.; Mao, Y.P.; He, Q.M.; Yang, X.J.; et al. Development and validation of a gene expression-based signature to predict distant metastasis in locoregionally advanced nasopharyngeal carcinoma: A retrospective, multicentre, cohort study. *Lancet Oncol.* **2018**, *19*, 382–393. [CrossRef] [PubMed]
36. Jakobsen, J.C.; Gluud, C.; Wetterslev, J.; Winkel, P. When and how should multiple imputation be used for handling missing data in randomised clinical trials—A practical guide with flowcharts. *BMC Med. Res. Methodol.* **2017**, *17*, 162. [CrossRef]
37. Gong, J.; Ou, J.; Qiu, X.; Jie, Y.; Chen, Y.; Yuan, L.; Cao, J.; Tan, M.; Xu, W.; Zheng, F.; et al. A Tool for Early Prediction of Severe Coronavirus Disease 2019 (COVID-19): A Multicenter Study Using the Risk Nomogram in Wuhan and Guangdong, China. *Clin. Infect. Dis.* **2020**, *71*, 833–840. [CrossRef] [PubMed]
38. Lindholm, D.; Lindbäck, J.; Armstrong, P.W.; Budaj, A.; Cannon, C.P.; Granger, C.B.; Hagström, E.; Held, C.; Koenig, W.; Östlund, O.; et al. Biomarker-Based Risk Model to Predict Cardiovascular Mortality in Patients With Stable Coronary Disease. *J. Am. Coll. Cardiol.* **2017**, *70*, 813–826. [CrossRef]
39. Pencina, M.J.; D'Agostino, R.B., Sr.; D'Agostino, R.B., Jr.; Vasan, R.S. Evaluating the added predictive ability of a new marker: From area under the ROC curve to reclassification and beyond. *Stat. Med.* **2008**, *27*, 157–172; discussion 207–112. [CrossRef]
40. Diblasio, C.J.; Kattan, M.W. Use of nomograms to predict the risk of disease recurrence after definitive local therapy for prostate cancer. *Urology* **2003**, *62* (Suppl. 1), 9–18. [CrossRef]
41. Akobeng, A.K. Understanding diagnostic tests 3: Receiver operating characteristic curves. *Acta Paediatr.* **2007**, *96*, 644–647. [CrossRef]
42. Steyerberg, E.W.; Vergouwe, Y. Towards better clinical prediction models: seven steps for development and an ABCD for validation. *Eur. Heart J.* **2014**, *35*, 1925–1931. [CrossRef]
43. Steyerberg, E.W.; Harrell, F.E., Jr.; Borsboom, G.J.; Eijkemans, M.J.; Vergouwe, Y.; Habbema, J.D. Internal validation of predictive models: Efficiency of some procedures for logistic regression analysis. *J. Clin. Epidemiol.* **2001**, *54*, 774–781. [CrossRef]
44. Vickers, A.J.; Elkin, E.B. Decision curve analysis: A novel method for evaluating prediction models. *Med. Decis. Mak. Int. J. Soc. Med. Decis. Mak.* **2006**, *26*, 565–574. [CrossRef]
45. Huang, Y.Q.; Liang, C.H.; He, L.; Tian, J.; Liang, C.S.; Chen, X.; Ma, Z.L.; Liu, Z.Y. Development and Validation of a Radiomics Nomogram for Preoperative Prediction of Lymph Node Metastasis in Colorectal Cancer. *J. Clin. Oncol. Off. J. Am. Soc. Clin. Oncol.* **2016**, *34*, 2157–2164. [CrossRef]
46. Kerr, K.F.; Brown, M.D.; Zhu, K.; Janes, H. Assessing the Clinical Impact of Risk Prediction Models with Decision Curves: Guidance for Correct Interpretation and Appropriate Use. *J. Clin. Oncol. Off. J. Am. Soc. Clin. Oncol.* **2016**, *34*, 2534–2540. [CrossRef]
47. Qaisar, R.; Qayum, M.; Muhammad, T. Reduced sarcoplasmic reticulum Ca(2+) ATPase activity underlies skeletal muscle wasting in asthma. *Life Sci.* **2021**, *273*, 119296. [CrossRef] [PubMed]
48. Ramos, E.; de Oliveira, L.V.; Silva, A.B.; Costa, I.P.; Corrêa, J.C.; Costa, D.; Alves, V.L.; Donner, C.F.; Stirbulov, R.; Arena, R.; et al. Peripheral muscle strength and functional capacity in patients with moderate to severe asthma. *Multidiscip. Respir. Med.* **2015**, *10*, 3. [CrossRef] [PubMed]
49. Moon, J.H.; Kong, M.H.; Kim, H.J. Implication of Sarcopenia and Sarcopenic Obesity on Lung Function in Healthy Elderly: Using Korean National Health and Nutrition Examination Survey. *J. Korean Med. Sci.* **2015**, *30*, 1682–1688. [CrossRef]

50. Kelly, M.M.; Leigh, R.; Jayaram, L.; Goldsmith, C.H.; Parameswaran, K.; Hargreave, F.E. Eosinophilic bronchitis in asthma: A model for establishing dose-response and relative potency of inhaled corticosteroids. *J. Allergy Clin. Immunol.* **2006**, *117*, 989–994. [CrossRef] [PubMed]
51. Steensberg, A.; Fischer, C.P.; Keller, C.; Møller, K.; Pedersen, B.K. IL-6 enhances plasma IL-1ra, IL-10, and cortisol in humans. *Am. J. Physiol. Endocrinol. Metab.* **2003**, *285*, E433–E437. [CrossRef]
52. Nielsen, A.R.; Hojman, P.; Erikstrup, C.; Fischer, C.P.; Plomgaard, P.; Mounier, R.; Mortensen, O.H.; Broholm, C.; Taudorf, S.; Krogh-Madsen, R.; et al. Association between interleukin-15 and obesity: Interleukin-15 as a potential regulator of fat mass. *J. Clin. Endocrinol. Metab.* **2008**, *93*, 4486–4493. [CrossRef] [PubMed]
53. Wang, G.; McDonald, V.M.; Gibson, P.G. Management of severe asthma: From stepwise approach to therapy to treatable traits? *Precis. Clin. Med.* **2021**, *4*, 293–296. [CrossRef]
54. Eckardt, K.; Görgens, S.W.; Raschke, S.; Eckel, J. Myokines in insulin resistance and type 2 diabetes. *Diabetologia* **2014**, *57*, 1087–1099. [CrossRef]
55. Levin, O.S.; Polunina, A.G.; Demyanova, M.A.; Isaev, F.V. Steroid myopathy in patients with chronic respiratory diseases. *J. Neurol. Sci.* **2014**, *338*, 96–101. [CrossRef]
56. Joassard, O.R.; Durieux, A.C.; Freyssenet, D.G. β2-Adrenergic agonists and the treatment of skeletal muscle wasting disorders. *Int. J. Biochem. Cell Biol.* **2013**, *45*, 2309–2321. [CrossRef]
57. Boneva-Asiova, Z.; Boyanov, M.A. Body composition analysis by leg-to-leg bioelectrical impedance and dual-energy X-ray absorptiometry in non-obese and obese individuals. *Diabetes Obes. Metab.* **2008**, *10*, 1012–1018. [CrossRef] [PubMed]
58. Stewart, S.P.; Bramley, P.N.; Heighton, R.; Green, J.H.; Horsman, A.; Losowsky, M.S.; Smith, M.A. Estimation of body composition from bioelectrical impedance of body segments: Comparison with dual-energy X-ray absorptiometry. *Br. J. Nutr.* **1993**, *69*, 645–655. [CrossRef] [PubMed]
59. Rusticus, S.A.; Lovato, C.Y. Impact of Sample Size and Variability on the Power and Type I Error Rates of Equivalence Tests: A Simulation Study. 2014. Available online: https://scholarworks.umass.edu/cgi/viewcontent.cgi?article=1323&context=pare (accessed on 2 December 2022).
60. Cohen, J. A power primer. *Psychol. Bull.* **1992**, *112*, 155–159. [CrossRef] [PubMed]

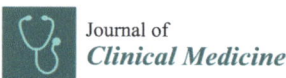
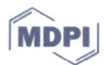

Article

Exhaled Breath Analysis for Investigating the Use of Inhaled Corticosteroids and Corticosteroid Responsiveness in Wheezing Preschool Children

Michiel A. G. E. Bannier [1,*], Sophie Kienhorst [1], Quirijn Jöbsis [1], Kim D. G. van de Kant [1], Frederik-Jan van Schooten [2], Agnieszka Smolinska [2,†] and Edward Dompeling [1,†]

[1] Department of Paediatrics, Division of Paediatric Respiratory Medicine, School for Public Health and Primary Care (CAPHRI), Maastricht University Medical Centre+, 6229 HX Maastricht, The Netherlands

[2] Department of Pharmacology and Toxicology, School of Nutrition and Translational Research in Metabolism (NUTRIM), Maastricht University, 6229 ER Maastricht, The Netherlands

* Correspondence: michiel.bannier@mumc.nl

† These senior authors contributed equally to this work.

Abstract: Exhaled breath analysis has great potential in diagnosing various respiratory and non-respiratory diseases. In this study, we investigated the influence of inhaled corticosteroids (ICS) on exhaled volatile organic compounds (VOCs) of wheezing preschool children. Furthermore, we assessed whether exhaled VOCs could predict a clinical steroid response in wheezing preschool children. We performed a crossover 8-week ICS trial, in which 147 children were included. Complete data were available for 89 children, of which 46 children were defined as steroid-responsive. Exhaled VOCs were measured by GC-*tof*-MS. Statistical analysis by means of Random Forest was used to investigate the effect of ICS on exhaled VOCs. A set of 20 VOCs could best discriminate between measurements before and after ICS treatment, with a sensitivity of 73% and specificity of 67% (area under ROC curve = 0.72). Most discriminative VOCs were branched $C_{11}H_{24}$, butanal, octanal, acetic acid and methylated pentane. Other VOCs predominantly included alkanes. Regularised multivariate analysis of variance (rMANOVA) was used to determine treatment response, which showed a significant effect between responders and non-responders ($p < 0.01$). These results show that ICS significantly altered the exhaled breath profiles of wheezing preschool children, irrespective of clinical treatment response. Furthermore, exhaled VOCs were capable of determining corticosteroid responsiveness in wheezing preschool children.

Keywords: preschool wheezing; asthma; exhaled breath; volatile organic compounds; inhaled corticosteroids; treatment response; children

1. Introduction

Exhaled breath analysis has shown great potential in diagnosing various respiratory and non-respiratory diseases [1]. In children, volatile organic compounds (VOCs) in exhaled breath were able to differentiate wheezing preschool children and children with asthma from healthy controls [2,3]. Exhaled VOCs could also indicate asthma exacerbations at an early stage [4,5] and predict future asthma in wheezing preschool children [6].

Currently, two methods are being used for exhaled breath analysis: an "offline" method using gas chromatography mass spectrometry (GC-MS) to identify VOCs and an "online" method, which mainly comprises electronic nose (eNose) technology. Although both techniques have their own methodological and analytical strengths and limitations [1], an exhaled breath analysis by means of GC-MS is considered the golden standard technique. In addition to the different methods, many potential confounding factors exist, including diet, exercise and pharmacological treatment [7]. To date, the latter has been insufficiently investigated, and it is yet unclear to what extent medication influences exhaled VOCs' patterns.

Moreover, exhaled VOCs might have the potential to predict a clinical corticosteroid response in wheezing preschool children. In adults with asthma, previous studies have shown the ability to predict oral steroid responsiveness [8] and loss-of-control after inhaled corticosteroid (ICS) withdrawal [9]. However, these studies have been performed in adults with confirmed asthma. The treatment of preschool wheezing has been debated for years, and it is yet unclear which wheezing preschool children might benefit from inhaled corticosteroids. Aeroallergen sensitisation and blood eosinophilia have been suggested as potential biomarkers to justify ICS prescription in wheezing preschool children [10]. However, in a recent randomised trial, blood eosinophilia-guided ICS prescription did not improve preschool wheezing management compared to standard care [11]. Hence, there is an urgent need for reliable biomarkers to predict steroid responsiveness in wheezing preschool children.

In the present study, we investigated the influence of ICS on the exhaled breath profiles of wheezing preschool children. We hypothesised that ICS significantly alter exhaled VOCs. Furthermore, we investigated whether exhaled VOCs could predict a clinical steroid response in wheezing preschool children.

2. Materials and Methods

2.1. Study Design

This study was part of the Asthma Detection and Monitoring (ADEM) study (clinicaltrial.gov: NCT 00422747), in which 202 wheezing children aged 2 to 4 years were prospectively followed until 6 years of age [12]. The primary goal of the ADEM study was to develop a non-invasive test for an early asthma diagnosis, including exhaled breath analysis and early lung function measurements. A detailed study protocol with in- and exclusion criteria was previously published [12,13].

Figure 1 shows the study flowchart of the current study. Children who experienced respiratory symptoms in the preceding month were included for a crossover ICS trial. If applicable, earlier prescribed ICS were stopped 4 weeks before the first study visit. During the initial visit, exhaled breath was collected, symptoms were assessed and lung function was measured (see details below). Children were instructed to refrain from solid foods and physical exercise 1 h before the measurement. Study visits were postponed in case of an airway infection. Atopy was determined by using the Phadiatop Infant test® (Phadia, Uppsala, Sweden). Subsequently, children were randomly allocated to 8 weeks of ICS (Beclomethasone extrafine 100 µg twice daily, via the Aerochamber®, Teva Pharma NL, Haarlem, The Netherlands) followed by 8 weeks without ICS, or vice versa. No asthma medication other than salbutamol (Airomir®, Teva Pharma, Haarlem, The Netherlands, for symptom relief) was allowed during the study period. Compliance with the study medication was measured by weighing the ICS canisters before and after therapy. Children were excluded if less than 80% of the prescribed study medication was used. After 8 and 16 weeks, all measurements were repeated. Children were followed until the age of 6 years, when a clinical diagnosis (healthy, transient wheeze or true asthma) was made by two experienced paediatric pulmonologists and a computer-based algorithm [6].

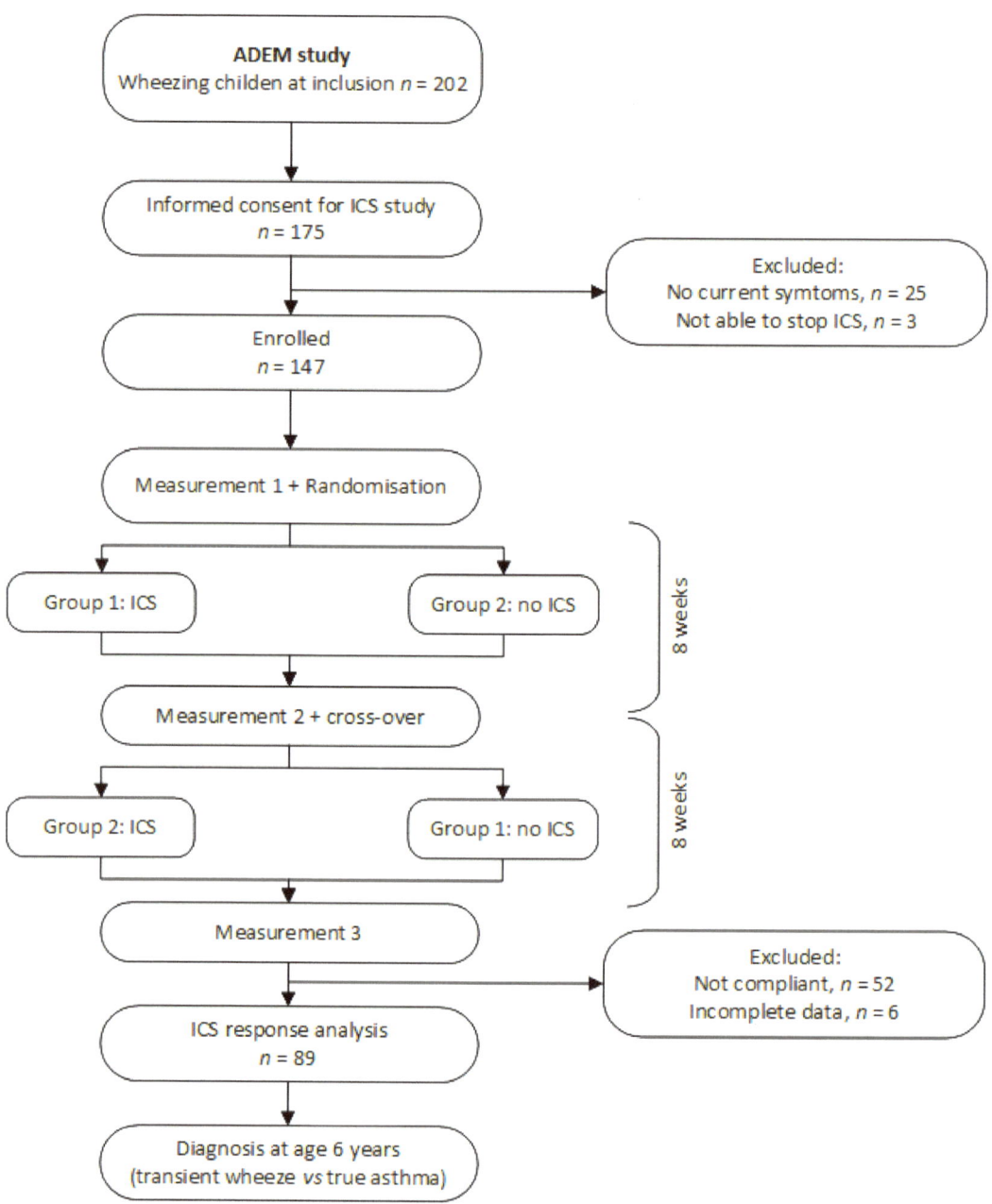

Figure 1. Study flowchart.

2.2. Response to ICS

Children were considered responsive to ICS when there was a decrease in respiratory symptoms of ≥30% and/or an improvement in airway resistance of ≥10% [13].

Airway resistance was determined by using the interrupter technique (MicroRint®, Micro Medical Ltd., Rochester, UK). Respiratory symptoms were assessed by a short questionnaire evaluating symptoms of cough, wheezing and dyspnoea. A total symptom score before and after treatment was calculated, ranging from six points (most severe symptoms) to thirty points (no symptoms) [13].

2.3. Exhaled Breath Sampling and Measurements

Subjects were asked to breathe through a face mask connected to a valve of a resistance-free 1 L plastic bag (Tedlar bag, SKC Ltd., Dorset, UK). Within an hour of collection, the content of the sampling bag was transferred onto carbon-filled, stainless-steel desorption tubes (carbograph 1TD/Carbopack X, Markes International, Llantrisant, UK).

The exhaled breath samples were measured by means of GC-*tof*-MS, as described before [14]. The first steps consisted of releasing volatile compounds from the sorption tubes by thermal desorption using the Markes International Ultra-Unity automated thermal desorption equipment (Markes International). In the next step, 10% of the mixture of vapour was loaded onto a cold (5 °C) sorption trap, while the remaining 90% of the mixture was recollected into an identical sample tube. The vapour mixture was then reloaded from trap into the GC-*tof*-MS analysis. The temperature of the GC was programmed as follows: first, 40 °C for 5 min; then, increased by 10 °C every minute until 270 °C was reached. This temperature was maintained for 5 min. Electron ionisation at 70 eV was used with a 5 Hz scanning rate over a range of m/z 35–350.

2.4. Data Pre-Processing

The raw, original GC-*tof*-MS spectra were pre-processed before an actual statistical analysis. This consisted of noise removal, baseline correction and alignment, as previously described [14]. Each step of data pre-processing was performed to increase the quality of the data and to allow multivariate statistical analysis to focus on information of interest. For each peak in the total ion current chromatogram, the peak picking was performed, which consisted of calculating the area under the peaks by taking into account the corresponding mass spectra at specific retention time. Note that these areas are proportional to relative amounts of measured compounds. The absolute concentrations of the compounds were not determined. Finally, the area under the peaks for each sample was merged by combining the corresponding compounds based on retention time and similarities in mass spectra. To make the spectra comparable, the final step of pre-processing involved normalisation by probabilistic quotient normalisation.

The data were analysed by means of Random Forest (RF) and regularised multivariate analysis of variance (rMANOVA) [15]. RF was used to determine the effect of ICS on volatile metabolites in exhaled breath.

RF is a machine learning algorithm that creates many uncorrelated decision trees that predict samples into the appropriate class (here, pre-ICS and post-ICS). RF combines these decision trees to produce a general classification model. The RF model was validated using an internal test set, which was selected using the Kennard and Stone algorithm (20% of samples per class) [16]. This algorithm is based on Euclidian distance and allows for selecting a representative training set. The training set was used for optimisation steps (i.e., variable selection and selecting model complexity) and for developing a classification RF model. The test set was subsequently used to validate the constructed model. In the case of the RF model, an extra validation was employed using the so-called out-of-bag (oob) error. For each RF tree, one-third of the training samples was left out and not used in the construction of the classification model. These left-out cases were next used to establish the prediction error. Compound selection was based on the variable importance as assessed by RF in combination with an internal validation procedure in which the training set was iteratively split up into a training and validation set. This process was run using 1000 trees and 1000 iterations. The RF model provides a measure of the importance of a compound that gives the most important compound the highest value. Based on this value, a set of compounds that can discriminate between pre-ICS and post-ICS was selected. It is important to state that the discriminatory RF model was first constructed and optimised on a training set, containing 80% of samples of each group, and the final, optimised model containing only discriminatory VOCs was validated using an internal independent test set. Note that RF looks for patterns, i.e., sets of compounds that allow for predicting the class of interest, i.e., pre-ICS or post-ICS.

To visualise the results, a Principal Coordinate Analysis (PCoA) was performed on the proximity matrix obtained from the RF model. The model performance was demonstrated using receiver operating characteristics (ROC) curve. The statistical significance of responsiveness to the therapy was investigated by means of rMANOVA.

Lastly, the set of discriminating VOCs was putatively identified using the National Institute of Standards and Technology (NIST) library in combination with expert interpretation.

3. Results

Of 150 eligible children, 147 (98%) were able to stop taking ICS and were included in the trial. Unfortunately, only 65% of children appeared to be adherent to ICS treatment. Complete data were available for 89 children (Figure 1), of which 46 children were defined as steroid-responsive (52%). Subject baseline characteristics are given in Table 1. Baseline characteristics showed a clinically not relevant but statistically significant difference in airway resistance between responders and non-responders. The other characteristics were not significantly different between groups.

Table 1. Baseline characteristics of responders and non-responders.

	Responders	Non-Responders
Study population (N)	46	43
Age (years), mean (SD)	3.2 (0.7)	3.4 (0.6)
Sex: male/female, n/n	20/26	25/18
Wheezing episodes, n (IQR)	8 (3–8)	8 (3–8)
Atopy, n/n (%)	12/45 (27)	9/41 (22)
Allergic rhinitis, n/n (%)	3/45 (7)	3/42 (7)
Eczema, n/n (%)	15/44 (34)	12/43 (28)
Positive API, n (%)	5/44 (11)	4/43 (9)
Inhaled corticosteroids, n/n (%)	12/45 (27)	9/42 (21)
Short acting β_2-agonists, n/n (%)	23/46 (50)	19/42 (45)
Long acting β_2-agonists, n/n (%)	1/46 (2)	0/42 (0)
Total symptom score, mean (SD)	24.7 (5.2)	26.4 (3.1)
Airway resistance (kPa s/L), mean (SD) *	1.6 (0.4)	1.4 (0.3)

Atopy is defined as a positive Phadiatop Infant test®. SD: standard deviation; IQR: interquartile range; API: stringent asthma predictive index. * $p = 0.005$ between responders and non-responders (Mann–Whitney U test). All other characteristics were statistically not significant ($p > 0.05$).

3.1. Influence of ICS on Exhaled VOCs

To identify the VOCs' pattern related to ICS, the RF model compared individuals before and after ICS treatment. The RF model was first optimised on the training set and consequently validated using the test set. A set of 20 VOCs was selected as being the most discriminative. The final RF model, built on the data containing individuals before and after ICS treatment, and the set of 20 discriminative VOCs yielded a sensitivity and specificity of 73% (95% confidence interval 64–82%) and 67% (95% confidence interval 57–77%) for internal test samples, respectively. The corresponding ROC curve is shown in Figure 2.

The groups' visualisation is shown in Figure 3A,B, where PCoA score plots are shown for training and projected test samples. The difference between pre- and post-ICS samples is observed between the first three principal coordinates (PCos), which explains 43.4% of the variance. The test samples are projected into the space of the corresponding training samples, which confirms the sensitivity and specificity of the RF model.

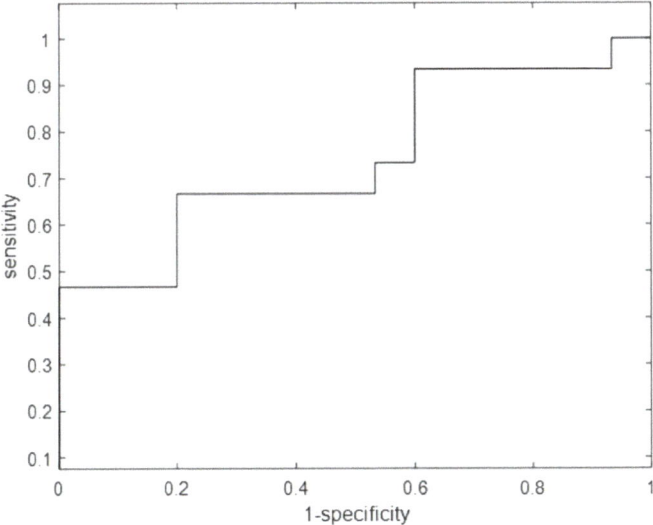

Figure 2. Receiver Operating Characteristics curve for the test set of the random forest model comparing individuals before and after ICS treatment using 20 discriminatory VOCs. The sensitivity and specificity were found to be 73% and 67%, respectively, with an area under the curve equal to 0.72. ICS: inhaled corticosteroids; VOCs: volatile organic compounds.

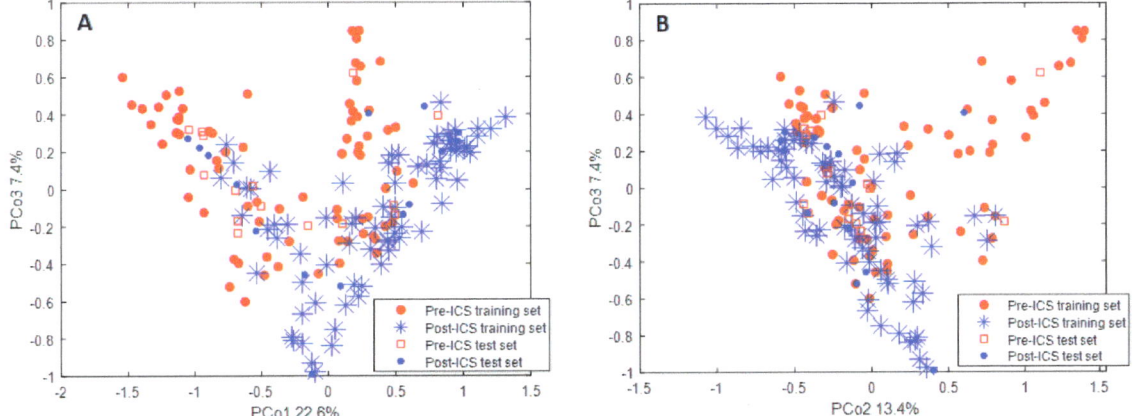

Figure 3. Principal Coordinate Analysis score plot for (**A**) PCo1 and PCo3, and (**B**) PCo2 and PCo3 on a proximity matrix obtained from the Random Forest model performed on the training set and 20 of the most discriminatory volatile organic compounds. The test set was projected into the space defined by the training samples. Every point belongs to a single breath fingerprint (blue stars: post-ICS training set; red circles: pre-ICS training set; blue circles: post-ICS test set; red squares: pre-ICS test set). The separation is observed on Principle Component 1, explaining 22.6% of the variance. PCo: Principal Coordinate; ICS: inhaled corticosteroids.

In Appendix A Figure A1, responsiveness to ICS treatment is visualised in the PCoA score plots. This figure demonstrates no natural clustering with respect to clinical treatment response.

The top five compounds contributing to the discrimination between the pre- and post-ICS treatments were putatively identified using the NIST library (Table 2). Interestingly, the levels of four compounds were reduced after ICS treatment and the level of only one compound was increased after ICS treatment. The remaining VOCs were identified only in a general way as the following family of compounds: two terpenes, seven alkanes and four branched alkanes. The remaining two compounds could not be identified due to insufficient mass spectrum, overlap in the retention time or absence of mass spectrum in the NIST library.

Table 2. Putative identification of the top 5 volatile organic compounds contributing to differentiation of individuals before and after treatment with ICS. ↓ indicates reduced level of a VOC in post-ICS individuals in reference to pre-ICS; ↑ indicates increased level of a VOC in post-ICS individuals in reference to pre-ICS.

Nr.	Compound Name	Concentration Changes in Post-ICS
1	Branched $C_{11}H_{24}$	↓
2	Butanal	↓
3	Octanal	↓
4	Acetic acid (ester)	↑
5	Methylated pentane	↓

ICS: inhaled corticosteroids; VOC: volatile organic compound.

3.2. Exhaled VOCs and Clinical Response to ICS

Due to the limited number of subjects, it was not feasible to create a reliable prediction model to discriminate between ICS responders and non-responders. Moreover, the study design included both children later diagnosed as transient wheezers and children later diagnosed as true asthmatics, for which treatment response might be different. As a result, discriminatory models for each group need to be built separately. Therefore, rMANOVA was used to demonstrate the usefulness of exhaled VOCs in determining steroid responsiveness. In this multivariate model, definitive diagnosis at an age of 6 years, i.e., true asthma or transient wheeze, as well as responsiveness to ICS were used as the main factors. Since airway resistance at baseline was statistically significantly different between responders and non-responders, it was included in the rMANOVA model as a potential confounder. The rMANOVA analysis yielded significant differences in VOCs' profiles for responders and non-responders and for later-diagnosed true asthma and transient wheeze as individual factors, as well as the interaction between them with a p-value < 0.01. This significant interaction effect indicates that the variation is dependent on both factors simultaneously, and thus, the commonly encountered One-Variable at a Time approach for investigating treatment responsiveness would not necessarily result in the best overall optimal outcomes.

4. Discussion

This study showed that exhaled VOCs in wheezing preschool children were significantly influenced by an 8-week trial of ICS, irrespective of a clinical treatment response. Our classification model showed that 20 VOCs were the most discriminative, with a sensitivity of 73% and specificity of 67%. The majority of these VOCs were alkanes, but the top five discriminative VOCs (Table 2) also included aldehydes. Furthermore, exhaled VOCs before the start of ICS treatment were significantly different between wheezing children who were later classified as ICS-responsive compared to those classified as non-responsive. To the best of our knowledge, this is the first study investigating ICS-induced changes in exhaled VOCs in children, as determined by GC-MS. Moreover, this is also the first study that used exhaled VOCs to assess a clinical ICS response in wheezing preschool children.

Our findings significantly contribute to the knowledge of clinically applying exhaled breath analysis. Despite the 2017 ERS Task Force statement on exhaled biomarkers in lung disease [7], exhaled breath sampling and analysis is still not standardised and large heterogeneity between studies exists. One important factor in standardising breath sampling is the potential confounding role of pharmacological treatment. Only a few studies have focused on this topic. The study by Gaugg et al. showed significantly altered breath prints in adults, as assessed by SESI-HRMS, 10 and 30 min after inhalation of salbutamol, which was not shown after inhalation of the placebo [17]. However, in most studies, subjects are instructed to not use their medication 2 to 4 h prior to breath sampling. Unfortunately, that time window was not used in the study by Gaugg et al.; however, Brinkman and colleagues investigated the association of exhaled VOCs, as measured by GC-*tof*-MS, with urinary levels of salbutamol and oral corticosteroids in adults with severe asthma [18]. Their study showed that exhaled breath profiles can be linked to recent medication use, with fairly good accuracies. However, an important limitation of this study was that the specific time and dose of medication intake were uncertain.

In children, no similar studies have been performed to date. In a previous study from our research group, performed in the same study population, markers in exhaled breath condensate (EBC) showed no differences before and after ICS treatment [13]. Two other studies from the same research group, performed a metabolomic analysis of EBC in children with asthma [19,20]. In non-severe asthma, this method was not able to detect differences between steroid-naïve children and children using regular ICS [19]. Furthermore, EBC profiles showed no differences after a 3-week course of ICS, despite significant clinical improvements [20]. Probably, as also suggested by the authors, their approach was not capable of detecting the subtle differences in exhaled breath profile potentially caused by ICS.

By using GC-*tof*-MS, we were able to detect 20 VOCs that were most discriminative for ICS use, of which the top 5 discriminative VOCs are shown in Table 2. The majority of these identified VOCs were alkanes. Exhaled alkanes and, to a lesser extent, exhaled aldehydes have been identified as significant markers for airway inflammation in various asthma studies [21]. Interestingly, four out of our top five most discriminative VOCs, of which two are alkanes and two are aldehydes, decreased after 8 weeks ICS. These findings might suggest that the changes found in breath profiles were caused by the down-regulation of airway inflammation. However, we cannot exclude that the differences in exhaled VOCs were solely and directly induced by ICS, as we did not investigate drug levels or metabolites in blood and urine to compare our findings. Moreover, the ICS-induced changes in breath profiles were irrespective of a clinical treatment response, as shown in Figure A1. Of interest, in the study by Brinkman et al., octanal in exhaled breath was associated with urinary levels of oral steroids [18]. In our study, octanal was identified at the baseline visit, when subjects were steroid-naïve for 4 weeks. Moreover, after the 8-week ICS trial, octanal levels reduced, which implies that octanal is not a biomarker for ICS use.

In summary, we cannot fully conclude whether the ICS-induced changes in exhaled VOCs were directly caused by the drugs or whether it truly reflected anti-inflammatory changes in wheezing children. Nevertheless, our findings indicate that pharmacological treatment should be taken into account when performing breath analysis. Most importantly, when breathomics is used for diagnostic purposes, timing and dose of medication could be important confounding factors as it is unclear how long the metabolic effects persist. The common prohibition to use drugs 2–4 h prior to exhaled breath sampling might not be sufficient to reduce the impact on exhaled VOCs. In our study, we were fairly sure about medication use as we only included children in the final analysis when they were both steroid-naïve at inclusion and considered treatment-adherent after the trial. As mentioned before, exact medication intake was uncertain in the study by Brinkman et al. [18], and the effects of salbutamol were only investigated until 30 min after inhalation in the study by Gaugg et al. [17]. An extension of the latter study, including a longer follow-up duration and the use of various drugs, is of pivotal importance to improving the standardisation and reliability of exhaled breath analysis.

Another research aim of this study was the prediction of a clinical response to ICS in wheezing preschool children. Unfortunately, due to the high number of insufficiently adherent children, the sample size was too small to create a prediction model that could be properly validated. Nonetheless, our results showed significant differences in exhaled

VOC profiles between ICS responsive and non-responsive wheezing preschool children. Moreover, this effect was dependent on the future diagnosis of these children at an age of 6 years: transient wheezing or true asthma. These results suggest that wheezing preschool children who eventually developed asthma had a higher chance of being steroid-responsive. Naturally, these results need validation and replication. However, the prediction of ICS responsiveness could be a unique and innovative potential application of exhaled breath analysis, as the treatment of wheezing preschool children has been debated for years [22]. Our findings are in line with a previous study in adults with asthma, in which an eNose was able to predict a clinical corticosteroid response with a good accuracy [8]. In children, most studies have focused on the use of fractional exhaled nitric oxide (FeNO) to predict a treatment response, with mixed findings [23]. In an earlier part of the ADEM study, we showed that FeNO and inflammatory markers in EBC could not predict a steroid response in wheezing preschool children [13]. Finally, in the study by Cavaleiro Rufo et al., an eNose analysis of EBC in children was able to identify children with asthma in need of ICS therapy [24]. Response to treatment was not investigated in this study. Our findings could implicate that exhaled breath analysis is able to better guide clinicians in identifying which wheezing children might benefit from ICS, potentially preventing both overtreatment and undertreatment with ICS and thereby reducing side effects as well as healthcare costs. The potential of exhaled VOCs as a diagnostic tool for 'personalised medicine' in this age group is highly interesting.

This study has several strengths. To the best of our knowledge, this is the first study to investigate the effect of ICS maintenance therapy on exhaled VOCs' profiles in children at preschool age. Furthermore, this is the first study using exhaled VOCs, as measured by GC-MS, in determining clinical steroid responsiveness in preschool children. Our study was performed in a real-life setting, which makes it highly suitable for clinical practice. Moreover, our subjects were clinically well characterised, including details on medication use and treatment response.

Our study also had some limitations. First, weighing inhaler canisters is considered a suboptimal strategy to identify treatment adherence [25]. However, in this real-life clinical setting, we considered it to be the most optimal strategy. Second, as we were very strict in identifying adherence, 35% of participating children were excluded from analysis. As a result, the sample size was too small to create a reliable prediction model of treatment response. Another limitation is that we did not assess blood eosinophils in this study. However, we did measure FeNO, which is related to airway eosinophilia. In a previous study, FeNO could not predict a steroid response in the same population [13]. Finally, we did not investigate drug levels or metabolites in blood or urine to compare our findings.

5. Conclusions

An 8-week trial of ICS significantly influenced the exhaled breath profiles of wheezing preschool children, irrespective of a clinical treatment response. Moreover, exhaled VOCs were capable of determining corticosteroid responsiveness in wheezing preschool children. These results highlight the urgent need for further standardisation of exhaled breath analysis and its potential to guide therapy in a 'personalised medicine' approach.

Author Contributions: Conceptualization, M.A.G.E.B., S.K., Q.J. and E.D.; methodology and analysis, M.A.G.E.B., A.S. and E.D.; investigation, K.D.G.v.d.K., Q.J. and E.D.; data curation, M.A.G.E.B. and A.S.; writing—original draft preparation, M.A.G.E.B.; writing—review and editing, S.K., Q.J., K.D.G.v.d.K., F.-J.v.S., A.S. and E.D.; visualization, M.A.G.E.B. and A.S.; supervision, A.S. and E.D. All authors have read and agreed to the published version of the manuscript.

Funding: This research received no external funding.

Institutional Review Board Statement: The study was conducted in accordance with the Declaration of Helsinki and approved by the Dutch National Medical Ethical Committee (Centrale Commissie Mensgebonden Onderzoek, CCMO): identifier number: NL17407.000.07/2007-001817-40, date of approval 12 June 2007.

Informed Consent Statement: Informed consent was obtained from all subjects involved in the study.

Data Availability Statement: The data presented in this study are available from the corresponding author upon request.

Conflicts of Interest: The authors declare no conflict of interest.

Appendix A

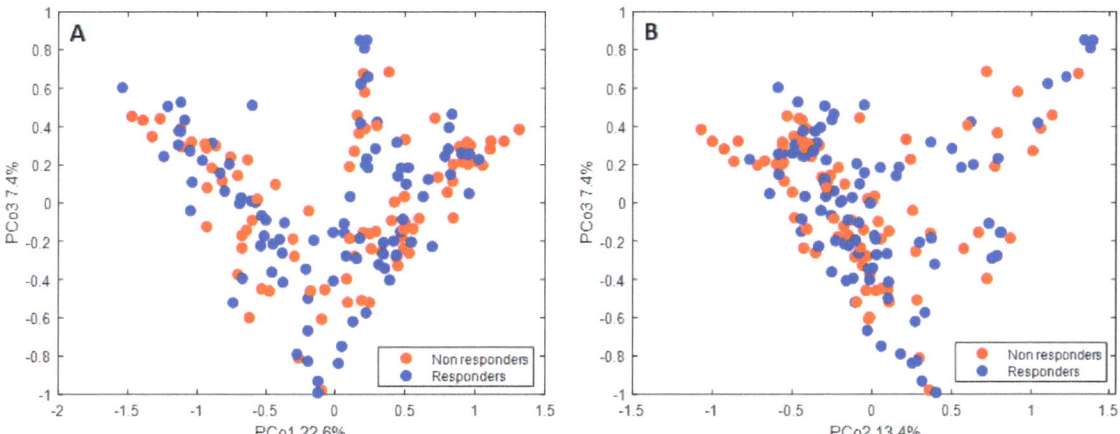

Figure A1. Principal Coordinate Analysis score plot for (**A**) PCo1 and PCo3, and (**B**) PCo2 and PCo3 on a proximity matrix obtained from the Random Forest model performed on training set and 20 most discriminatory volatile organic compounds. The samples are color-coded with respect to the responsiveness to ICS treatment, with blue dots being responders and red ones being non-responders. The figure demonstrates no natural clustering with respect to ICS responsiveness. PCo: Principal Coordinate; ICS: inhaled corticosteroids.

References

1. Ibrahim, W.; Carr, L.; Cordell, R.; Wilde, M.J.; Salman, D.; Monks, P.S.; Thomas, P.; Brightling, C.E.; Siddiqui, S.; Greening, N.J. Breathomics for the clinician: The use of volatile organic compounds in respiratory diseases. *Thorax* **2021**, *76*, 514–521. [CrossRef]
2. Van De Kant, K.D.G.; Van Berkel, J.J.B.N.; Jöbsis, Q.; Passos, V.L.; Klaassen, E.M.M.; Van Der Sande, L.; Van Schayck, O.C.P.; De Jongste, J.C.; Van Schooten, F.J.; Derks, E.; et al. Exhaled breath profiling in diagnosing wheezy preschool children. *Eur. Respir. J.* **2013**, *41*, 183–188. [CrossRef] [PubMed]
3. Dallinga, J.W.; Robroeks, C.M.H.H.T.; Van Berkel, J.J.B.N.; Moonen, E.J.C.; Godschalk, R.W.L.; Jöbsis, Q.; Dompeling, E.; Wouters, E.F.M.; Van Schooten, F.J. Volatile organic compounds in exhaled breath as a diagnostic tool for asthma in children. *Clin. Exp. Allergy* **2010**, *40*, 68–76. [CrossRef]
4. Robroeks, C.M.; van Berkel, J.J.; Jöbsis, Q.; van Schooten, F.-J.; Dallinga, J.W.; Wouters, E.F.; Dompeling, E. Exhaled volatile organic compounds predict exacerbations of childhood asthma in a 1-year prospective study. *Eur. Respir. J.* **2013**, *42*, 98–106. [CrossRef]
5. Van Vliet, D.; Smolinska, A.; Jöbsis, Q.; Rosias, P.; Muris, J.; Dallinga, J.; Dompeling, E.; Van Schooten, F.-J. Can exhaled volatile organic compounds predict asthma exacerbations in children? *J. Breath Res.* **2017**, *11*, 16016. [CrossRef]
6. Klaassen, E.M.M.; van de Kant, K.D.G.; Jöbsis, Q.; van Schayck, O.C.P.; Smolinska, A.; Dallinga, J.W.; van Schooten, F.J.; den Hartog, G.J.M.; de Jongste, J.C.; Rijkers, G.T.; et al. Exhaled Biomarkers and Gene Expression at Preschool Age Improve Asthma Prediction at 6 Years of Age. *Am. J. Respir. Crit. Care Med.* **2015**, *191*, 201–207. [CrossRef]
7. Horvath, I.; Barnes, P.J.; Loukides, S.; Sterk, P.J.; Hogman, M.; Olin, A.C.; Amann, A.; Antus, B.; Baraldi, E.; Bikov, A.; et al. A European Respiratory Society technical standard: Exhaled biomarkers in lung disease. *Eur. Respir. J.* **2017**, *49*, 1600965. [CrossRef]
8. van der Schee, M.P.; Palmay, R.; Cowan, J.O.; Taylor, D.R. Predicting steroid responsiveness in patients with asthma using exhaled breath profiling. *Clin. Exp. Allergy* **2013**, *43*, 1217–1225. [CrossRef] [PubMed]
9. Brinkman, P.; Van De Pol, M.A.; Gerritsen, M.G.; Bos, L.; Dekker, T.; Smids, B.S.; Sinha, A.; Majoor, C.; Sneeboer, M.M.; Knobel, H.H.; et al. Exhaled breath profiles in the monitoring of loss of control and clinical recovery in asthma. *Clin. Exp. Allergy* **2017**, *47*, 1159–1169. [CrossRef]

10. Fitzpatrick, A.M.; Jackson, D.J.; Mauger, D.T.; Boehmer, S.J.; Phipatanakul, W.; Sheehan, W.J.; Moy, J.N.; Paul, I.M.; Bacharier, L.B.; Cabana, M.D.; et al. Individualized therapy for persistent asthma in young children. *J. Allergy Clin. Immunol.* **2016**, *138*, 1608–1618.e12. [CrossRef]
11. Saglani, S.; Bingham, Y.; Balfour-Lynn, I.; Goldring, S.; Gupta, A.; Banya, W.; Moreiras, J.; Fleming, L.; Bush, A.; Rosenthal, M. Blood eosinophils in managing preschool wheeze: Lessons learnt from a proof-of-concept trial. *Pediatr. Allergy Immunol.* **2022**, *33*, e13697. [CrossRef] [PubMed]
12. Van De Kant, K.D.; Klaassen, E.M.; Jöbsis, Q.; Nijhuis, A.J.; Van Schayck, O.C.; Dompeling, E. Early diagnosis of asthma in young children by using non-invasive biomarkers of airway inflammation and early lung function measurements: Study protocol of a case-control study. *BMC Public Health* **2009**, *9*, 210. [CrossRef] [PubMed]
13. Van De Kant, K.D.G.; Koers, K.; Rijkers, G.T.; Passos, V.L.; Klaassen, E.M.M.; Mommers, M.; Dagnelie, P.C.; Van Schayck, C.P.; Dompeling, E.; Jöbsis, Q. Can exhaled inflammatory markers predict a steroid response in wheezing preschool children? *Clin. Exp. Allergy* **2011**, *41*, 1076–1083. [CrossRef]
14. Smolinska, A.; Klaassen, E.M.M.; Dallinga, J.W.; Van De Kant, K.D.G.; Jobsis, Q.; Moonen, E.J.C.; Van Schayck, O.C.P.; Dompeling, E.; Van Schooten, F.J. Profiling of Volatile Organic Compounds in Exhaled Breath as a Strategy to Find Early Predictive Signatures of Asthma in Children. *PLoS ONE* **2014**, *9*, e95668. [CrossRef]
15. Engel, J.; Blanchet, L.; Bloemen, B.; van den Heuvel, L.P.; Engelke, U.H.; Wevers, R.A.; Buydens, L.M. Regularized MANOVA (rMANOVA) in untargeted metabolomics. *Anal. Chim Acta* **2015**, *899*, 1–12. [CrossRef] [PubMed]
16. DDaszykowski, M.; Walczak, B.; Massart, D.L. Representative subset selection. *Anal. Chim. Acta* **2002**, *468*, 91–103. [CrossRef]
17. Gaugg, M.T.; Engler, A.; Nussbaumer-Ochsner, Y.; Bregy, L.; Stöberl, A.S.; Gaisl, T.; Bruderer, T.; Zenobi, R.; Kohler, M.; Sinues, P.M.-L. Metabolic effects of inhaled salbutamol determined by exhaled breath analysis. *J. Breath Res.* **2017**, *11*, 46004. [CrossRef]
18. Brinkman, P.; Ahmed, W.M.; Gómez, C.; Knobel, H.H.; Weda, H.; Vink, T.J.; Nijsen, T.M.; Wheelock, C.E.; Dahlen, S.-E.; Montuschi, P.; et al. Exhaled volatile organic compounds as markers for medication use in asthma. *Eur. Respir. J.* **2020**, *55*, 1900544. [CrossRef]
19. Carraro, S.; Giordano, G.; Reniero, F.; Carpi, D.; Stocchero, M.; Sterk, P.; Baraldi, E. Asthma severity in childhood and metabolomic profiling of breath condensate. *Allergy* **2013**, *68*, 110–117. [CrossRef]
20. Ferraro, V.A.; Carraro, S.; Pirillo, P.; Gucciardi, A.; Poloniato, G.; Stocchero, M.; Giordano, G.; Zanconato, S.; Baraldi, E. Breathomics in Asthmatic Children Treated with Inhaled Corticosteroids. *Metabolites* **2020**, *10*, 390. [CrossRef]
21. Rufo, J.C.; Madureira, J.; Fernandes, E.O.; Moreira, A. Volatile organic compounds in asthma diagnosis: A systematic review and meta-analysis. *Allergy* **2016**, *71*, 175–188. [CrossRef]
22. Bush, A.; Saglani, S. Medical algorithm: Diagnosis and treatment of preschool asthma. *Allergy* **2020**, *75*, 2711–2712. [CrossRef]
23. Di Cicco, M.; Peroni, D.G.; Ragazzo, V.; Comberiati, P. Application of exhaled nitric oxide (FeNO) in pediatric asthma. *Curr. Opin. Allergy Clin. Immunol.* **2021**, *21*, 151–158. [CrossRef] [PubMed]
24. Rufo, J.C.; Paciencia, I.; Mendes, F.C.; Farraia, M.; Rodolfo, A.; Silva, D.; de Oliveira Fernandes, E.; Delgado, L.; Moreira, A. Exhaled breath condensate volatilome allows sensitive diagnosis of persistent asthma. *Allergy* **2019**, *74*, 527–534. [CrossRef] [PubMed]
25. Klok, T.; Kaptein, A.A.; Brand, P.L.P. Non-adherence in children with asthma reviewed: The need for improvement of asthma care and medical education. *Pediatr. Allergy Immunol.* **2015**, *26*, 197–205. [CrossRef] [PubMed]

MDPI AG
Grosspeteranlage 5
4052 Basel
Switzerland
Tel.: +41 61 683 77 34

Journal of Clinical Medicine Editorial Office
E-mail: jcm@mdpi.com
www.mdpi.com/journal/jcm

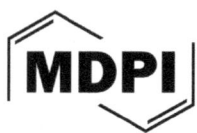

Disclaimer/Publisher's Note: The title and front matter of this reprint are at the discretion of the Guest Editor. The publisher is not responsible for their content or any associated concerns. The statements, opinions and data contained in all individual articles are solely those of the individual Editor and contributors and not of MDPI. MDPI disclaims responsibility for any injury to people or property resulting from any ideas, methods, instructions or products referred to in the content.

www.ingramcontent.com/pod-product-compliance
Lightning Source LLC
LaVergne TN
LVHW072355090526
838202LV00019B/2549